Advances in Infant and Pediatric Feeding and Nutrition

Advances in Infant and Pediatric Feeding and Nutrition

Guest Editor

Jann Foster

MDPI

Basel • Beijing • Wuhan • Barcelona • Belgrade • Novi Sad • Cluj • Manchester

Guest Editor
Jann Foster
School of Nursing and
Midwifery
Western Sydney University
Penrith
Australia

Editorial Office
MDPI AG
Grosspeteranlage 5
4052 Basel, Switzerland

This is a reprint of the Special Issue, published open access by the journal *Nutrients* (ISSN 2072-6643), freely accessible at: https://www.mdpi.com/journal/nutrients/special_issues/8YA8BJD73Z.

For citation purposes, cite each article independently as indicated on the article page online and as indicated below:

Lastname, A.A.; Lastname, B.B. Article Title. *Journal Name* **Year**, *Volume Number*, Page Range.

ISBN 978-3-7258-5089-1 (Hbk)
ISBN 978-3-7258-5090-7 (PDF)
https://doi.org/10.3390/books978-3-7258-5090-7

Contents

About the Editor

Jann Foster

Jann Foster is a Senior Lecturer at the School of Nursing and Midwifery, Western Sydney University. Jann holds a master's in health science education and completed her PhD in 2011. She has substantial experience as a researcher, educator, and coordinator of research projects at the local, state, national, and international levels. She undertakes research projects that investigate the practical aspects of neonatal care, and has over 70 peer-reviewed nursing and medical journal publications. Her work in undertaking systematic reviews has also resulted in her providing recommendations critical to safe and effective neonatal and pediatric clinical practice. Her international standing as a researcher has been recognized by Stanford University through Elsevier's World Top 2% Scientists List 2024, a yearly ranking of the world's most influential researchers, including those who have had a significant impact in a single year.

Preface

The purpose of this Reprint, "Advances in Infant and Pediatric Feeding and Nutrition", is to explore the latest evidence regarding the impact of feeding and nutrition on both the short- and long-term health of infants.

Early life nutrition plays a pivotal role in shaping future health, so this collection aims to highlight original research and reviews examining how specific feeding and nutrition approaches influence growth, body composition, and neurodevelopment, from breastfeeding through to complementary feeding during the first years of life.

Jann Foster
Guest Editor

nutrients

Editorial

Advances in Infant and Pediatric Feeding and Nutrition

Jann Foster [1,2,3,4]

1 School of Nursing & Midwifery, Western Sydney University, Locked Bag 1797, Penrith, NSW 2751, Australia; j.foster@westernsydney.edu.au
2 School of Nursing and Midwifery, University of Canberra, Bruce, ACT 2617, Australia
3 Ingham Research Institute, Liverpool, NSW 2170, Australia
4 NSW Centre for Evidence-Based Health Care: A JBI Centre of Excellence, Parramatta, NSW 2751, Australia

This Special Issue presents original works and reviews that delve into how specific feeding strategies, spanning from lactation to complementary feeding in infancy, impact growth and neurofunctional development.

The twelve articles cover a broad spectrum of topics, ranging from the epigenetic effects of human milk on the ongoing neurodevelopment of infants and children, the impact of milk oligosaccharides, maternal fish consumption, and the use of bovine colostrum or infant formula from hydrolyzed whey protein to the validation of an instrument for evaluating parental feeding behaviors, breastfeeding, and childhood caries. These articles provide novel insights into the complex nature of infant feeding and nutrition.

Feeding infants human milk has many benefits that are universally recognized, and human milk contains all the nutrients an infant requires in the first six months of life [1]. Gialeli et al., 2023, offer fresh perspectives in their narrative review, which explores how bioactive components in breast milk, such as microRNAs, long non-coding RNAs, stem cells, and the microbiome may impact the neurodevelopment of preterm and full-term infants through epigenetic mechanisms. The review establishes a compelling connection between early-life experiences and long-lasting health outcomes in preterm and term infants.

Fan et al., 2023, reviewed the impact of milk oligosaccharides, a group of complex carbohydrates, on the brain and on neurocognitive development in early life. The authors report that the benefits for cognitive development of human milk oligosaccharides (HMOs) may be due to sialic acid and fucose, which have been implicated in brain development. Ultimately, this review posits that there is a consistent connection between early life consumption of HMOs and cognitive developmental outcomes. The review also emphasizes the importance of clinical studies to explore the specific mechanisms through which milk oligosaccharides enhance learning and memory development in infants.

Kasamatsu et al.'s 2023 cross-sectional study examined the links between maternal diet, infant feeding practices, and serum levels of docosahexaenoic acid (DHA), a crucial n-3 long-chain polyunsaturated fatty acid (LCPUFA) important for infant brain development. Data were gathered through a maternal dietary questionnaire and serum fatty acid levels from the blood samples of infants. The study found significant positive associations between the infants' serum DHA levels and the consumption of "blue-back fish" and "white fish". These novel results suggest that lactating mothers who regularly consume these types of fish, while also prioritizing breastfeeding over DHA-supplemented cow's milk formula, could effectively boost their infants' serum DHA levels. The study was conducted in Tokyo, Japan, and the authors recognize that these findings may not apply to other populations.

 https://doi.org/10.3390/nu17142378

Whilst exclusive breastfeeding for the first 6 months of an infant's life is recommended by the WHO, human milk continues to provide significant nutritional and immunological value beyond 6 months. The American Academy of Pediatrics supports continued breastfeeding, along with complementary foods introduced at about 6 months [2]. The literature review by Froń & Orczyk-Pawilowicz, 2024, examines the evidence supporting extended breastfeeding beyond six months. A key takeaway from the review is that longer breastfeeding durations are linked to a variety of health benefits, such as a reduced risk of gastrointestinal and respiratory infections, enhanced growth and cognitive development, and a decreased likelihood of developing allergic diseases and obesity in later life. Moreover, breastfeeding has positive effects on metabolic syndrome, blood pressure regulation, otitis media, and malaria. Based on these findings, the authors advocate for encouraging mothers to breastfeed for longer periods.

The systematic review and meta-analysis by Shrestha et al. synthesized evidence to determine if there is an association between breastfeeding and early childhood caries (ECC), a significant chronic disease that affects infants and preschool children worldwide [3]. Whilst the review did not demonstrate an overall difference in dental caries between breastfed and non-breastfed infants, a significant increase in ECC was found for children who were breastfed for $\geq$6 months compared to those breastfed for <6 months, those who were breastfed for $\geq$12 months compared to those fed for <12 months, and those who were breastfed for $\geq$18 months compared to <18 months. Nocturnal breastfeeding also increases the risk of ECC. This review has improved our understanding of the effect of breastfeeding exposure time on ECC. The authors recommend that policy-makers develop an infant oral health promotion program and that healthcare professionals receive training on oral hygiene practices for infants.

Whilst human milk is regarded as the best source of nutrition during early life [4], it is not always possible to rely on it exclusively, and various infant formulas and/or supplements may be used to substitute human milk. Hill & Buck's (2023) double-blinded RCT explored the impact on serum metabolite levels of feeding formulas enriched with different levels of 2′-fucosyllactose (2′-FL) and galactooligosaccharides (GOSs), comparing them to a non-randomized group of breastfed infants. The control formula contained only GOS. The researchers hypothesized that, due to 2′-FL's known role as a prebiotic that can influence gut microbiome composition, its supplementation could significantly affect metabolic output, mimicking some of the systemic benefits associated with breastfeeding. Their results showed that fortifying infant formula with 2′-FL led to a dose-dependent increase in circulating metabolites produced by gut microbial metabolism. Specifically, 2′-FL supplementation was linked to higher levels of secondary bile acids and the activation of systemic immune mediators, when compared to the control formula, reaching concentrations akin to those seen in breastfed infants. The researchers also offer valuable recommendations for future investigations.

Canbolat et al.'s 2024 review examines the composition, benefits, and effects of bovine colostrum (BC), and concludes that bovine colostrum is the most viable alternative to human colostrum for infant feeding. With its anti-inflammatory, antioxidant, antibacterial, prebiotic, and antiviral properties, BC offers a distinct colostrum profile. However, the authors emphasize that BC should be regarded as a supplement rather than as a reliable treatment, and its use must be guided by a healthcare professional, especially in preterm infants or those with medical conditions. The review also suggests that future research should focus on identifying the optimal dosages, formulations, and safety profiles of BC, particularly regarding allergic reactions in infants with cow's milk protein allergies or lactose intolerance.

Protein is essential for the growth and development of infants [5]. Fleddermann et al., 2023, assess the nutritional safety and suitability of an infant formula manufactured from extensively hydrolyzed protein (HP) compared to infant formula manufactured from intact protein (IP—with a low or standard protein content). The authors conduct a combined analysis of raw data from two randomized infant feeding studies. The results show no significance in weight gain between the two formulas, and secondary growth measures such as weight, length, and head circumference were generally similar across both the HP and IP formula groups, at both protein levels. However, the HP formula group showed greater monthly gains in head circumference (for the low-protein formula, both in the per-protocol set (PPS) and the full-analysis set (FAS)) and in length (for the standard protein formula, FAS) compared to the IP formula groups. The authors note a higher occurrence of adverse events for the HP formula group, though these events were transient and mild, leading them to conclude that there were no safety concerns.

Inappropriate complementary feeding (CF) can result in childhood illness and affect a child's growth and development [6]. The cross-sectional study by Ashraf et al. investigates the prevalence of inappropriate CF and the factors influencing early feeding patterns among mothers in Pakistan. This crucial research reveals that 47.0% of caregivers began CF before 4 months of age, which negatively impacts infant health. In contrast, 39.7% followed guidelines by introducing CF between 4 and 6 months, potentially enhancing infant health outcomes, and 30.9% started complementary feeding after 7 months. This study identifies several factors, such as birth order, mother's employment status, parental education, the number of children, household income, maternal knowledge, and maternal health, as significant influencers of CF practices. The findings contribute to existing knowledge and highlight the need for targeted interventions and policy changes to improve CF practices in Pakistan.

Unhealthy eating behaviors in childhood contribute to the obesity epidemic [7,8]. González-Torres et al. investigated the effectiveness of the self-administered Scale on Parental Feeding Behaviors in terms of its ability to assess various parental feeding practices among Mexican caregivers, grounded in theoretical concepts of coercive control, structure, and autonomy support. The authors found that the scale is effective at measuring both the positive and negative parental eating behaviors that influence the development of healthy eating habits in childhood. Notably, the scale was deemed valuable for designing interventions aimed at preventing health issues linked to poor nutrition and childhood obesity.

Guevara et al. reviewed the nutritional composition of cereal-based foods offered to infants (from 4 months) and toddlers in Spain and Ecuador. A total of 127 products were included, with 105 from Spain and 22 from Ecuador. The study revealed that, in Ecuador, commercial companies recommend starting the consumption of cereals at 6 months, while in Spain, the recommendation is from 4 months. Only 39 products in Spain and 2 products in Ecuador could be classified as "low in sugar". There was noticeable variation in the declaration of vitamin content between the two countries and, regarding mineral content, cereals in Ecuador had higher reported calcium levels, while Ecuadorian cereals and cookies also had higher iron content. Cookies in both countries were found to have high sodium levels. The authors highlight some differences in the nutritional composition of cereals for breastfeeding infants between those from Spain and those from Ecuador. Importantly, the authors highlight the lack of studies on the nutritional quality of infant foods in Ecuador, suggesting their research could serve as a foundation for future investigations.

This editorial summarizes the twelve articles that comprise the Special Issue further advancing our knowledge of infant and pediatric feeding and nutrition. The findings from these articles deepen our understanding of issues related to feeding and nutrition and pave the way for practical applications and future research.

Conflicts of Interest: The author declares no conflict of interest.

List of Contributions

1. Gialeli, G.; Panagopoulou, O.; Liosis, G.; Siahanidou, T. Potential Epigenetic Effects of Human Milk on Infants' Neurodevelopment. *Nutrients* **2023**, *15*, 3614. https://doi.org/10.3390/nu15163614.
2. Fan, Y.; McMath, A.L.; Donovan, S.M. Review on the Impact of Milk Oligosaccharides on the Brain and Neurocognitive Development in Early Life. *Nutrients* **2023**, *15*, 3743. https://doi.org/10.3390/nu15173743.
3. Kasamatsu, A.; Tachimoto, H.; Urashima, M. Impact of Maternal Fish Consumption on Serum Docosahexaenoic Acid (DHA) Levels in Breastfed Infants: A Cross-Sectional Study of a Randomized Clinical Trial in Japan. *Nutrients* **2023**, *15*, 4338. https://doi.org/10.3390/nu15204338.
4. Froń, A.; Orczyk-Pawiłowicz, M. Breastfeeding Beyond Six Months: Evidence of Child Health Benefits. *Nutrients* **2024**, *16*, 3891.https://doi.org/10.3390/nu16223891.
5. Shrestha, S.K.; Arora, A.; Manohar, N.; Ekanayake, K.; Foster, J. Association of Breastfeeding and Early Childhood Caries: A Systematic Review and Meta-Analysis. *Nutrients* **2024**, *16*, 1355. https://doi.org/10.3390/nu16091355.
6. Hill, D.R.; Buck, R.H. Infants Fed Breastmilk or 20-FL Supplemented Formula Have Similar Systemic Levels of Microbiota-Derived Secondary Bile Acids. *Nutrients* **2023**, *15*, 2339. https://doi.org/10.3390/nu15102339.
7. Canbolat, A.A.; Lombardo, M.; Mondragon, A.d.C.; López, J.M.M.; Bechelany, M.; Karav, S. Bovine Colostrum in Pediatric Nutrition and Health. *Nutrients* **2024**, *16*, 4305. https://doi.org/10.3390/nu16244305.
8. Fleddermann, M.; Knoll, A.; Koletzko, B. Safety and Suitability of Infant Formula Manufactured from Extensively Hydrolyzed Whey Protein Compared to Intact Protein: A Combined Analysis of Two Randomized Controlled Studies. *Nutrients* **2024**, *16*, 245. https://doi.org/10.3390/nu16020245.
9. Ashraf, I.; Bestman, P.L.; Assiri, A.A.; Kamal, G.M.; Uddin, J.; Luo, J.; Orayj, K.M.; Ishaqui, A.A. Status of Inappropriate Complementary Feeding and Its Associated Factors Among Infants of 9–23 Months. *Nutrients* **2024**, *16*, 4379. https://doi.org/10.3390/nu16244379.
10. Guevara, D.; Marcos, A.; Ruiz, F.I.; Gómez-Martínez, S.; del Pozo, S. A Descriptive Study of Spanish and Ecuadorian Commercial Infant Cereals: Are They in Line with Current Recommendations? *Nutrients* **2024**, *16*, 1992. https://doi.org/10.3390/nu16131992.
11. González-Torres, M.L.; Garza-Olivares, X.; Navarro-Contreras, G.; González-Orozco, L.A. Validation of the Scale on Parental Feeding Behaviors (ECOPAL) for Caregivers of Mexican Children. *Nutrients* **2023**, *15*, 3698. https://doi.org/10.3390/nu15173698.
12. Białek-Dratwa, A.; Kowalski, O. Prevalence of Feeding Problems in Children and Associated Factors—A Cross-Sectional Study among Polish Children Aged 2–7 Years. *Nutrients* **2023**, *15*, 3185. https://doi.org/10.3390/nu15143185.

References

1. World Health Organization, WHO. Infant and Young Child Feeding. 2023. Available online: https://www.who.int/news-room/fact-sheets/detail/infant-and-young-child-feeding (accessed on 20 June 2025).
2. Meek, J.Y.; Noble, L. Section on Breastfeeding. Policy Statement: Breastfeeding and the Use of Human Milk. *Pediatrics* **2022**, *150*, e2022057988. [CrossRef] [PubMed]
3. American Academy of Pediatric Dentistry (AAP). Policy on early childhood caries (ECC): Classifications, consequences, and preventive strategies. In *The Reference Manual of Pediatric Dentistry*; American Academy of Pediatric Dentistry: Chicago, IL, USA, 2020; pp. 79–81.
4. Lugonja, N.; Marinković, V.; Pucarević, M.; Miletić, S.; Stojić, N.; Crnković, D.; Vrvić, M. Human Milk—The Biofluid That Nourishes Infants from the First Day of Life. *Foods* **2024**, *13*, 1298. [CrossRef] [PubMed]

5. Das, J.K.; Lassi, Z.S.; Hoodbhoy, Z.; Salam, R.A. Nutrition for the Next Generation: Older Children and Adolescents. *Ann. Nutr. Metab.* **2018**, *72* (Suppl. S3), 56–64. [CrossRef] [PubMed]
6. Berhanu, Z.; Alemu, T.; Argaw, D. Predictors of inappropriate complementary feeding practice among children aged 6 to 23 months in Wonago District, South Ethiopia, 2017: Case control study. *BMC Pediatr.* **2019**, *19*, 146. [CrossRef] [PubMed]
7. Qiu, C.; Hatton, R.; Li, Q.; Xv, J.; Li, J.; Tian, J.; Yuan, S.; Hou, M. Associations of parental feeding practices with children's eating behaviors and food preferences: A Chinese cross-sectional study. *BMC Pediatr.* **2023**, *23*, 84. [CrossRef] [PubMed]
8. Kininmonth, A.R.; Herle, M.; Haycraft, E.; Farrow, C.; Croker, H.; Pickard, A.; Edwards, K.; Blissett, J.; Llewellyn, C. Prospective associations between parental feeding practices used in toddlerhood and preschool children's appetite vary according to appetite avidity in toddlerhood. *Appetite* **2023**, *185*, 106541. [CrossRef] [PubMed]

nutrients

MDPI

Article

Status of Inappropriate Complementary Feeding and Its Associated Factors Among Infants of 9–23 Months

Iqra Ashraf [1], Prince L. Bestman [1], Abdullah A. Assiri [2], Ghulam Mustafa Kamal [3], Jalal Uddin [4,*], Jiayou Luo [1,*], Khalid M. Orayj [2] and Azfar A. Ishaqui [2]

1 Department of Maternal and Child Health, Xiangya School of Public Health, Central South University, Changsha 410083, China; 216919002@csu.edu.cn (I.A.); plbestman@csu.edu.cn (P.L.B.)
2 Department of Clinical Pharmacy, College of Pharmacy, King Khalid University, Abha 61441, Saudi Arabia; aalabdullah@kku.edu.sa (A.A.A.); korayg@kku.edu.sa (K.M.O.); amianishaqui@kku.edu.sa (A.A.I.)
3 Institute of Chemistry, Khwaja Fareed University of Engineering & Information Technology, Rahim Yar Khan 64200, Pakistan; mustafa.kamal@kfueit.edu.pk
4 Department of Pharmaceutical Chemistry, College of Pharmacy, King Khalid University, Abha 61441, Saudi Arabia
* Correspondence: jalaluddinamin@gmail.com (J.U.); jiayouluo@126.com (J.L.)

Abstract: Background: Inappropriate complementary feeding during the first two years of life significantly impacts children's health, increasing risks of malnutrition and illness. **Methods**: This study investigates factors influencing early feeding patterns among 600 mothers of children aged 9–23 months in selected hospitals in Punjab, Pakistan. Using a structured questionnaire, data were collected and analyzed, with associations measured by odds ratios (ORs) and 95% confidence intervals (CIs). **Results:** The results showed the key indicators of inappropriate complementary feeding among young children, including timely complementary feeding, minimum meal frequency, dietary diversity, and acceptable diet. The rates for these factors were found to be 60.3%, 32.7%, 24.6%, and 48.5%, respectively. The study identified several significant factors influencing these practices. Key predictors of inappropriate feeding included the order of birth, the mother's employment status, parental education, the number of children, household income, maternal knowledge, and maternal health. **Conclusion:** The findings underscore that maternal education, employment, and health significantly influence complementary feeding. Targeted interventions and education programs are essential to support healthy feeding behaviors, especially for mothers facing challenges related to education, work, or health conditions. Addressing these practices can improve child health outcomes, contributing to economic growth and a healthier future for Pakistan's youngest population.

Keywords: inappropriate complementary feeding; associated factors; minimum meal frequency; minimum dietary diversity; minimum acceptable diet

1. Introduction

The period from birth to two years is a "critical window" for promoting optimal growth, health, and development, being mainly dependent on nutrition [1]. The World Health Organization (WHO) recommends exclusive breastfeeding until six months of age. Complementary feeding (CF), which involves introducing other foods and liquids alongside breast milk when breast milk alone can no longer meet the nutritional needs of infants, should begin at this time [2]. Specifically, the WHO recommends introducing complementary foods at six months of age [3]. In line with this, similar guidelines have been recommended by ESPGHAN, NASPGHAN, and the European Academy of Allergy and Clinical Immunology (EAACI), which advise introducing complementary foods between 17 and 26 weeks of age [4].

WHO identifies four indicators for appropriate CF: the timing of introduction, minimum meal frequency, dietary diversity, and acceptable diet. Failure to meet these criteria signifies inappropriate CF, while meeting them all indicates proper practice [5,6].

From around six months, a newborn's nutritional needs increase, requiring CF to provide vital energy and nutrients necessary for growth and development. If complementary foods are introduced improperly or not at all, a child's growth may be affected. The period from 6 to 23 months is a critical time for the onset of growth faltering, micronutrient deficiencies, and infectious diseases [7]. Additionally, there has been a rise in food allergies, particularly to eggs, shellfish, and nuts, in Western children. The early introduction of allergenic foods, such as oats, fish, and eggs, has been shown to reduce the risk of asthma, allergic rhinitis, and atopic dermatitis [8]. The introduction of gluten between 4 and 6 months may reduce the risk of celiac disease, with a gradual introduction being recommended while breastfeeding [9]. CF is vital for providing essential nutrients like iron, zinc, and vitamin A, with early inclusion of foods like meat, eggs, and liver being beneficial to address common deficiencies [10,11].

Malnutrition is characterized by an imbalance of energy and nutrients in the body, which negatively impacts the physical health of both children and adults [12]. One form of malnutrition, undernutrition, occurs when there is an insufficient intake of essential nutrients, including energy, high-quality protein, essential amino acids, vitamins, and minerals. This deficiency prevents the body from meeting its nutritional needs for proper growth, maintenance, and function [13]. Undernutrition accounts for almost one-third of all deaths in children under the age of five worldwide, with Asia accounting for the greatest percentage [14]. Approximately 21.3% of children under the age of five are stunted (too short for their height), 13% are underweight (too thin for their age), and 6.9% are wasting (low weight for their height) [15]. Malnutrition accounts for 60 percent of all under-five fatalities in underdeveloped nations [16]. Inadequate feeding habits, including a lack of dietary diversity, infrequent feeding, and improper timing of CF (either before 4 months or after 7 months), account for approximately 66% of all fatal accidents among children under five [17]. South Asia has a disproportionately high malnutrition burden compared to other areas, with the greatest rates of stunting (33.2%, about 60 million children) and wasting (14.8%, approximately 27 million children).

The Pakistan Demographic and Health Survey found that 45% of children under 5 were stunted, 11% were wasting, and 30% were underweight. The report also discovered that among babies aged 6 to 9 months, only 5.3% were solely breastfed, 10.3% received breast milk with water, 11% received breast milk with cow's milk, and only 56.6% received CF in addition to breastmilk [18]. The existing literature on the determinants of child eating patterns, including minimal dietary diversity and meal frequency, showed that feeding practices are associated with the mother's education, maternal profession, the child's gender, and postnatal care [19]. Furthermore, the residence, family size, financial status, child age, the mother's health (emotional and mental health) [20], and delivery site are important predictors of child feeding behaviors [21–23]. Recent research has also indicated that the birth interval, mother's independence, and exposure to media are important determinants of dietary diversification [24].

Nutrition-related research in Pakistan and other low and middle-income countries generally focuses on improving breastfeeding patterns, with minimal focus on improving CF practices. However, one notable exception is the work by Muzi et. at. [25] which employed multi-level regressions to analyze the factors influencing CF practices in Pakistan, using data from the 2012–2013 Demographic and Health Survey. However, their analysis relies on data that are now eight years old, so the objective of this study is to provide fresh evidence of the knowledge of child-feeding practices in Pakistan and examine the relationship between child-feeding practices and individual-, household-, and community-level indicators using the most recent data.

This study is expected to provide valuable insights into the factors that influence early CF practices among children aged 9–23 months in Punjab, Pakistan. The anticipated results aim to identify key predictors of inappropriate feeding, including maternal education, employment, and health status, as well as socio-economic factors such as household income and family size. It is expected that the study will reveal a significant association between these factors and the rates of timely CF, meal frequency, dietary diversity, and acceptable diets. These findings are expected to underscore the importance of targeted interventions and education programs to improve maternal knowledge and promote healthier feeding behaviors, ultimately contributing to better child health outcomes and supporting economic growth in Pakistan. The results will also provide a foundation for future research and policy recommendations focused on enhancing child nutrition and health in the region.

2. Methodology

2.1. Study Design and Setting

This cross-sectional study examined the prevalence of inappropriate CF among infants aged 9–23 months. The study was conducted in multiple hospitals located in multiple cities across Pakistan, including both public and private sector healthcare facilities. The selected cities, namely Lahore, Multan, Islamabad, Gujranwala, and Faisalabad, were randomly chosen to ensure the representation of diverse geographical regions and populations within the country. The reason for choosing the hospital setting rather than a community setting was to ensure a diverse participant pool, as hospitals provide access to caregivers from various socio-economic backgrounds, including both urban and rural populations. Hospitals are frequently visited for routine check-ups and vaccinations, facilitating easier participant's recruitment. Additionally, hospitals offer better infrastructure for data collection, such as access to medical records, which enhances the reliability of participant selection.

2.2. Study Participants and Eligibility Criteria

The target population for this study were infants between 9 and 23 months and their caregivers, primarily mothers, while the study population were only infants of 9–23 months. We mainly targeted this age group because appropriate CF is crucial during this developmental stage. Only those mothers who could read and write properly and signed the consent form were selected. Infants with congenital disorders or diseases that could potentially impact their diet, such as heart defects or autism, were excluded from the study.

2.3. Sample Size and Sampling Technique

The sample size for this study was determined using Cochran's formula, resulting in a sample size of 600 participants. For the sampling technique, as the study was conducted in a hospital setting, a clinical survey approach was employed. Convenient sampling was used to select the hospitals, and participants were selected based on convenience, ensuring ease of access and recruitment from the available patient pool.

2.4. Instrument

The data collection for the study used structured and semi-structured questionnaire, consisting of both close-ended (multiple choice) and open-ended questions. It was organized into eight main sections with sub-questions focusing on gathering information from mothers regarding inappropriate CF. The first section collected demographic information about the child, including age, weight, height, gender, and birth order.

The second section of the questionnaire gathered parents' information, including age, weight, education level, and employment status. The third section focused on household details, such as the number of children, place of delivery, monthly income, and healthcare access. The fourth section assessed mothers' knowledge of CF through 12 questions, with responses of "Yes", "No", or "Don't know". Scores ranged from 0 to 12, categorizing knowledge as low (<4), moderate (4–8), or high (>9).

The fifth section addressed the child's feeding history, including breastfeeding duration and the introduction of complementary foods. Section six covered the infant's health status, such as gastrointestinal and respiratory issues. Section seven focused on access to clean water and hygiene practices, while section eight explored maternal health during various phases. The final section used a Food Frequency Questionnaire (FFQ) to assess dietary diversity, categorizing infants' food intake based on eight food groups. A score of 1 was assigned for consuming four or fewer food groups, and 0 for more than four, helping evaluate the infant's nutrition and dietary variety.

2.5. Data Collection

The researcher underwent training to conduct interviews and surveys with caregivers at various hospitals to collect data on CF practices and knowledge. Topics covered in the training included appropriate food types, feeding frequency, portion sizes, and hygiene. Data collection involved initial online Google forms and face-to-face interviews with mothers based on the form responses. Mothers who agreed to participate signed a form, and this process continued until the desired number of participants was achieved, ensuring all participants' voluntary involvement in the study.

2.6. Operational Definitions

Timely introduction of complementary foods: It is recommended to start between 4 and 6 months. Mothers were asked about the introduction of solid foods to their children. Based on their responses, the introduction of complementary food was categorized into early (<4 months), timely (4–6 months), and late (>7 months) stages of CF. This categorization helped us to assess if the introduction of solid foods is aligned with the recommended guidelines.

Minimum dietary diversity: Minimum dietary diversity refers to the percentage of children aged 6–23 months who have consumed at least four of the eight food groups. There are eight dietary groups: breast milk, cereals, roots, and tubers, legumes and nuts, dairy products (infant formula, milk, yogurt, and cheese), flesh foods (meat, fish, and organ meats), eggs, vitamin A-rich fruits and vegetables, and other fruits and vegetables.

Dietary variety scores range from 0 to 7, where a score of zero means the child did not eat from any food group and a score of 7 indicates they ate from all food groups. We applied the minimum dietary diversity measure based on WHO recommendation. If a child consumed foods from four or more food categories, we gave them a score of "1" for minimum dietary variety. If they ate from less than four food groups, they received a score of "0", indicating low dietary diversity.

Minimum meal frequency: The minimum meal frequency is defined as how many times a child receives complementary food in a day. According to WHO, it is twice for 6–8 months, three times for 9–11 months, three times for breastfed children aged 12–23 months, and four times for non-breastfed children. Appropriate feeding frequency was categorized as 1 (minimum meal frequency), whereas incorrect was recorded as 0 (low meal frequency).

Minimum acceptable diet: This is the combination of both the minimum dietary diversity and meal frequency.

2.7. Inappropriate Complementary Feeding Practice

CF methods that fail to meet the requirements for either a timely introduction or the minimum acceptable diet were assessed.

2.8. Statistical Analysis

Descriptive data of children, parents, and households were presented as frequencies and percentages. In addition, a chi-square test was used to determine the association between categorical variables, while a *t*-test was applied for continuous variables. Associations between inappropriate CF practices and other characteristics was examined using logistic regression. WHO guidelines were used to evaluate appropriate meal frequency, diversity, and acceptability. Dietary diversity was classified into seven WHO food groups to calculate the minimum nutritional variety. The odds ratios (ORs) were reported with 95% confidence intervals (CIs). A p-value of <0.05 was considered statistically significant. The SPSS version (26.0, IBM, Armonk, NY, USA) was used to conduct all the analyses.

3. Results

3.1. Socio-Demographic Characteristics of Participants

Among the demographic characteristics assessed in the study, a notable proportion of children fell within the age range of 13–18 months, comprising 45.4% of the total sample. This age range had the highest number of participants indicating a critical developmental period for infants. Regarding gender distribution, slightly more than half of the children (51%) were female. When examining body height, most children (57.5%) measured between 69 and 79 cm, indicating a relatively even distribution within this height range.

Moreover, the Body Mass Index (BMI) distribution revealed that a significant portion of children (45.5%) fell within the healthy weight category, while a smaller proportion were classified as underweight (18.2%), overweight (8.3%), or obese (2.5%). These findings emphasize the importance of monitoring growth parameters and nutritional status in early childhood, with implications for interventions promoting healthy development and preventing adverse health outcomes.

3.2. Complementary Feeding Indicators

This study reveals that a significant proportion (47.0%) of caregivers introduced CF before the recommended age of 4 months, compromising the health of infants. However, 39.7% adhered to guidelines by initiating CF between 4 and 6 months, which may improve infant health outcomes. Conversely, 30.9% started feeding after 7 months.

According to the results, 196 infants (32.7%) did not fulfill the WHO guidelines for CF instead of consuming the recommended 3–4 feeds appropriate for their age, these infants exhibited varied feeding patterns, including once a day, 12 times a day, or more than 4 times a day. Conversely, 67.2% of infants aged 9–23 months received appropriate CF, meeting this age group's recommended frequency of 3–4 times daily. The prevalence of inappropriate complementary feeding and its key indicators are shown in Figure 1.

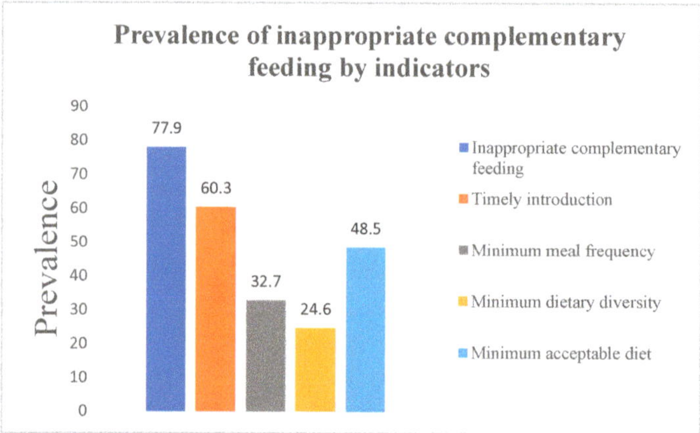

Figure 1. Prevalence of inappropriate complementary feeding by indicators.

The study assessed dietary diversity among children aged 9–23 months across various food groups. The results indicate varying levels of dietary diversity across age groups. Among infants aged 9–13 months, wheat (18.2%), fruits (18.2%), and vegetables (33.4%) were the most commonly consumed food groups, while dairy products (44.5%) and rice (41.5%) were also prevalent. In the 14–18 months' age group, fruits (44.5%) and dairy products (54.9%) exhibited higher consumption rates, with rice (33.2%) and white meat

(35.5%) also significant. In the oldest age group (19–23 months), fruits (36.9%) and white meat (45.8%) remained popular choices, along with dairy products (51.4%) and vegetables (58.9%), indicating a broader dietary diversity among older infants.

The study found that 48.5% of the sample met the Minimum Acceptable Diet (MAD) criteria. This indicates that nearly half of the infants aged 6–23 months received a diet meeting the minimum standards for adequate nutrition.

3.3. *Monovariate Factor Analysis of Inappropriate Complementary Feeding*

The monovariate factor analysis of inappropriate complementary feeding in children, as presented in Table 1, reveals several significant associations between various demographic and socioeconomic factors and the practice of CF. Firstly, maternal employment status was significantly associated with CF practices ($\chi^2 = 8.423$, $p = 0.038$), with employed mothers exhibiting a lower prevalence of incomplete feeding compared to unemployed or retired mothers. Similarly, the father's education level showed a significant association with CF practices ($\chi^2 = 12.07$, $p = 0.017$), with higher education levels correlating with lower rates of incomplete feeding.

Table 1. Summarized demographic characteristics and monovariate factor analysis of inappropriate complementary feeding in children.

Variables	N (%)	Inappropriate Complementary Feeding Yes (%)	No (%)	Test Statistics	*p* Value
Age (month)				1.725	0.42
7–9	109 (18.2%)	28 (25.7)	81 (74.3)		
10–18	273 (45.4%)	61 (22.3)	212 (77.7)		
19–23	218 (36.3%)	42 (19.3)	176 (80.7)		
Gender				0.128	0.72
Male	294 (49%)	66 (22.4)	228 (77.6)		
Female	306 (51%)	65 (21.2)	241 (78.8)		
Body height (cm)				1.799	0.40
Mean ± SD	75.7 ± 9.4	76.1 ± 9.8	75.6 ± 9.2	0.523	0.60
54–68 cm	101 (16.8%)	26 (25.7)	75 (74.3)		
69–79 cm	345 (57.5%)	69 (20)	276 (80)		
89 and above	154 (25.7%)	36 (23.4)	118 (76.6)		
Body weight (kg)				1.725	0.422
Mean ± SD	11.8 ± 2.6	11.7 ± 2.7	11.9 ± 2.6	0.756	0.451
7–9 kg	314 (52.3%)	68 (21.7)	246 (78.3)		
10–12 kg	125 (20.8%)	23 (18.4)	102 (81.6)		
9–23 kg	161 (26.8%)	40 (24.8)	121 (75.2)		
BMI (kg/m^2)				4.718	0.194
Mean ± SD	20.8 ± 3.6	20.7 ± 3.3	20.9 ± 3.7	0.597	0.55
Less than 18.5 (underweight)	140 (18.2%)	26 (18.6)	114 (81)		
Btw 18.5–24.9 (healthy weight)	395 (45.5%)	96 (24.3)	299 (75.7)		
Among 25–29.9 (overweight)	50 (36.3%)	7 (14)	43 (86)		
30.0 or higher above (obese)	15 (2.5%)	2 (13.3)	13 (86.7)		
Birth's Order				1.452	0.693
First-born	72 (12%)	16 (22.2)	56 (77.8)		
Second-born	225 (37.5%)	51 (22.7)	174 (77.3)		
Third-born	256 (42.7%)	57 (22.3)	199 (77.7)		
Fourth and above	47 (7.8%)	7 (14.9)	40 (85.1)		
Parents Information					

Table 1. *Cont.*

Variables	N (%)	Inappropriate Complementary Feeding Yes (%)	No (%)	Test Statistics	p Value
Age of the mother (year)				7.006	0.072
20–30	341 (56.8%)	76 (26.3)	213 (73.7)		
31–40	213 (35.5%)	42 (18.6)	184 (81.4)		
41–50	40 (6.7%)	12 (15.8)	64 (84.4)		
51–60	6 (1%)	1 (11.1)	8 (88.9)		
Height of the mother (cm)				0.885	0.829
Mean ± SD	165.6 ± 7.3	164.2 ± 3.5	165.8 ± 6.7	0.231	0.82
150 cm	2 (0.3%)	20 (22.2)	70 (77.8)		
152–165 cm	312 (52%)	65 (21.7)	235 (78.3)		
167–180 cm	285 (47.5%)	45 (22.5)	155 (77.5)		
182–193 cm	1 (0.2%)	1 (10)	9 (90)		
Body weight (kg)				0.252	0.969
Mean ± SD	81.2 ± 10.3	81.5 ± 9.9	81.1 ± 10.1	0.405	0.69
60–70 kg	99 (16.5%)	20 (20.2)	79 (79.8)		
71–80	181 (30.2%)	40 (22.1)	141 (77.9)		
81–90	189 (31.5%)	41 (22.7)	148 (78.3)		
Above	131 (21.8%)	30 (22.9)	101 (77.1)		
Mothers Education				2.552	0.635
None	171 (28.5%)	38 (22.2)	133 (77.8)		
Secondary school	316 (52.7%)	73 (23.1)	243 (76.9)		
FSC	93 (15.5%)	15 (16.1)	78 (83.9)		
University Level	14 (2.5%)	3 (21.4)	11 (78.6		
Postgraduate	10 (1%)	2 (33.3)	4 (66.7)		
Employment of Mother				8.423	0.038 *
Employed	28 (4.7%)	1 (3.6)	27 (96.4)		
Not employed	13 (2.2%)	5 (38.5)	8 (61.5)		
Retired	408 (68%)	95 (23.3)	313 (76.7)		
Own business	151 (25.2)	30 (19.9)	121 (80)		
Age of the Father (year)				2.611	0.625
20–30		9 (32.1)	19 (67.9)		
31–40		63 (21.6)	228 (78.4)		
41–50		32 (20)	127 (79.9)		
51–60		27 (22.5)	93 (77.5)		
Above 60		0 (0)	2 (100)		
Father's Education				12.07	0.017 *
None		2 (50)	2 (50)		
Secondary school		0 (0)	1 (100)		
high school		28 (19.7)	114 (80.3)		
Undergraduate		58 (18.4)	258 (81.6)		
Graduation		43 (31.4)	94 (68.6)		
Employment of Father				2.149	0.542
Employed		75 (22.3)	262 (77.7)		
Not employed		3 (16.7)	15 (83.3)		
Retired		1 (7.1)	13 (92.9)		
Own business		52 (22.5)	179 (77.5)		
Household Information					

Table 1. *Cont.*

Variables	N (%)	Inappropriate Complementary Feeding Yes (%)	No (%)	Test Statistics	*p* Value
Number of Children				22.64	<0.001 *
1 Child		0 (0)	1 (100)		
2 Child		6 (7.2)	77 (92.8)		
3 Child		54 (19.1)	229 (80.9)		
4 Child		62 (31.3)	136 (68.7)		
5 or above		9 (25.7)	26 (74.3)		
Have enough food for children				1.799	0.180
Yes		78 (20.2)	309 (79.8)		
No		53 (24.9)	160 (75)		
Place of Delivery				0.123	0.726
Home		46 (22.7)	157 (77.3)		
Health Institution		85 (21.4)	312 (78.3)		
Sex of Household				0.178	0.673
Male		127 (22)	451 (78)		
Female		4 (18.2)	18 (81.8)		
Average Monthly Income				9.809	0.007 *
<50k PKR		49 (16.5)	248 (83.5)		
50k–100k PKR		75 (27.1)	202 (72.9)		
>100k PKR		7 (26.9)	19 (73.1)		
Difficulty in accessing healthcare facilities				0.590	0.443
Yes		77 (23)	258 (77)		
No		54 (20.4)	211 (79.6)		
The score of Maternal knowledge In complementary feeding practice					
Mean overall score				8.571	0.014 *
<4		40 (16.4)	204 (83.)		
4–8		87 (26.3)	244 (73.3)		
9–12		4 (16)	21 (84)		
Child Feeding					
Has your child been fed by their mother's milk?				1.489	0.223
Yes		112 (21.1)	419 (78.9)		
No		19 (27.5)	50 (72.5)		
Still breastfeeding your child?				1.062	0.588
Yes		85 (22.2)	298 (77.8)		
No		45 (20.9)	170 (79.1)		
Age at which the child stops breastfeeding?				**0.984**	**0.805**
<6 months		15 (22.4)	52 (77.6)		
6–12 months		34 (24.6)	104 (75.4)		
>12 months		54 (20.4)	211 (79.6)		
Skip		28 (21.5)	102 (78.50		
Age of the child when complementary feeding was started?				**150.3**	**<0.001**
<4 months		23 (8.2)	259 (91)		
4–6 months		98 (52.7)	88 (47.3)		
>7 months		10 (7.6)	122 (92.4)		

Table 1. *Cont.*

Variables	N (%)	Inappropriate Complementary Feeding Yes (%)	No (%)	Test Statistics	p Value
Reason for starting complementary food at the chosen age?				**0.627**	**0.890**
Baby seemed interested in food		16 (21.1)	60 (78.9)		
Healthcare recommendation		36 (23.8)	115 (76.2)		
Family or cultural tradition		47 (20.5)	182 (79.5)		
I was unsure when to start		32 (22.2)	112 (77.8)		
Number of times you fed your child per day				**13.45**	**0.004**
Once only		19 (15.6)	103 (84.4)		
2–3 times		48 (19.2)	202 (80)		
3–4 times		58 (30.7)	131 (69.3)		
4+ times		6 (15.4)	33 (84.5)		
Information on Clean Water					
Access to clean water				**1.245**	**0.264**
Yes		16 (27.6)	42 (72.4)		
No		115 (21.2)	427 (78.8)		
Does your domestic setup has the facilities to cook clean food?				**2.341**	**0.126**
Yes		110 (20.9)	417 (79.1)		
No		21 (28.8)	52 (71.2)		
Mothers Health					
Have you experienced any of these changes when started CF				**5.715**	**0.335**
Weight gain		42 (89.4)	5 (10.6)		
Weight loss		47 (72.3)	18 (27.7)		
Digestive problems		85 (77.3)	25 (22.7)		
Fatigue		112 (80.6)	27 (19.4)		
Emotional changes		105 (77.2)	31 (22.8)		
Skin changes		78 (75.7)	25 (24.3)		
Have you experienced any emotional changes when starting CF				**6.498**	**0.039**
Felt more emotionally stable		94 (86.2)	15 (13.8)		
Yes, my stress increases		276 (77.7)	79 (22.3)		
No Its same		99 (72.8)	37 (27.2)		
Have you experienced any physical changes when starting CF				**5.084**	**0.079**
I have noticed Positive changes		49 (27.7)	128 (72.3)		
I have noticed negative changes		49 (19.8)	199 (80.2)		
No its same		33 (18.9)	142 (81.1)		

* The value is statistically significat at $p < 0.05$.

Bivariate factor analysis of Inappropriate Complementary feeding

Furthermore, the number of children in the household was strongly associated with CF practices ($\chi^2 = 22.64$, $p < 0.001$), with households having more children showing higher rates of incomplete feeding. Additionally, average monthly income was significantly associated with CF practices ($\chi^2 = 9.809$, $p = 0.007$), with lower-income households exhibiting a higher prevalence of incomplete feeding.

Maternal knowledge scores regarding infant feeding practices also showed a significant association with CF practices ($\chi^2 = 8.571$, $p = 0.014$), with higher knowledge scores correlating with lower rates of incomplete feeding. The age of the child when CF was initiated also emerged as a significant factor ($\chi^2 = 150.3$, $p < 0.001$), with earlier initiation associated with higher rates of incomplete feeding.

Furthermore, the daily feeding frequency was significantly associated with CF practices ($\chi^2 = 13.45$, $p = 0.004$), with higher-frequency feeding correlating with lower rates of incomplete feeding. Lastly, emotional changes experienced by mothers when starting CF showed a significant association with CF practices ($\chi^2 = 6.498$, $p = 0.039$), with increased stress levels linked to higher rates of incomplete feeding.

Emotional changes during CF initiation were significantly associated with maternal stress levels. Mothers experiencing increased stress had a higher prevalence of incomplete feeding, with 22.3% reporting elevated stress levels compared to 13.8% who felt more emotionally stable and 27.2% whose emotional state remained unchanged.

In this study, several factors were found to be non-significant considering inappropriate CF practices. Demographic characteristics such as the age and gender of the children, as well as parental factors including maternal age, education level, and body characteristics (height and weight), did not show significant associations with CF practices. Similarly, household characteristics such as access to clean water, facilities for cooking clean food, and difficulty in accessing healthcare facilities were not significantly associated with inappropriate CF. Additionally, factors related to child-feeding practices such as breastfeeding initiation, frequency, and duration did not demonstrate significant associations with inappropriate CF practices.

To promote optimal infant feeding practices, socioeconomic, demographic, and emotional factors must be addressed, as these factors influence CF practices in multiple ways.

The logistic regression analysis provided insights into factors associated with inappropriate CF practices in infants (Table 2). Several demographic and socioeconomic variables showed significant associations. Infants born first in the birth order displayed notably higher odds of inappropriate CF (OR: 3.118, $p = 0.048$) compared to those born later in the birth order. Maternal employment status also appeared to be a significant factor, with unemployed mothers showing lower odds of inappropriate CF than employed counterparts (OR: 16.875, $p = 0.015$).

Table 2. The multivariate factor analysis of inappropriate complementary feeding in children.

Variables	OR (95%CI)	*p*-Value
Body weight (kg)		
7–9	1.451 (0.56–3.7)	0.44
10–18	1.094 (0.6–1.8)	0.74
19–23 (ref)		
Gender		
Male	1.197 (0.7–1.8)	0.419
Female (ref)		
Body height (cm)		
54–68	0.765 (0.2–2.5)	0.661
69–79	0.668 (0.3–1.3)	0.250
89 and Above (ref)		
Body weight (kg)		
7–9	0.784 (0.3–1.5)	0.493
10–12	0.791 (0.4–1.5)	0.488
9–23 (ref)		
BMI (kg/m^2)		
Less than 18.5 (underweight)	0.936 (1.4–5.9)	0.944
Btw 18.5–24.9 (healthy weight)	1.496 (0.2–8.3)	0.647
Among 25–29.9 (overweight)	0.875 (0.13–5.6)	0.889
30.0 or higher above (obese) (ref)		

Table 2. *Cont.*

Variables	OR (95%CI)	*p*-Value
Birth's order		
First-born	3.118 (1.0–9.6)	0.048 *
Second-born	2.537 (0.9–6.7)	0.063
Third-born	1.954 (0.7–5.07)	0.169
Fourth-born (ref)		
Parents Information		
Age of the mother (year)		
20–30	2.854 (0.3–23)	0.327
31–40	1.826 (0.2–14)	0.575
41–50	1.500 (1.7–13)	0.714
51–60 (ref)		
Height of the mother (cm)		
150	2.571 (0.3–21)	0.384
152–165	2.489 (0.3–20)	0.391
167–180	2.613 (0.3–21)	0.368
182–193 (ref)		
Body weight (kg)		
60–70	0.680 (0.3–1.4)	0.299
71–80	0.966 (0.5–1.7)	0.914
81–90	1.052 (0.5–1.9)	0.870
Above (ref)		
Mothers Education		
None	0.589 (0.1–3.4)	0.556
Metric	0.624 (0.1–3.5)	0.595
FSC	0.388 (0.06–2.3)	0.308
University Level	0.535 (0.06–4.6)	0.569
Postgraduate (ref)		
Employment of mother		
Unemployed	16.875 (1.7–166)	0.015 *
Retired	8.195 (1–61)	0.040 *
Self employed	6.694 (0.8–51)	0.067
Employed (ref)		
Age of the Father (year)		
20–30	0.987 (0.5–1.8)	0.968
31–40	1.067 (0.5–2.0)	0.842
41–50	0.910 (0.4–1.9)	0.804
Above 60 (ref)		
Father's Education		
None	2.186 (0.2–16)	0.442
FSC	0.537 (0.3–0.9)	0.026 *
Postgraduate	0.491 (0.3–0.77)	0.002 *
University Level (ref)		
Employment of Father		
Employed	1.143 (0.7–1.7)	0.562
Not employed	0.986 (0.2–4.2)	0.985
Retired	0.245 (0.02–2.1)	0.208
Self-employed (ref)		
Household Information		

Table 2. *Cont.*

Variables	OR (95%CI)	*p*-Value
Number of Children		
2	0.194 (0.50.6)	0.008 *
3	0.621 (0.2–1.5)	0.310
4	1.249 (0.5–3.1)	0.633
5 or above (ref)		
Have enough food for children		
Yes	0.720 (0.4–1.1)	0.147
No (ref)		
Place of Delivery		
Home	1.020 (0.6–1.6)	0.931
Health Institution (ref)		
Sex of Household		
Male	0.832 (0.2–2.8)	0.772
Female (ref)		
Average Monthly Income (×1000 PKR)		
<50	1.879 (1.2–2.8)	0.002 *
50–100	1.865 (0.7–4.6)	0.184
>100 (ref)		
Difficulty in accessing healthcare facilities		
Yes	1.080 (0.6–1.6)	0.735
No (ref)		
Maternal knowledge		
<4	1.818 (1.1–2.7)	0.005 *
4–8	0.971 (0.3–2.9)	0.960
9–12 (ref)		
Child Feeding		
Has your child been fed by their mother's milk?		
Yes	0.639 (0.3–1.2)	0.177
No (ref)		
Still breastfeeding your child?		
Yes	0.443 (0.02–7.6)	0.576
No	0.360 (0.02–6)	0.476
Age at which the child stops breastfeeding? (Months)		
<6	1.051 (0.5–2.1)	0.891
6–12	1.191 (0.6–2.1)	0.548
>12	0.932 (0.5–1.5)	0.789
Skip (ref)		
Age of the child when complementary feeding was started? (Months)		
<4	1.041 (0.4–2.2)	0.919
4–6	13.91 (6.8–28.4)	<0.001 *
>7 (ref)		
Reason for starting complementary food at the chosen age?		
Baby seemed interested in food	0.964 (0.4–1.9)	0.916
Healthcare recommendation	1.117 (0.6–1.9)	0.693
Family or cultural tradition	0.917 (0.5–1.5)	0.740
I was unsure when to start (ref)		

Table 2. *Cont.*

Variables	OR (95%CI)	*p*-Value
Number of times you fed your child per day		
Once only	1.093 (0.3–3.3)	0.876
2–3 times	1.426 (0.5–4.0)	0.503
3–4 times	3.021 (1.0–8.5)	0.038 *
4+ times (ref)		
Information about clean water		
Access to clean water		
Yes	0.1443 (0.7–2.6)	0.241
No (ref)		
Does your domestic setup have the facilities to cook clean food?		
Yes	0.644 (0.3–1.11)	0.117
No (ref)		
Mothers Health		
Have you experienced any of these changes when started CF		
Weight gain	0.371 (1.1–1.04)	0.061
Weight loss	1.285 (0.6–2.5)	0.494
Digestive problems	0.968 (0.5–1.8)	0.922
Fatigue	0.750 (0.4–1.3)	0.365
Emotional changes	0.962 (0.5–1.7)	0.902
Skin changes (ref)		
Have you experienced any emotional changes when starting CF		
Felt more emotionally stable	1.679 (1–2.7)	0.047 *
Yes, my stress increases	1.024 (0.6–1.6)	0.925
It's the same (ref)		
Have you experienced any emotional changes when starting CF		
I have noticed positive changes	0.404 (0.2–0.7)	0.008 *
I have noticed negative changes	0.747 (0.4–1.1)	0.214
It's the same (ref)		

* The value is statistically significat at $p < 0.05$.

Moreover, certain parental characteristics and household dynamics were linked to inappropriate CF practices. For instance, fathers with postgraduate education displayed decreased odds of inappropriate CF (OR: 0.491, $p = 0.002$) compared to those with university-level education. Additionally, households with two children exhibited significantly lower odds of inappropriate CF (OR: 0.194, $p = 0.008$) than those with five or more children. Furthermore, financial factors played a role, with households earning less than 50k PKR per month having higher odds of inappropriate CF (OR: 1.879, $p = 0.002$) than those earning above 100k PKR per month.

Health-related factors also showed associations with inappropriate CF. For instance, infants introduced to CF between 4 and 6 months had substantially higher odds of inappropriate CF (OR: 13.91, $p < 0.001$) than those introduced after 7 months. Additionally, infants fed three to four times daily had higher odds of inappropriate CF (OR: 3.021, $p = 0.038$) compared to those fed four or more times daily.

The findings emphasize the complicated nature of factors influencing CF practices in infants, highlighting the need for targeted interventions that address socioeconomic, demographic, and health factors.

4. Discussion

This study aims to assess the prevalence of inappropriate CF among infants in Pakistan and identify factors associated with it while examining its impact on health outcomes. It is recommended to introduce CF at six months of age, as feeding before or after six months may lead to adverse health consequences.

In this study, questionnaire data were used to examine minimum dietary diversity, meal frequency, and acceptable diet among Pakistani children aged 9 to 23 months. However, according to this study, the practices of timely initiation of CF, minimum meal frequency, minimum dietary diversity, and minimum acceptable diet were 60.3%, 32.7%, 24.6%, and 48.5%, respectively, among mothers of children aged 9–23 months. The rate of timely CF initiation in our study is lower compared to regional countries, where 71% and 70% of children in Bangladesh [26] and Nepal [27]. However, Sri Lanka has the highest CF rate in South Asia, i.e., 84% [28]. The proportion of 6–23-month-old children who met the Minimum Meal Frequency (MMF) criteria in the current study was 32.7%. This is lower than the findings from Sri Lanka (88.3%), Bangladesh (81%), Nepal (82%), coastal South India (77.5%), Derashe, Southern Ethiopia (95%), and the Amibara district, Northeast Ethiopia (69.2%) [29–34]. However, it is nearly comparable to the results from Nagle Arsi (67.3%) and the Bale Zone, Ethiopia (68.4%) [35,36].

The disparity in MMF proportions among these studies may be attributed to differences in caregivers' sociocultural, educational, and employment conditions. The current study found that 24.6% of children met the Minimum Dietary Diversity (MDD), which indicates that these children were fed from at least four out of the seven food groups: grains, roots and tubers; legumes and nuts; dairy products; flesh foods; vitamin A-rich foods; eggs; and other fruits and vegetables. When comparing this figure to other studies, the percentage in the current study is somewhat similar to Bangladesh, where 42% of children met the MDD. However, it is higher than the figures reported from the Nagle Arsi region (18.8%), Damota Sore (16%), India (15%), and Nepal (34%). On the other hand, the percentage is significantly lower than in Sri Lanka, where 71% of children met the MDD [37–39].

This study shows that the significant factors of inappropriate CF are the order of birth, mother's employment status, parental education, number of children, household income, maternal knowledge, and maternal health. The findings show that maternal education, employment, and health significantly influence CF.

The work situation of mothers significantly influences the appropriateness of CF. Mothers working part-time have a reduced risk of adopting inappropriate CF compared to non-working mothers. This finding is consistent with a study conducted in Nepal [40], where working mothers, due to their increased empowerment and decision-making role in the household, are better able to manage their child's feeding. On the other hand, in developed countries, working mothers often initiate CF before 6 months, which is considered inappropriate. This early initiation is linked to their work schedules and the belief that breastfeeding is outdated [41]. In Ethiopia, some studies have shown that working mothers may wean breastfeeding too early to return to work, while non-working mothers are more likely to start CF at the recommended 6 months. Various studies have revealed that a lack of knowledge of the mother was the primary reason for the early introduction of CF [42].

Our study shows a positive correlation between mothers' education and inappropriate CF practices. Mothers with limited knowledge are less likely to know about CF, which aligns with findings from other studies [43–45]. Memon et al. described a positive relationship between maternal education and nutritional status, noting that some uneducated mothers delayed CF until their child was 1 year old [46]. Our qualitative research findings indicate that a significant number of mothers lack awareness regarding the appropriate age to initiate CF for their children. In their explanations, they cited various reasons for delaying the introduction of CF. Some expressed concerns that semi-solid and solid foods were too harsh for their children's delicate digestive systems, fearing potential adverse reactions such as vomiting or diarrhea. Despite being the primary caregivers, many mothers reported that decisions regarding feeding practices, including the introduction of CF, are often made by their husbands and mothers-in-law. Additionally, mothers acknowledged that their mothers-in-law possess greater knowledge about the nutritional requirements of children and the importance of providing them with nutrient-rich foods.

Regarding household characteristics, the monthly income also positively showed an association with inappropriate CF, similar to a published study, which showed that the percentage of timely CF at 6–8 months was higher in richer and richest households, at 51.3 and 70.9%, respectively, compared with poorest, poorer, and middle households, which achieved rates of 28.0, 33.7, and 23.1%, respectively [47]. This association are in accordance with other studies [3,28,47,48], where they also highlighted how women perceived poverty as a barrier to adequately feeding their children [48], while Liaqat et al. identified poverty as a primary factor contributing to inappropriate feeding practices [49].

In Pakistan, the timing of CF is a significant challenge, as the percentage of timely introductions of complementary food is lower than in some other South Asian nations. One of the studies conducted by Shamim et al. [50] indicates that the premature initiation of CF has been linked to an elevated risk of infections, and study [51] showed that a delayed introduction of CF negatively impacts growth and may contribute to problematic eating behaviors such as food rejection and difficulty in learning to chew. Late or early intake of complementary foods in Pakistani children is a critical concern, as a diverse diet is connected to an optimal micronutrient intake and a decreased risk of stunted development among children in underdeveloped countries.

Unlike previous research in Pakistan and other low- and middle-income countries that has primarily focused on breastfeeding, our study uniquely emphasized improving CF practices. While other study [25] like that of analyzed CF practices using data from the 2012–2013 Demographic and Health Survey, our research provides fresh, up-to-date evidence on child-feeding behaviors. Our findings reveal that factors such as childbirth order, the mother's employment, parental education, number of children, income, maternal knowledge, and maternal health significantly influence CF practices. Specifically, maternal education, employment, and health were found to have a strong impact on appropriate feeding behaviors. This highlights the importance of these socio-economic and maternal factors in improving child nutritional outcomes. Our study fills existing gaps in the literature and offers valuable insights for targeted interventions and policy recommendations to enhance CF practices in Pakistan.

Limitations of the Study

The study has several limitations that need to be considered. First, the cross-sectional nature of the data limits our ability to draw causal conclusions. Additionally, the questionnaire was administered only once, which may introduce respondent biases, such as socially desirable answers. The survey did not include detailed information on the quantity and quality of food consumed, making it difficult to assess nutritional adequacy. Furthermore, the data were collected in a hospital setting, which may not be fully representative of the general population. This setting requires participants to have access to Google and literacy skills, limiting the sample to those with these resources. A community center could have provided a broader and more diverse sample.

5. Conclusions

Our research found that the inappropriate CF practices of infants are strongly related to maternal education, job, number of children, maternal knowledge, birth order, and the mother's health. As a result, efforts must be made in laws and regulations to promote safe breastfeeding and CF, female education, and the availability of inexpensive, nutritious, and diversified meals.

Author Contributions: I.A. designed the study, acquired the data, conducted the analysis, and wrote the manuscript. P.L.B. jointly replicated the analysis and provided input on the methodology and manuscript. G.M.K. and J.U. provided insight into the refinement and improvement of the manuscript. A.A.A., A.A.I. and K.M.O. provided financial support for APC and help in revising the manuscript. J.L. provided support and project administration as the supervisor. All authors have read and agreed to the published version of the manuscript.

Funding: The authors extend their appreciation to the Deanship of Research and Graduate Studies at King Khalid University for funding this work through large Research project grant number RGP1/370/45.

Institutional Review Board Statement: This project received ethical approval from Xiang Ya School of Public Health, through "Letter No. XYGW-2023-83, 14 September 2023".

Informed Consent Statement: Informed consent was obtained from all subjects involved in the study.

Data Availability Statement: Complementary feeding and its associated factors among infants' data will be made available on demand.

Conflicts of Interest: The authors declare no conflict of interest.

References

1. Dewey, K.G.; Adu-Afarwuah, S. Systematic review of the efficacy and effectiveness of complementary feeding interventions in developing countries. *Matern. Child Nutr.* **2008**, *4*, 24–85. [CrossRef] [PubMed]
2. Ahmed, I.; Farooq, N.; Jadoon, H.; Khan, K.; Seema, N.; Saleem, S. Lactation, breast-feeding supplementation and nutrition. *J. Ayub Med. Coll. Abbottabad* **2001**, *13*, 34–37. [PubMed]
3. Dykes, F.; Lhussier, M.; Bangash, S.; Zaman, M.; Lowe, N. Exploring and optimising maternal and infant nutrition in North West Pakistan. *Midwifery* **2012**, *28*, 831–835. [CrossRef] [PubMed]
4. Pallás-Alonso, C.R. *Controversias del Nuevo Documento de la ESPGHAN Sobre Alimentación Complementaria y Lactan-Cia Maternal*; Asociación Española de Pediatría: Madrid, Spain, 2009.
5. Guiding Principles for Complementary Feeding of the Breastfed Child WHO Recomendation. Available online: https://iris.paho.org/handle/10665.2/752 (accessed on 12 September 2020).
6. Agostoni, C.; Decsi, T.; Fewtrell, M.; Goulet, O.; Kolacek, S.; Koletzko, B.; Michaelsen, K.F.; Moreno, L.; Puntis, J.; Rigo, J.; et al. Complementary Feeding: A Commentary by the ESPGHAN Committee on Nutrition. *J. Pediatr. Gastroenterol. Nutr.* **2008**, *46*, 99–110. [CrossRef]
7. WHO. *The Optimal Duration of Exclusive Breastfeeding: Report of an Expert Consultation*; World Health Organization: Geneva, Switzerland, 2001; WHO/NHD/01.09, WHO/FCH/CAH 01.24.
8. Perkin, M.R.; Logan, K.; Tseng, A.; Raji, B.; Ayis, S.; Peacock, J.; Brough, H.; Marrs, T.; Radulovic, S.; Craven, J.; et al. Randomized Trial of Introduction of Allergenic Foods in Breast-Fed Infants. *N. Engl. J. Med.* **2016**, *374*, 1733–1743. [CrossRef]
9. Grote, V.; Theurich, M.; Koletzko, B. Do complementary feeding practices predict the later risk of obesity? *Curr. Opin. Clin. Nutr. Metab. Care* **2017**, *15*, 293–297. [CrossRef]
10. Jimenez-Cruz, A.; Bacardi-Gascon, M.; Pichardo-Osuna, A.; Mandujano-Trujillo, Z.; Castillo-Ruiz, O. Infant and toddlers' feeding practices and obesity amongst low-income families in Mexico. *Asia Pac. J. Clin. Nutr.* **2010**, *19*, 316–323. [PubMed]
11. Kimani-Murage, E.W.; Madise, N.J.; Fotso, J.-C.; Kyobutungi, C.; Mutua, M.K.; Gitau, T.M.; Yatich, N. Patterns and determinants of breastfeeding and complementary feeding practices in urban informal settlements, Nairobi Kenya. *BMC Public Health* **2018**, *11*, 396.
12. Kimiywe, J.; Chege, P. Determinants of Com-plementary Feeding and Nutrition Status of Children 6–23 Months in Vihiga County, Kenya. *BAOJ* **2017**, *3*, 032.
13. Kitui, J.; Lewis, S.; Davey, G. Factors influencing place of delivery for women in Kenya: An analysis of the Kenya demographic and health survey, 2008/2009. *BMC Pregnancy Childbirth* **2013**, *13*, 40. [CrossRef]
14. Ali, M.; Arif, M.; Shah, A.A. Complementary feeding practices and associated factors among children aged 6–23 months in Paki-stan. *PLoS ONE* **2021**, *16*, e0247602. [CrossRef] [PubMed] [PubMed Central]
15. de Onis, M.; Monteiro, C.; Clugston, G. The worldwide magnitude of protein energy malnutrition: An overview from the WHO global database on child growth. *Bull. World Health Organ.* **1993**, *71*, 703–712. [PubMed]
16. Black, R.E.; Allen, L.H.; Bhutta, Z.A.; Caulfield, L.E.; De Onis, M.; Ezzati, M.; Mathers, C.; Rivera, P.J.; for the Maternal and Child Undernutrition Study Group. Maternal and child undernutrition: Global and regional exposures and health consequences. *Lancet* **2008**, *371*, 243–260. [CrossRef] [PubMed]
17. de Onis, M.; Brown, D.; Blossner, M.; Borghi, E. Levels and Trends in Child Malnutrition. In *UNICEF-WHO-The World Bank Joint Child Malnutrition Estimates*; UNICEF-WHO: New York, NY, USA, 2019.

18. Wuneh, A.G.; Ahmed, W.; Bezabih, A.M.; Reddy, P.S. Dietary Diversity and Meal Frequency Practices among Children Aged 6–23 Months in Agro Pastoral Communities in Afar Region, Ethiopia: A Cross-sectional Study. *Ecol. Food Nutr.* **2019**, *58*, 575–596. [CrossRef] [PubMed]
19. International Food Policy Research Institute. *Global Nutrition Report*; International Food Policy Research Institute: Washington, DC, USA, 2014.
20. Mekonen, E.G.; Zegeye, A.F.; Workneh, B.S. Complementary feeding practices and associated factors among mothers of children aged 6 to 23 months in Sub-saharan African countries: A multilevel analysis of the recent demographic and health survey. *BMC Public Health* **2024**, *24*, 115. [CrossRef] [PubMed] [PubMed Central]
21. Alemu, S.F.; Zerga, A.A.; Yimer, R.D.; Tadesse, S.E. Time to complementary feeding initiation and its predictors among children aged 9–23 months in Meket District, Northeast Ethiopia: A Cox Weibull regression. *J. Nutr. Sci.* **2023**, *12*, e98. [CrossRef] [PubMed] [PubMed Central]
22. Anato, A.; Baye, K.; Tafese, Z.; Stoecker, B.J. Maternal depression is associated with child undernutrition: A cross-sectional study in Ethiopia. *Matern. Child Nutr.* **2020**, *16*, e12934. [CrossRef]
23. Beyene, A.D. Determinants of off-farm participation decision of farm households in Ethiopia. *Agrekon* **2008**, *47*, 140–161. [CrossRef]
24. Krebs, N.F.; Hambidge, K.M. Complementary feeding: Clinically relevant factors affecting timing and composition. *Am. J. Clin. Nutr.* **2007**, *85*, 639S–645S. [CrossRef] [PubMed]
25. Na, M.; Aguayo, V.M.; Arimond, M.; Stewart, C.P. Risk factors of poor complementary feeding practices in Pakistani children aged 6–23 months: A multilevel analysis of the Demographic and Health Survey 2012–2013. *Matern. Child Nutr.* **2017**, *13*, e12463. [CrossRef]
26. Tessema, M.; Belachew, T.; Ersino, G. Feeding patterns and stunting during early childhood in rural communities of Sidama, South Ethiopia. *Pan Afr. Med. J.* **2013**, *14*, 75. [PubMed]
27. Black, R.E.; Victora, C.G.; Walker, S.P.; Bhutta, Z.A.; Christian, P.; De Onis, M.; Ezzati, P.M.; Grantham-McGregor, P.S.; Katz, P.J.; Martorell, P.R.; et al. Maternal and child undernutrition and overweight in low-income and middle-income countries. *Lancet* **2013**, *382*, 427–451. [CrossRef] [PubMed]
28. Senarath, U.; Godakandage, S.S.; Jayawickrama, H.; Siriwardena, I.; Dibley, M.J. Determinants of inappropriate complementary feeding practices in young children in Sri Lanka: Secondary data analysis of Demographic and Health Survey 2006–2007. *Matern. Child Nutr.* **2012**, *8* (Suppl. S1), 60–77. [CrossRef] [PubMed]
29. Manzoor, I.; Bukhari, F.S.A.; Daud, S.; Munir, M.K.; Hashmi, N.R.; Sameer, S.; Idrees, J. Weaning. *Prof. Med. J.* **2009**, *16*, 27984. [CrossRef]
30. Marandi, A.; Afzali, H.M.; Hossaini, A.F. The reasons for early weaning among mothers in Teheran. *Bull. World Health Organ.* **1993**, *71*, 561. [PubMed Central]
31. Senarath, U.; Agho, K.E.; Akram, D.; Godakandage, S.S.; Hazir, T.; Jayawickrama, H.; Joshi, N.; Kabir, I.; Khanam, M.; Patel, A.; et al. Comparisons of complementary feeding indicators and associated factors in children aged 6–23 months across five south Asian countries. *Matern. Child Nutr.* **2012**, *8* (Suppl. S1), 89–106. [CrossRef] [PubMed]
32. Senarath, U.; Dibley, M.J. Complementary feeding practices in South Asia: Analyses of recent national survey data by the South, Asia Infant Feeding Research Network. *Matern. Child Nutr.* **2012**, *8* (Suppl. S1), 5–10. [CrossRef] [PubMed]
33. Melkam, A.; Molla, M.; Zelalem, B.; Azeb, A. Dietary diversity and meal frequency practices among infant and young children aged 6–23 months in Ethiopia: A secondary analysis of Ethiopian demographic and health survey 2011. *J. Nutr. Metab.* **2013**, *2013*, 782931.
34. Rao, S.; Swathi, P.M.; Unnikrishan, B.; Hegre, A. Study of complementary feeding practices among mothers of child aged 6 months to two years- A study from coastal south India. *Australas. Med. J.* **2011**, *4*, 252–257. [CrossRef]
35. Wondafrash, M.; Amsalu, T.; Woldie, M. Feeding styles of caregivers of children 6–23 months of age in Derashe special district, Southern Ethiopia. *BMC Public Health* **2012**, *12*, 235. [CrossRef] [PubMed]
36. Wagris, M.; Seid, A.; Kahssay, M.; Ahmed, O. Minimum Meal Frequency Practice and Its Associated Factors among Children Aged 6–23 Months in Amibara District, North East Ethiopia. *J. Environ. Public Health* **2019**, *2019*, 8240864. [CrossRef] [PubMed]
37. Kassa, T.; Meshesha, B.; Haji, Y.; Ebrahim, J. Appropriate complementary feeding practices and associated factors among mothers of children age 6–23 months in southern Ethiopia, 2015. *BMC Pediatr.* **2016**, *16*, 131. [CrossRef] [PubMed]
38. Tegegne, M.; Sileshi, S.; Benti, T.; Teshome, M.; Woldie, H. Factors associated with minimal meal frequency and dietary diversity practices among infants and young children in the predominantly agrarian society of Bale zone, Southeast Ethiopia: A community based cross sectional study. *Arch. Public Health* **2017**, *75*, 53. [CrossRef] [PubMed]
39. Ergib, M.; Shumey, A.; Ferede, S.; Haile, F. Magnitude and factors associated with appropriate complementary feeding among mothers having children 6–23 months-of-age in Northern Ethiopia; A Community-Based Cross-Sectional Study. *J. Food Nutr. Sci.* **2014**, *2*, 36.
40. Areja, A.; Yohannes, D.; Yohannis, M. Determinants of appropriate complementary feeding practice among mothers having children 6–23 months of age in rural Damot sore district, Southern Ethiopia. *BMC Nutr.* **2017**, *3*, 82. [CrossRef] [PubMed]
41. UNICEF. *Infant and Young Child Feeding; Current Status Progress*; UNICEF: New York, NY, USA, 2016.

42. Joshi, N.; Agho, K.E.; Dibley, M.J.; Senarath, U.; Tiwari, K. Determinants of inappropriate complementary feeding practices in young children in Nepal: Secondary data analysis of demographic and Health Survey 2006. *Matern. Child Nutr.* **2012**, *8*, 45–59. [CrossRef]
43. Gardner, H.; Green, K.; Gardner, A.; Scott, J.; Binns, C. Infant Feeding Practices of Emirati Women in the rapidly developing City of Abu Dhabi, United Arab Emirates. *Int. J. Environ. Res. Public Health* **2015**, *12*, 10923–10940. [CrossRef]
44. Shumey, A.; Demissie, M.; Berhane, Y. Timely initiation of complementary feeding and associated factors among children aged 6 to 12 months in Northern Ethiopia: An institution-based cross-sectional study. *BMC Public Health* **2013**, *13*, 1050. [CrossRef]
45. Shamim, S. Weaning practices in peri-urban low socioeconomic groups. *J. Coll. Physicians Surg. Pak.* **2005**, *15*, 129–132.
46. Memon, S.; Shaikh, S.; Kousar, T.; Memon, Y. Assessment of infant feeding practices at a tertiary care hospital. *J. Pak. Med. Assoc.* **2010**, *60*, 1010–1015.
47. Hazir, T.; Senarath, U.; Agho, K.; Akram, D.S.; Kazmi, N.; Abbasi, S.; Dibley, M.J. Determinants of inappropriate timing of introducing solid, semi-solid or soft food to infants in Pakistan: Secondary data analysis of Demographic and Health Survey 2006–2007. *Matern. Child Nutr.* **2012**, *8*, 78–88. [CrossRef] [PubMed]
48. Lingam, R.; Gupta, P.; Zafar, S.; Hill, Z.; Yousafzai, A.; Iyengar, S.; Sikander, S.; Haq, Z.U.; Mehta, S.; Skordis-Worrel, J.; et al. Understanding care and feeding practices: Building blocks for a sustainable intervention in India and Pakistan. *Ann. N. Y. Acad. Sci.* **2014**, *1308*, 204–217. [CrossRef] [PubMed]
49. Liaqat, P.; Rizvi, M.A.; Qayyum, A.; Ahmed, H. Association between complementary feeding practice and mothers education status in Islamabad. *J. Hum. Nutr. Diet.* **2007**, *20*, 340–344. [CrossRef] [PubMed]
50. Shamim, S.; Naz, F.; Jamalvi, S.W.; Ali, S.S. Effects of weaning period on nutritional status of children. *J. Coll Physicians Surg. Pak.* **2006**, *16*, 529–531.
51. Sarwar, T. Infant feeding practices of Pakistani mothers in England and Pakistan. *J. Hum. Nutr. Diet.* **2002**, *15*, 419–428. [CrossRef]

nutrients

MDPI

Article

A Descriptive Study of Spanish and Ecuadorian Commercial Infant Cereals: Are They in Line with Current Recommendations?

Debby Guevara [1], Ascensión Marcos [2], Fátima Isabel Ruiz [3], Sonia Gómez-Martínez [2,*] and Susana del Pozo [1]

[1] Department of Nutrition and Food Science, Faculty of Pharmacy, Complutense University of Madrid, 28040 Madrid, Spain; debbygue@ucm.es (D.G.); spozocal@ucm.es (S.d.P.)
[2] Immunonutrition Research Group, Department of Metabolism and Nutrition, Institute of Food Science and Technology and Nutrition (ICTAN)—CSIC, 28040 Madrid, Spain; amarcos@ictan.csic.es
[3] Retiro Social Services Center, Madrid City Council, 28007 Madrid, Spain; ruizgfa.ext@madrid.es
* Correspondence: sgomez@ictan.csic.es; Tel.: +34-699523142

Abstract: Cereals are an important source of nutrients, especially used in complementary feeding. The objective of this study is to review the nutritional composition of cereal-based foods for infants from 4 months and toddlers that are offered in Spain and Ecuador, countries selected because of the opportunity to work in them, and due to their socio-economic differences (industrialized and developing countries, respectively). The number of these products was 105 cereals in Spain and 22 in Ecuador. The products were classified as gluten-free cereals, five cereals, eight cereals, multigrain cereals, and cookies. A 25 g serving was used to determine the percentage in which the samples analyzed can cover the Reference Nutrient Intake (RNI) for micronutrients in infants from 7 months and toddlers according to the European Food Safety Authority (EFSA). Nutritional information per 100 g of dry product was collected according to medium, minimum, and maximum units, and nutrient density was calculated. The age range in which these products are recommended is different in both countries. The nutritional composition presents some differences; Spanish cereals show a lower content of sodium, added sugars, hydrolyzed cereals, and maltodextrin than Ecuadorian cereals. Commercialized cereals could contribute to satisfying the nutritional needs of infants and toddlers; however, they can also be a source of non-recommended components.

Keywords: Spain; Ecuador; cereals; cookies; infants; toddler; complementary feeding; macronutrients; micronutrients

1. Introduction

Diet quality can be influenced by characteristics of the country of residence, such as socio-economic status. Indicators such as Gross Domestic Product (GDP) can give us information about differences between countries. In this sense, Spain and Ecuador, with different GDPs (USD 52.01 thousand per capita and USD 14.48 thousand per capita, respectively), are examples of industrialized and developing countries, respectively [1].

An optimal diet, leading to a nutritional situation that prevents alterations by excess or defect during the first 1000 days of human life (from pregnancy to 2 years of age), is the key to maintaining a good state of health throughout life [2].

Under this premise, the introduction of new foods for "infants", understood as "children under 12 months of age" [3], is a crucial moment to initiate healthy feeding practices [4]. The introduction of foods other than breastmilk or infant formula as a complement to, rather than a substitute for, breastfeeding is called complementary feeding (CF), or Beikost [5]. According to the current evidence base, the World Health Organisation (WHO) supports the initiation of CF from the sixth month, with particular emphasis on not delaying initiation beyond this time to avoid nutritional deficiencies, especially iron and zinc deficiencies [6]. This initiation of CF at 6 months is also indicated by the Ecuadorian Ministry of Public

Health (MSP) [7] and the Spanish Paediatric Association (AEP) [5]. The AEP allows the introduction of foods from 4 months of age in non-breastfed children [5].

The European Society for Pediatric Gastroenterology, Hepatology, and Nutrition (ESPGHAN) also agrees with this recommendation [4]. According to the European Food Safety Authority (EFSA) recommendations, the introduction of foods before 6 months of age is not necessary, except in infants at risk of iron deficiency, when introducing iron-rich foods before 6 months of age could be beneficial [8]. In the LAyDI study, which included 1200 Spanish children born between April 2017 and March 2018, it was observed that the average iron intake was lower than the EFSA recommendations, possibly due to a decrease in the consumption of processed infant foods enriched with iron among children aged 18 to 24 months [9]. Other studies in Spain indicate deficiencies of micronutrients in the diets of more than half of children, particularly in vitamins E and D, calcium, folate, and magnesium [10,11]. Meanwhile, in Ecuador, 9.9% of children under five years of age and 1.8% of school-aged children have iron deficiency [12]. Furthermore, zinc deficiency is present in 27.5% of children under 5 years old and in 28.1% of school-aged children [12].

To initiate this transition between exclusive breastfeeding and Beikost, the latest recommendations of the AEP state that CF can be initiated with any food that does not pose a risk of choking [5], as does the MSP, which suggests starting CF with soft foods [13]. These guidelines in both countries are in line with the infant feeding method called "Baby Led Weaning (BLW)", which involves the baby leading their own feeding [14], choosing from a variety of soft food offered by the parents/guardians [5,15]. This may lead to better energy self-regulation [16] like the BLISS method, which, in addition to promoting energy self-regulation, aims to prevent iron deficiency by offering foods that meet their nutritional needs [17].

For decades, this initiation of CF has mainly been carried out with the cereal group [18], as it serves as an excellent vehicle for enriching the diet with iron [18], thus covering the needs for this mineral, which are increased in infants from 6 months of age [19]. Cereals are also a good source of phosphorus and potassium, as well as vitamins, including those of the B group, except B_{12} [18,20]. However, it should be remembered that these micronutrients are found in the bran, so their final contribution will depend on the degree of grain processing [18,20]. A frequent practice in the industry is subsequent enrichment [21]. Other reasons for the use of cereals to initiate CF are its mild taste, semi-solid consistency, and texture [22].

All of the above-mentioned benefits led to the popularization of cereal products in infant feeding during the 19th century, resulting in their commercialization [18]. According to the Spanish Agency of Food Safety and Nutrition (AESAN), "Cereal-based foods are those intended to meet the specific needs of infants (children under 12 months of age) and toddlers (children from 1 to 3 years of age) in good health, as a supplement to their diet and/or for their progressive adaptation to the family diet" [3]. The presentation of these products has evolved over time. Initially, infant cereals consisted of a mixture of cereal flour and water. By the mid-19th century, the first infant formulas containing cow's milk, wheat flour, and malt flour appeared. Subsequently, modified starches became a common component in the preparation of baby foods [18] through the process of hydrolysis, which involves improved starch digestibility and its dispersibility in liquids, resulting in an enhancement of sensory properties, including an increase in sweetness due to the release of sugar [23]. Considering the ESPGHAN recommendations to avoid sugar in CF [4], this practice is not recommended [24]. The European Childhood Obesity Project found that over 95% of Spanish infants aged 9 to 12 months included in its study cohort consumed at least one sugary commercial complementary food [25].

Based on the aforementioned considerations, the aim of this study is to review the nutritional composition of cereal-based foods that are offered to infants from 4 months and toddlers in Spain and Ecuador, countries selected because of the opportunity to work in them and their socio-economic differences (industrialized and developing countries, respectively).

2. Materials and Methods

For the present study, nutritional information and ingredient labeling of 212 processed cereal-based foods were collected in 2021. However, in 2022, the database of this sample was updated to visualize changes in the market of these CF products, incorporating new products and eliminating those that were no longer sold, resulting in a total of 127 processed cereal-based foods. Thus, in Spain, a sample of 192 products was selected between January and March 2021. However, the sample was updated between May and June 2022, resulting in a final sample of 105 products (70 non-updated, 18 updated, and 17 new): 96 commercial infant cereals and 9 cookies (Figure 1). In Ecuador, a sample of 20 products was selected between February and March 2021 and subsequently updated in July 2022, resulting in a sample of 22 products (13 non-updated, 4 updated, and 5 new): 16 commercial infant cereals and 6 cookies (Figure 1). For the selection of these products, researchers included infant cereals for children up to two years of age and infant cookies commercialized in pharmacies, supermarkets, and websites from Spain and Ecuador, excluding cereal-based products for children over two years of age.

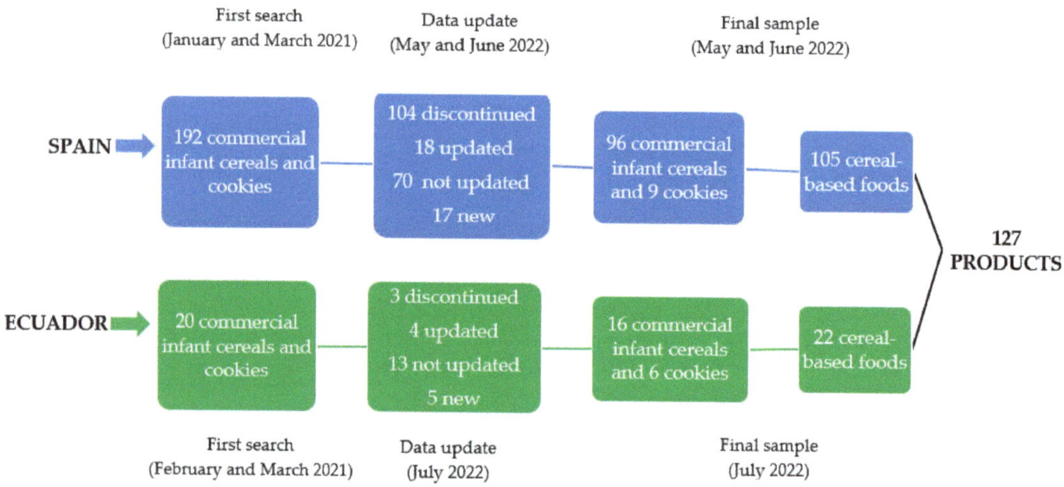

Figure 1. Sample selection.

The samples were classified using the commercial names of the cereals (gluten-free cereals, 5 cereals, 8 cereals, multigrain cereals, and cookies), as well as the type and number of cereals, mentioning that the "multigrain" category included products that contained more than one cereal, but could not be grouped in either the "5 cereals" or the "8 cereals" categories due to the number of cereals present.

The following data were recorded: the recommended age of consumption by the manufacturer, the types of cereals present in each category, and the number of products with whole grains and added sugars (including glucose, fructose, sucrose, glucose syrup, and those naturally present in honey and fruit juices), using AESAN as a reference [26], and hydrolyzed cereals (when the ingredients indicated hydrolyzed or dextrinized cereal).

The sugar content was examined based on the AESAN criteria, which state that "A food may only be declared as having a low sugar content, as well as any other declaration that may have the same meaning for the consumer, if the product does not contain more than 5 g of sugars per 100 g in the case of solids" [27].

Along these lines, the fiber content indicated on the labeling was also reviewed to determine whether it met the AESAN criteria for declaring a food high in fiber (≥6 g of fiber per 100 g or 3 g of fiber per 100 kcal) [27].

In addition, since the nutritional labeling of the Spanish products only indicated the salt content, the sodium content was calculated by converting salt to sodium (salt in g = sodium in g × 2.5) [28]. However, in Ecuador, this calculation was omitted, as the Ecuadorian products do indicate the sodium content.

Considering the serving size suggested by most manufacturers, a 25 g serving was used to determine the percentage in which the samples analyzed cover the Reference Nutrient Intake (RNI) for vitamins and minerals of infants (7 months to 1 year) and toddlers (1 to 3 years) according to the EFSA [29]. Importantly, the 4- to 6-month-old group was excluded from the analysis due to the absence of commercial cereals targeting children under 6 months in Ecuador, as they are not recommended for this age range [7]. The current study reviewed various nutritional variables, including energy, protein, total fat, saturated fat, carbohydrates, total sugars, and fiber. Additionally, water-soluble vitamins such as vitamin C (ascorbic acid), vitamin B_1 (thiamin), vitamin B_2 (riboflavin), vitamin B_3 (niacin), vitamin B_5 (pantothenic acid), vitamin B_6 (pyridoxine), vitamin B_9 (folic acid), and vitamin B_{12} (cobalamin), as well as fat-soluble vitamins, such as vitamin A (retinol), vitamin D (cholecalciferol), and vitamin E (tocopherol), were reviewed. Minerals such as calcium, iron, zinc, and sodium were also reviewed. For the statistical analysis, nutritional information of these variables was collected per 100 g of dry product according to medium, minimum, and maximum units, and nutrient density (the amount of nutrient/unit of energy, in our case calculated per 1000 kcal) was calculated using Excel 2021.

3. Results

3.1. Characteristics of the Sample

A total of 127 cereal-based foods were included from Spain (105) and from Ecuador (22). These products were categorized based on their commercial denomination as follows: gluten-free cereals (27), five cereals (13), eight cereals (43), multigrain cereals (29) and cookies (15) (Table 1).

Table 1. Description of products from Spain and Ecuador.

Commercial Cereal Categories	Country	Total	Gluten	Whole Grains	Added Sugar	Hydrolyzed Cereals
		Number of Products				
GLUTEN-FREE CEREALS	Spain	23	0	6	1	11
	Ecuador	4	0	0	0	3
5 CEREALS	Spain	7	7	5	0	5
	Ecuador	6	6	3	1	2
8 CEREALS	Spain	39	39	22	19	21
	Ecuador	4	4	1	1	3
MULTIGRAIN CEREALS	Spain	27	27	12	6	10
	Ecuador	2	2	1	1	1
COOKIES	Spain	9	7	1	9	0
	Ecuador	6	4	1	5	0

Regarding the recommended age for the consumption of infant cereals, the commercial companies in Ecuador suggest their 22 products from 6 months of age. In contrast, 25 infant cereals from Spain are recommended from 4 months of age, with only one product containing gluten in this group.

3.2. Description of Ingredients

The samples were categorized based on the number of cereals they contain, with Spain predominantly featuring products from the "8-cereals" category (n = 39), while Ecuador had products from the "5-cereals" category (n = 6) and "cookies" (n = 6). Additionally, the cereals comprising each category were examined. In both countries, the "gluten-free" category mainly consists of rice and corn. Conversely, the "5-cereals" category is characterized by wheat, barley, oats, and rice, with corn in Ecuador and rye in Spain. The "8-cereals" category typically includes wheat, corn, rice, oats, barley, rye, sorghum, and millet in both countries, also featuring products with triticale and spelt in Spain. In the "multigrain" category, products usually contain wheat, rice, and oats in both countries, while Spain additionally offers products with corn, quinoa, barley, rye, and spelt. Cookies in both countries commonly contain wheat, rice, and oats; meanwhile, often in Spain, corn, barley, and rye are also included.

Table 1 shows the number of products containing gluten, whole grains, added sugars, and hydrolyzed grains. The "5-cereals" category has the highest percentage of products that include whole grains.

It is worth noting that, with the exception of one cookie in Ecuador, all of them mention the presence of added sugars, but none of these products contain hydrolyzed cereals (Table 1).

3.3. *Energy and Nutrient Content per 100 g of Product*

In terms of energy content, children's cereals offered in Spain (377–438 kcal/100 g) and Ecuador (377–420 kcal/100 g) show similar values. Notably, cookies have the highest caloric content among the categories (Table 2).

Regarding macronutrient content, the samples showed similar amounts of proteins, carbohydrates, and fats. The labeling also indicated the presence of saturated fatty acids, which were found in greater quantities in the cookies compared to the other categories (Table 2).

Following the AESAN criteria [27], 39 products in Spain and 2 products in Ecuador can be classified as "low in sugar" ($\leq$5 g of sugars per 100 g) (Table 2).

The fiber content indicated on the labeling was also examined, revealing that cereals marketed in Spain contain a higher amount (2–8 g/100 g) of fiber compared to those offered in Ecuador (1–4.3 g/100 g), with gluten-free cereals and cookies having the lowest amount of fiber in both countries. Additionally, some products meet the criteria set by AESAN for declaring a food as high in fiber ($\geq$6 g of fiber per 100 g or 3 g of fiber per 100 kcal) [27], despite not explicitly stating it in their commercial name (Table 2).

Regarding the declaration of vitamin content in nutrition labeling, in Ecuador, products in the category of multigrain cereals do not declare the amount of any vitamin and cookies only declare the content of vitamin B_1. In Spain, on the other hand, multigrain cereals declare the presence of all the vitamins studied and cookies declare vitamins B_1, B_2, B_3, B_5, B_6 and C (Table 2).

Among the cereals that report their micronutrient content, Table 2 shows that vitamin C is found in greater quantities in the five-cereal category.

Regarding minerals, the calcium content indicated on the label is higher in the cereals offered in Ecuador. In relation to iron, cereal products and cookies marketed in Ecuador have the highest amount of this mineral. With regard to sodium, cookies are the products with the highest content in both countries (Table 2).

Table 2. Energy and nutrient content per 100 g of Spanish and Ecuadorian products (median).

	Country	Gluten-Free Cereals	5 Cereals	8 Cereals	Multigrain Cereals	Cookies
Number of products	Spain	23	7	39	27	9
	Ecuador	4	6	4	2	6
				Median (minimum–maximum)		
Energy kcal/100 g	Spain	382 (277–416)	379 (368–388)	377 (366–416)	382 (362–414)	438 (423–466)
	Ecuador	380 (380–382)	380 (374–420)	376.5 (370–420)	385 (380–390)	420 (357.1–420)
Proteins g/100 g	Spain	7.5 (3.9–13.6)	9.6 (5.7–12.4)	9.4 (4.6–14.8)	9.3 (4.6–15.3)	6.8 (1.1–11.2)
	Ecuador	7.3 (7–8.5)	10 (7–16)	9.5 (7–15)	8 (6–10)	8 (7.1–10)
* Fats g/100 g	Spain	1.5 (0.6–8.1)	1.8 (1.3–4)	2 (0.9–8.6)	2.4 (1.2–8.5)	12.2 (10–14.3)
	Ecuador	1.4 (0.5–1.5)	2.5 (1.6–25)	2.2 (1.6–9)	2.8 (1.5–4)	8 (8–10)
** SFA g/100 g	Spain	0.2 (0–3)	0.4 (0.2–0.8)	0.4 (0.17–3.1)	0.5 (0.2–3.1)	4.5 (1.2–7.6)
	Ecuador	0.3 (0.2–0.5)	0.2 (0–4)	0.3 (0.2–2.9)	1 (1–1)	1 (0.9–1)
Carbohydrates g/100 g	Spain	83 (72–91)	73.8 (72.8–87.2)	76.5 (68.4–88.5)	76.7 (68–87.1)	75.4 (68.9–81)
	Ecuador	84.6 (84–86)	81.5 (68–84)	80.5 (66–84)	83 (82–84)	80 (73–95.2)
* Sugar g/100 g	Spain	3.2 (0.3–29)	18 (1.5–28)	20.2 (1–39.1)	7.5 (0.6–35)	24 (12–32.5)
	Ecuador	18 (12–28)	22 (1–28)	26.5 (22–37)	23 (22–24)	23 (3–23.8)
Fiber g/100 g	Spain	2 (0.1–8.5)	8 (1.9–10.5)	6.1 (2.2–11)	6 (1–10.6)	2.3 (0.6–5.3)
	Ecuador	1.1 (0.5–5)	4 (2–4)	4.3 (3.3–11)	4.3 (3–5.5)	1 (0.7–4)
				VITAMINS		
Vitamin C mg/100 g	Spain	30 (25–70)	50 (30–71)	30 (30–85)	30 (25–93)	35 (35–35)
	Ecuador	42.5 (35–50)	50 (25–60)	35 (25–50)	-	-
Vitamin B_1 mg/100 g	Spain	0.5 (0.5–1.6)	0.5 (0.5–0.8)	0.5 (0.5–1.3)	0.8 (0.5–1.8)	0.5 (0.48–1.2)
	Ecuador	0.5 (0.4–0.5)	0.5 (0.4–0.5)	0.4 (0.4–0.5)	-	0.8 (0.8–0.8)
Vitamin B_2 mg/100 g	Spain	0.6 (0.32–0.6)	0.6 (0.6–0.6)	0.6 (0–0.6)	0.6 (0.32–0.6)	0.6 (0.3–1)
	Ecuador	0.6 (0.6–0.6)	0.5 (0.3–0.5)	0.6 (0.3–0,6)	-	-
Vitamin B_3 mg/100 g	Spain	6 (3–8.9)	6 (5–6.5)	6 (3–8.5)	7.25 (3–8.9)	5.9 (4.1–10)
	Ecuador	5.5 (5–6)	3.6 (3.3–3.6)	5 (3.3–6)	-	-
Vitamin B_5 mg/100 g	Spain	2.8 (2–3)	2.8 (2.5–2.8)	2.7 (2–2.8)	2.8 (2–3)	2.4 (1.8–5)
	Ecuador	2.9 (2.8–3)	2 (0.2–2)	2.8 (1.5–3)	-	-
Vitamin B_6 mg/100 g	Spain	0.4 (0.3–0.8)	0.6 (0.3–0.8)	0.4 (0.25–0.8)	0.4 (0.3–0.8)	0.6 (0.4–1)
	Ecuador	0.7 (0.6–0.8)	0.3 (0.3–0.43)	0.6 (0.4–0.8)	-	-
Vitamin B_9 µg/100 g	Spain	50 (30–70)	45 (40–56)	50 (30–80)	70 (30–100)	-
	Ecuador	52.5 (40–65)	80 (22–80)	40 (22–65)	-	-

Table 2. *Cont.*

	Country	Gluten-Free Cereals	5 Cereals	8 Cereals	Multigrain Cereals	Cookies
Vitamin B_{12} µg/100 g	Spain	1 (0.5–1.1)	1 (1–1)	1 (1–1.1)	0.5 (0.5–1)	-
	Ecuador	1 (0.9–1)	0.7 (0.5–0.7)	0.9 (0.5–1)	-	-
Vitamin A µg/100 g	Spain	420 (255–450)	435 (300–450)	420 (255–450)	375 (255–450)	-
	Ecuador	410 (370–450)	500 (394–500)	394 (370–450)	-	-
Vitamin D µg/100 g	Spain	7.5 (5–10)	7.5 (7.5–9)	7.5 (5–11.5)	7.5 (5–11)	-
	Ecuador	7.3 (7–7.5)	6.6 (6.6–6.6)	7 (6.6–7.5)	-	-
Vitamin E mg/100 g	Spain	4.4 (2.8–5.4)	4.7 (4.4–5)	4.4 (2.8–6)	4.7 (3–7.3)	-
	Ecuador	3.5 (2.5–4.4)	4 (2.4–4)	2.5 (2.4–4.4)	-	-
				MINERALS		
Calcium mg/100 g	Spain	160 (132–678)	256 (145–430)	176.5 (144–669)	179.5 (133–666)	310 (290–329)
	Ecuador	324.5 (160–489)	310 (310–435)	420 (160–470)	-	310 (310–310)
Iron mg/100 g	Spain	7.5 (5.2–8)	7 (5.2–9)	7.5 (2–10.5)	7.5 (5.5–11)	5.9 (5–8.3)
	Ecuador	6.5 (6–7)	32 (5.8–31.9)	6 (5.8–7)	-	24 (24–24)
Zinc mg/100 g	Spain	1.2 (1–4.4)	2.8 (1.1–4.4)	1.2 (1–4.4)	1.3 (1.1–5.3)	-
	Ecuador	2.5 (2.5–2.5)	2.8 (2.8–2.8)	2.5 (2.5–2.5)	-	11 (11–11)
* Sodium mg/100 g	Spain	16 (8–224)	24 (8–40)	20 (8–240)	16 (8–240)	88 (32–360)
	Ecuador	26.5 (12–30)	27.5 (20–150)	32.5 (12–140)	32.5 (30–35)	134.5 (2.5–250)

* Critical nutrients. ** SFA: saturated fatty acid. - No information is provided or the detailed micronutrient composition is not available.

3.4. The Nutrient Density of Infant Cereals

To assess the nutritional quality of infant cereals, their nutrient density (amount of nutrients per 1000 kcal) was calculated. Based on this measure, it was observed that the "5-cereals" category exhibits the highest protein density (Table 3).

Regarding fiber density, cereals available in Spain (5–20.7 g/1000 kcal) demonstrate higher levels compared to those in Ecuador (2–11 g/1000 kcal) (Table 3).

From these findings, it is notable that vitamins D and E, in products where they are specified, tend to be higher in cereals from Spain (Table 3).

Based on the minerals most frequently declared in the products reviewed (calcium, iron, zinc, and sodium), we can highlight that, in terms of the nutritional density of iron, the greatest differences between both samples are observed in the "5-cereals" and "cookies" categories, with higher levels in the products commercialized in Ecuador. Additionally, the nutritional density of zinc and sodium was higher in the cereals offered in Ecuador (Table 3).

3.5. Results of the Contribution of 25 g of Product to the EFSA Recommended Nutrient Intakes for Infants and Toddlers

Table 4 presents the percentage by which these products can meet the EFSA RNIs for micronutrients of infants (7 months to 1 year) and toddlers (1 to 3 years) in an average serving of 25 g. It is important to note that Table 4 only displays the percentages of RNIs for vitamins and minerals declared in the nutritional labeling. Upon closer examination of the data, it is notable that products in the "5-cereals" category, in a 25 g serving, can meet more than 60% of the RNI for vitamin C. It is worth mentioning that the reviewed sample contributes a higher percentage towards meeting the RNI for vitamin C, while it provides a lower percentage to fulfill the RNI for vitamin B_9 and sodium.

In terms of the RNI for vitamin A, it can be observed that a 25 g serving of cereals offered in Spain and Ecuador provides more than 39% of the RNI (Table 4).

Considering the percentage contribution of all categories to the RNI for iron, significant differences are noted between the minimum and maximum values in the cereals offered in Ecuador. For instance, products in the "5-cereals" category contribute up to 114% of the recommendations (Table 4).

Table 3. The nutrient density of the products ***.

		Gluten-Free Cereals	5 Cereals	8 Cereals	Multigrain Cereals	Cookies
Number of products	Spain	23	7	39	27	9
	Ecuador	4	6	4	2	6
				Median (minimum–maximum)		
Proteins g/1000 kcal	Spain	19.8 (9.9–32.7)	25.8 (15–32.5)	25.1 (11.9–35.6)	24.9 (11.9–39.3)	14.6 (2.4–26.3)
	Ecuador	19 (18.4–22.4)	25.7 (18.7–38.1)	25.3 (18.9–35.7)	20.9 (15.4–26.3)	20 (19.1–23.8)
Fiber g/1000 kcal	Spain	5.1 (0.2–22.9)	20.7 (4.9–28.5)	16 (5.5–30.1)	15.7 (2.5–28.8)	5 (1.3–12.1)
	Ecuador	2.9 (1.3–13.2)	10.5 (4.8–10.5)	10.7 (8.6–29.7)	11 (7.9–14.1)	2 (2–9.5)
				VITAMINS		
Vitamin C mg/1000 kcal	Spain	79.4 (67–179)	134.6 (77.3–184)	80.4 (72.1–217)	78.1 (65.5–245)	82.2 (82.2–82.2)
	Ecuador	112 (91.6–132)	132 (65.8–158)	91.4 (59.5–135)	-	-
Vitamin B_1 mg/1000 kcal	Spain	1.5 (1.3–4.2)	1.4 (1.3–2.1)	1.4 (1.3–3.1)	2.1 (1.3–4.9)	1.2 (1.1–2.7)
	Ecuador	1.2 (1.1–1.3)	1.2 (1.1–1.3)	1 (1–1.4)	-	2 (1.9–1.9)
Vitamin B_2 mg/1000 kcal	Spain	1.6 (0.8–1.6)	1.6 (1.6–1.6)	1.6 (0.8–1.6)	1.6 (0.8–1.7)	1.4 (0.7–2.3)
	Ecuador	1.6 (1.6–1.6)	1.3 (0.9–1.3)	1.6 (0.8–1.6)	-	-
Vitamin B_3 mg/1000 kcal	Spain	16 (7.2–30.7)	16.2 (12.9–16.8)	16 (7.2–22.7)	19 (7.3–24.6)	13.9 (9.7–23.4)
	Ecuador	14.4 (13.1–15.8)	9.5 (8.7–9.5)	13.1 (7.9–16.2)	-	-
Vitamin B_5 mg/1000 kcal	Spain	7.2 (4.8–8)	7.5 (6.4–7.6)	7 (4.8–7.7)	7.4 (4.8–8.3)	5.6 (4.1–11.8)
	Ecuador	7.6 (7.4–7.9)	5.3 (0.6–5.3)	7.6 (3.6–7.8)	-	-
Vitamin B_6 mg/1000 kcal	Spain	0.9 (0.7–2.2)	1.6 (0.8–2.2)	0.9 (0.6–2.2)	1.1 (0.7–2.1)	1.4 (0.9–2.3)
	Ecuador	1.8 (1.6–2.1)	0.8 (0.8–1.1)	1.6 (1–2.2)	-	-
Vitamin B_9 µg/1000 kcal	Spain	129 (72.1–253)	119 (108–145)	130 (72.1–204)	185 (72.5–264)	-
	Ecuador	138 (105–170)	211 (58–211)	108 (52.4–170)	-	-
Vitamin B_{12} µg/1000 kcal	Spain	2.7 (1.3–2.7)	2.7 (2.7–2.7)	2.7 (2.6–2.7)	1.3 (1.2–2.6)	-
	Ecuador	2.5 (2.4–2.6)	1.8 (1.3–1.8)	2.4 (1.2–2.7)	-	-
Vitamin A µg/1000 kcal	Spain	1084 (613–1354)	1159 (775–1223)	1097 (613–1230)	993 (616–1187)	-
	Ecuador	1076 (969–1184)	1316 (1037–1316)	966 (938–1216)	-	-
Vitamin D µg/1000 kcal	Spain	20 (12–36.1)	20.2 (19.3–23.3)	20.1 (12–29.3)	19.8 (0–29)	-
	Ecuador	19 (18.3–19.7)	17.4 (17.4–17.4)	18.3 (15.7–20.3)	-	-
Vitamin E mg/1000 kcal	Spain	11.7 (7.2–13.8)	12.4 (11.8–13.2)	11.9 (7.2–15.1)	12.2 (7.3–19.1)	-
	Ecuador	9 (6.5–11.6)	10.5 (6.3–10.5)	6.5 (5.7–11.9)	-	-
				MINERALS		
Calcium mg/1000 kcal	Spain	425 (336–1630)	679 (374–1156)	455 (363–1617)	477 (345–1609)	708 (678–778)
	Ecuador	853 (419–1287)	816 (816–1145)	768 (0–1135)	-	738 (738–738)
Iron mg/1000 kcal	Spain	19.5 (12.5–27.1)	19 (13.7–23.3)	19.8 (5.3–26.8)	20 (13.3–28.8)	13.9 (11.4–19.6)
	Ecuador	17.1 (15.7–18.4)	84 (15.3–84)	14.7 (0–18.9)	-	57 (57.1–57.1)
Zinc mg/1000 kcal	Spain	3.1 (2.7–11.5)	7.2 (2.8–11.6)	3.1 (2.5–11.7)	3.3 (2.8–13.7)	-
	Ecuador	6.5 (6.5–6.5)	7.4 (7.4–7.4)	6.5 (6.5–6.5)	-	26 (26.2–26.2)
Sodium mg/1000 kcal	Spain	42.2 (21.1–539)	64.5 (21.1–109)	51.7 (20.8–577)	43.2 (20.1–580)	208 (69.7–845)
	Ecuador	69.7 (31.4–78.9)	73 (52.6–357)	87.8 (67.6–67.6)	84.4 (79–89.7)	345 (6–595)

*** Nutrient density/1000 kcal. - No information is provided or the detailed micronutrient composition is not available.

Table 4. Results of the contribution of 25 g of product to the EFSA Recommended Nutrient Intakes for infants and toddlers.

	Age	Country	Gluten-Free Cereals	5 Cereals	8 Cereals	Multigrain Cereals	Cookies
					VITAMINS		
Vitamin C (%)	7–12 month	Spain	38	63	38	38	44
		Ecuador	53	63	44	-	-
	1–3 years	Spain	38	63	38	38	44
		Ecuador	53	63	44	-	-
Vitamin B_1 (%)	7–12 months	Spain	42	42	42	67	42
		Ecuador	42	42	33	-	67
	1–3 years	Spain	25	25	25	40	25
		Ecuador	25	25	20	-	40
Vitamin B_2 (%)	7–12 months	Spain	38	38	38	38	38
		Ecuador	38	31	38	-	-
	1–3 years	Spain	25	25	25	25	25
		Ecuador	25	21	25	-	-
Vitamin B_3 (%)	7–12 months	Spain	34	34	34	41	34
		Ecuador	31	20	28	-	-
	1–3 years	Spain	20	20	20	24	20
		Ecuador	19	12	17	-	-
Vitamin B_5 (%)	7–12 months	Spain	23	23	23	23	20
		Ecuador	24	17	23	-	-
	1–3 years	Spain	18	18	17	18	15
		Ecuador	18	13	18	-	-
Vitamin B_6 (%)	7–12 months	Spain	33	50	33	33	50
		Ecuador	58	25	50	-	-
	1–3 years	Spain	17	25	17	17	25
		Ecuador	29	13	25	-	-
Vitamin B_9 (%)	7–12 months	Spain	0.02	0.02	0.02	0.02	-
		Ecuador	0.02	0.03	0.01	-	-
	1–3 years	Spain	0.01	0.01	0.01	0.01	-
		Ecuador	0.01	0.02	0.01	-	-

Table 4. *Cont.*

	Age	Country	Gluten-Free Cereals	5 Cereals	8 Cereals	Multigrain Cereals	Cookies
Vitamin B_{12} (%)	7–12 months	Spain	17	17	17	8	-
		Ecuador	17	12	15	-	-
	1–3 years	Spain	17	17	17	8	-
		Ecuador	17	12	15	-	-
Vitamin A (%)	7–12 months	Spain	42	44	42	38	-
		Ecuador	41	50	39	-	-
	1–3 years	Spain	42	44	42	38	-
		Ecuador	41	50	39	-	-
Vitamin D (%)	7–12 months	Spain	19	19	19	19	-
		Ecuador	18	17	18	-	-
	1–3 years	Spain	13	13	13	13	-
		Ecuador	12	11	12	-	-
Vitamin E (%)	7–12 months	Spain	22	24	22	24	-
		Ecuador	18	20	13	-	-
	1–3 years	Spain	12	13	12	13	-
		Ecuador	10	11	7	-	-
					MINERALS		
Calcium (%)	7–12 months	Spain	14	23	16	16	28
		Ecuador	29	28	38	-	28
	1–3 years	Spain	9	14	10	10	17
		Ecuador	18	17	23	-	17
Iron (%)	7–12 months	Spain	17	16	17	17	13
		Ecuador	15	73	14	-	55
	1–3 years	Spain	27	25	27	27	21
		Ecuador	23	114	22	-	86
Zinc (%)	7–12 months	Spain	10	24	10	11	-
		Ecuador	22	24	22	-	95
	1–3 years	Spain	7	16	7	8	-
		Ecuador	15	16	15	-	64
Sodium (%)	7–12 months	Spain	2	3	2.5	2	11
		Ecuador	3	3.4	4	4	17
	1–3 years	Spain	0.4	0.5	0.5	0.4	2
		Ecuador	0.6	0.6	0.7	0.7	3

- No information is provided or the detailed micronutrient composition is not available.

4. Discussion

For the initiation of CF, both countries have developed their own guidelines regarding the age, presentation, and order of introduction of the different food groups [5,7]. These guidelines likely contribute to the notable disparity in the number of cereal-based products identified in Spain (105 products) and in Ecuador (22 products). Moreover, dietary recommendations for children under two years of age in Spain advocate for the consumption of cereals in different formats, including powdered cereals [5], whereas in Ecuador, the emphasis is solely on the consumption of cereals in their natural state [13], possibly influenced by socio-economic and cultural factors. Thus, in another Latin American country similar to Ecuador, such as Chile, a cross-sectional study was developed between August and December 2018 with a sample of 364 mothers of children under 24 months, of whom 11.4% reported having offered cereals as the first food to their infants during the first two years of life [30]. This finding is noteworthy, considering that 12.1% of health professionals in Latin America recommend initiating CF with cereals [31]. In contrast, a Spanish study carried out in 2018, which examined the most commonly used foods among children under two years old, found that 93% of respondents reported using other types of food. This category included cereals such as pasta (62%), bread (53%), semolina (20%), or rice (81%) [32].

According to the results in the current study, in Ecuador, all the cereal products reviewed (22) are recommended by the manufacturer for infants from the age of 6 months, while in Spain, less than a third are indicated for use from 4 months. This finding aligns with the Ecuadorian CF guidelines, which suggests initiating the introduction of foods, including cereals, from 6 months, and the Spanish feeding guide, which, in non-breastfed children, allows the introduction of food from 4 months of age [5,7], similarly to ESPGHAN [4]. The EFSA suggests not introducing food before 6 months unless there is a risk of iron deficiency, recommending in this case the incorporation of iron-rich foods [8]. The ESPGHAN committee notes that around 4 months of age, renal and gastrointestinal functions are mature enough to start CF from week 17 [33]. In contrast, the United States and Mexico recommend introducing cereals from 6 months of age [34,35]. Thus, it only seems to be agreed for the introduction of cereals "not to be ingested before four months of age" [24]. Therefore, further studies are needed to ensure and globally regulate the correct age for introducing cereals into an infant's diet, considering that the introduction of food requires the development of certain motor skills, physiological processes, and maturity of the various systems in the infant's body [36].

In relation to the labeling of these products, both countries comply with the mandatory declaration of nutrients and the voluntary declaration of vitamins and minerals. However, in Ecuador, the declaration of sodium is mandatory, while in Spain, the salt content must be declared directly. Below are detailed regulations that must be complied with in each market where infant cereals are commercialized. In Spain, the mandatory nutritional information to be declared in accordance with the provisions of Regulation (EU) No. 1169/2011 of the European Parliament and of the Council of 25 October 2011 includes the following: "The energy value, fats, saturated fats, carbohydrates, sugars, proteins, and salt must be declared "per 100 g or per 100 mL", which allows comparison between products and, on a voluntary basis, can be declared: monounsaturated and polyunsaturated fatty acids, polyols, starch, dietary fiber, vitamins, or minerals". This fact explains why cookies in Spain do not include information on all the vitamins and minerals listed in Tables 2 and 3 [37]. According to the Ecuadorian Technical Standard (NTE) 2618:2013 from the Ecuadorian Institute of Standardization (INEN) for cereal-based foods for infants and young children, the mandatory nutritional information for declaration is as follows: "The energy value, expressed in kilojoules (kJ) or optionally in calories (kcal), and the amount in grams (g) of protein, carbohydrates, and fat per 100 g of food or 100 mL of prepared food and, when appropriate, per serving. As for the declaration of vitamins and minerals, this should be done considering the reference values suggested by the regulations, highlighting that the declaration of these nutrients is not indicated as mandatory" [38]. In addition to the above, the NTE of INEN 1334-2:2011, for the labeling of food products for human consumption, indicates the following: **5.1.2** In addition to the mandatory nutrients, for those products whose total fat content is equal to or greater than 0.5 g per100 g (solids) or 100 mL (liquids), the amounts of saturated fatty acids and trans fatty acids, in grams, shall be declared in addition to the total fat. **5.1.3** The amount of any other nutrient for which a nutrition and health claim is made. **5.1.4** Where a claim is made with respect to the amount or type of carbohydrate, the total amount of sugars should be included, the amounts of starch and/or other carbohydrate constituent(s) may also be indicated. Where a claim is made for dietary fiber content, the amount of dietary fiber should be stated. This regulation also refers to the obligation to declare sodium [39]. All this information implies that the comparison is complicated because it depends on what the manufacturer has included in its label.

Another aspect reviewed in the current study was the type of ingredients, including gluten, which is present in commercial cereals recommended in Spain from 4 months of age and in Ecuador from 6 months of age. In this sense, there is no consensus among all the entities about when to introduce gluten; thus, the MSP of Ecuador recommends including it from 8 months of age [13], while the ESPGHAN suggests avoiding the early (before 4 months) or late (after 7 months) introduction of gluten [40]. On the other hand, the Enquiring About Tolerance (EAT) study found that recruited breastfed infants who consumed enough potentially allergenic foods (including wheat) from 3 months of age had a significant reduction in the prevalence of food allergies [41].

In terms of added sugars, among the samples analyzed, 35 products (33.3%) offered in Spain and 8 products in Ecuador contained added sugars, results similar to those reported in the European Union report based on the Global Novel Products Database, which states that out of 4196 infant foods (including 502 processed cereal-based foods), 1359 products (31.9%) had added or free sugars [42]. Similarly, a study conducted in Africa (Burkina Faso, Cameroon, Ghana, Nigeria, and Senegal) found that 49.4% of commercial baby foods (including cereals) contained added sugars [43]. Considering the request of the ESPGHAN to limit the addition of added sugars to CF products [44], manufacturers should comply with this recommendation and avoid adding any sugars and the hydrolysis process in the manufacture of commercial cereals for infants. This process is unjustified given infants' ability to digest starch, facilitated by enzymes such as salivary α-amylase and glucoamylase-maltase, which compensate for the deficiency of pancreatic α-amylase typical of their age [45].

In reviewing the number of products containing whole grains, it was established that almost half of the sample in Spain and less than a third of the products in Ecuador contain whole grains. Based on the data presented, we believe that manufacturers should incorporate this type of cereal into their products to contribute to the average fiber requirement, which according to EFSA for children between 1 and 3 years of age is 10 g/day [29]. It is worth emphasizing that in children under one year of age, there are no recommended dietary intakes of fiber, as breast milk (the primary food for this age group) covers their needs [46]. Additionally, studies on dietary habits show the necessity of increasing the consumption of whole-grain cereals in the infant population [47], due to their positive effects on controlling body weight and reducing the risk of diabetes and cerebrovascular diseases [48].

In terms of energy content, among the samples reviewed, "cookies" represent the category that meets the energy content recommended by the Codex Alimentarius, which stipulates that complementary foods consisting of a mixture of cereals should provide no less than 4 kcal/g in dry weight [49]. Moreover, the fat content complies with recommendations, as they contain less than 30% of the total energy from fats and less than 10% from saturated fatty acids, thus aligning with the nutrient profile model of the Pan American Health Organization (PAHO) [50]. However, based on these results, the quantity and quality of energy provided in general may not contribute to weight gain, a significant finding given the high prevalence of childhood obesity in Spain (14.2%) [51] and the double burden of malnutrition in Ecuador, where obesity affects 35.4% of children aged 5–11 [52], while chronic malnutrition affects 20.1% of children under two and 17.5% of children under five [53].

Regarding the presence of carbohydrates, according to AESAN criteria [27], 2 products in the Ecuadorian market and 39 (37%) products in the Spanish market can be classified as "low sugar" infant cereals, a finding similar to another Spanish study conducted in 2020 titled "Current Content of Infant Cereals and Possible Alternatives: Not Everything Counts in Childhood Nutrition". This study observed a decrease in the sugar content of cereal-based foods, with 18.3% to 30.9% of products with ≤5 g of sugar per 100 g [54]. While these findings indicate a reduction in the sugar content of infant cereals available in Spain, the percentage of products meeting the recommendations remains below 50% in both countries. In our opinion, this result highlights the need to review and modify regulations governing the manufacture and distribution of these foods in order to reduce sugar content.

Taking into account the fact that cereals typically have lower-quality protein compared to animal sources, ESPGHAN suggests that the protein content in cereal porridges should be between 1 and 3 g/100 kcal (excluding those enriched in protein) [55]. The products examined in both countries exhibit an optimal protein content. In terms of vitamin content, this group of products marketed for breastfeeding infants in both countries was found to contribute to meeting the requirements of vitamins such as C, B_6, and A. In a 25 g serving of product, some categories provide more than 40% of the recommended intakes by EFSA [29], indicating that cereal-based foods in both Spain and Ecuador have great potential to meet the needs of children under 2 years of age. The products examined serve as an important source of vitamin A, covering more than 38% of the needs of infants for this micronutrient, despite not indicating whether they are fortified. According to WHO recommendations, complementary foods can be fortified with micronutrients if necessary [56].

Regarding the recommendations for the intake of micronutrient supplements in the child population, in Spain, specialists often recommend the administration of vitamin D supplements in the form of drops to infants during the first 12 months of life as a preventive measure [57]. In Ecuador, the MSP recommends preventive supplementation with biannual megadoses of vitamin A and providing powdered micronutrients (iron, zinc, vitamin A, folic acid, and vitamin C) to children aged 6 to 24 months as a measure to prevent malnutrition and anemia [58,59]. It is important to highlight that 24.7% of children under five years of age residing in Ecuador receive this micronutrient supplementation to prevent anemia [59]. The OMS also suggests maintaining a varied and fortified diet in the infant population at risk of deficiency to meet vitamin A needs [60]. As reported by a study in Africa (Burkina Faso, Cameroon, Ghana, Nigeria and Senegal), 40.2% of a sample of commercial infant food products (including cereals) were fortified [43], with a higher percentage in Cambodia and Indonesia (72.1% and 65.9% of infant food products were fortified), in contrast to the Philippines, where only 28.4% were fortified with micronutrients [61].

Cereals are also a source of minerals such as zinc, magnesium, iron, and, to a lesser extent, calcium [62]. Regarding sodium content, the reviewed cereal sample meets the Codex Alimentarius specification (recommended sodium values ≤ 100 mg/100 kcal) [63], similar to commercial infant cereals in Germany (27 ± 7.0 mg/100 kcal). However, a Spanish study in 2015 analyzed commercial infant formula and found that they exceeded the maximum allowable level of sodium [64]. We consider that these studies show that the infant feeding industry has sought to adapt its products to the needs of infants, who, due to the immaturity of their kidneys, have a low sodium requirement, making it unnecessary to add salt to complementary feeding [5].

The cereal-based foods reviewed in both countries contribute more than 84% of the iron requirements for the 1–3-year-old age group as indicated by EFSA [29], based on a 100 g serving. In another Latin American country (Honduras), commercial cereals sold in this country were found to have an average content of >4 mg/100 g [65], contributing more than 50% of the EFSA recommendations. Given the importance of this mineral for motor, cognitive, and behavioral development [66], it is essential for cereal-based foods to report their iron content to assess the percentage of the requirement they cover. In Ecuador and Spain, 41% and 62% of products indicate the iron content on the label, whereas in Germany, less than a third of commercial cereals for breastfeeding infants provide this information, highlighting that most of these cereals are fortified [67].

Considering the EFSA zinc requirements [29], in a 25 g serving, the samples from Spain and Ecuador contribute up to 24% and 95% of the requirements for infants between 7 and 12 months. Meanwhile, in countries such as Burkina Faso, Cameroon, Ghana, Nigeria, and Senegal, a medium-sized serving covers between 34% and 58% of the RNI of zinc for infants between 6 and 36 months [43]. It is important to keep in mind that, to meet the needs of infants, fortified foods are an excellent option to avoid diarrhea, poor appetite, growth retardation, and other consequences of zinc deficiency [68].

Limitations of this research include the non-homogeneous sample of products, as the availability of these foods in Ecuador is lower than in Spain. In addition, the nutritional information of infant cereals marketed in Ecuador is not available online, so this study took into account the information provided in stores. Furthermore, due to the dynamic nature of the market for infant products, we had to update the nutritional information of the sample twice, resulting in a decrease in Spain and an increase in Ecuador.

On the other hand, this study is the first to look at the nutritional composition of infant cereals sold in Ecuador, distinguishing it from Spain, where similar analyses have already been carried out.

These studies are highly relevant for evaluating the nutritional quality of complementary foods for breastfeeding infants, given their specific nutritional needs and the potential impact on the health of this age group.

5. Conclusions

The recommended age for eating cereal-based foods differs between the two countries. In relation to the description of the nutritional content of cereals marketed in Spain and Ecuador, it shows that this type of product could contribute to meeting the nutritional needs of children under two years of age by being a vehicle for nutrients (carbohydrates, proteins, fats, vitamins, and minerals), mainly fortified products, for the prevention of malnutrition and the development of pathologies related to poor nutrition. In this sense, we consider it necessary to standardize the content of some nutrients such as iron to ensure that needs are met. On the other hand, these products can also be a source of components, such as added sugars, maltodextrin, and/or honey, which are not recommended during the first year of life. It is essential to minimize the content of undesirable components such as those described.

The nutritional composition of the cereals for breastfeeding infants offered in Spain and Ecuador presents some differences; Spanish cereals have a lower content of sodium, added sugars, hydrolyzed cereals, and maltodextrin than Ecuadorian cereals. So far, no studies have been developed in Ecuador to analyze the nutritional quality of infant products. The data obtained in this study may be an adequate starting point to work in this direction, allowing for the development of new research. Meanwhile, in Spain, despite the fact that similar studies have already been conducted, we have been able to update the information and determine the nutritional contribution that the described sample may provide.

Author Contributions: Conceptualization, D.G., A.M., S.G.-M. and S.d.P.; methodology, D.G., S.G.-M. and S.d.P.; formal analysis, D.G., S.G.-M. and S.d.P.; investigation, D.G. and F.I.R.; data curation, D.G.; writing—original draft preparation, D.G.; writing—review and editing, D.G., A.M., F.I.R., S.G.-M. and S.d.P.; funding acquisition, S.G.-M. All authors have read and agreed to the published version of the manuscript.

Funding: This research was funded by Special Intramural Proyects of the CSIC. ref 202270E089.

Institutional Review Board Statement: This study was approved by Ethics Committee of UCM (CE_20210715-4_SAL).

Informed Consent Statement: Not applicable.

Data Availability Statement: The raw data used in this study are available from the corresponding author upon request due to Privacy.

Conflicts of Interest: The authors declare no conflicts of interest.

References

1. International Monetary Fund. GDP per Capita, Current Prices. Available online: https://www.imf.org/external/datamapper/PPPPC@WEO/OEMDC/ADVEC/WEOWORLD (accessed on 17 June 2024).
2. Moreno Villares, J.M.; Collado, M.C.; Larqué, E.; Leis Trabazo, M.R.; Sáenz de Pipaon, M.; Moreno Aznar, L.A. The First 1000 Days: An Opportunity to Reduce the Burden of Noncommunicable Diseases. *Nutr. Hosp.* **2019**, *36*, 218–232.
3. Agencia Española de Seguridad Alimentaria y Nutrición (AESAN). Alimentos Para Grupos Específicos de Población. Available online: https://www.aesan.gob.es/AECOSAN/web/para_el_consumidor/ampliacion/productos_dieteticos.htm (accessed on 30 July 2023).
4. Fewtrell, M.; Bronsky, J.; Campoy, C.; Domellöf, M.; Embleton, N.; Mis, N.F.; Hojsak, I.; Hulst, J.M.; Indrio, F.; Lapillonne, A.; et al. Complementary Feeding: A Position Paper by the European Society for Paediatric Gastroenterology, Hepatology, and Nutrition (ESPGHAN) Committee on Nutrition. *J. Pediatr. Gastroenterol. Nutr.* **2017**, *64*, 119–132. [CrossRef]
5. Gómez, M. Recomendaciones de La Asociación Española de Pediatría Sobre Alimentación Complementaria. 2018. Available online: https://www.aeped.es/sites/default/files/documentos/recomendaciones_aep_sobre_alimentacio_n_complementaria_nov2018_v3_final.pdf (accessed on 30 July 2023).
6. Organización Mundial de la Salud (OMS). *La Alimentación del Lactante y del Niño Pequeño*; Ediciones la OMS: Washington, DC, USA, 2010; pp. 19–28.
7. Tello, B.; Gutiérrez, P.; Caicedo, R.; Mena, A.; Cuadrado, F.; Fernández, F.; Jarrín, E.; Coronel, E.; Vinueza, K.; Aguirre, A.; et al. *Paso a Paso por una Infancia Plena*, 1st ed.; Ministerio de Salud Pública, Ed.; Ministerio de Salud Pública: Quito, Ecuador, 2015; Volume 1, pp. 18–57.
8. European Food Safety Authority (EFSA). *Age to Start Complementary Feeding of Infants*; European Food Safety Authority: Parma, Italy, 2019.
9. Gómez-Martín, M.; Domínguez, B.; Gueimonde, M.; González, S. Identification of Nutritional Targets in Spanish Children Belonging to the LAyDI Cohort for the Development of Health Promotion Strategies in the First Two Years of Life. *Int. J. Environ. Res. Public Health* **2021**, *18*, 939. [CrossRef]
10. Cuadrado-Soto, E.; López-Sobaler, A.M.; Jiménez-Ortega, A.I.; Aparicio, A.; Bermejo, L.M.; Hernández-Ruiz, Á.; Villoslada, F.L.; Leis, R.; de Victoria, E.M.; Moreno, J.M.; et al. Usual Dietary Intake, Nutritional Adequacy and Food Sources of Calcium, Phosphorus, Magnesium and Vitamin D of Spanish Children Aged One to <10 Years. Findings from the EsNuPi Study. *Nutrients* **2020**, *12*, 1787. [CrossRef]
11. López-Sobaler, A.M.; Aparicio, A.; González-Rodríguez, L.G.; Cuadrado-Soto, E.; Rubio, J.; Marcos, V.; Sanchidrián, R.; Santos, S.; Pérez-Farinós, N.; Dal Re, M.Á.; et al. Adequacy of Usual Vitamin and Mineral Intake in Spanish Children and Adolescents: ENALIA Study. *Nutrients* **2017**, *9*, 131. [CrossRef]
12. Freir, W.B.; Ramírez-Luzuriaga, M.J.; Belmont, P.; Mendieta, M.J.; Silva-Jaramillo, K.; Romero, N.; Sáenz, K.; Piñeiros, P.; Gómez, L.F.; Monge, R. Encuesta Nacional de Salud y Nutrición ENSANUT-ECU 2012. Available online: https://www.ecuadorencifras.gob.ec/documentos/web-inec/Estadisticas_Sociales/ENSANUT/MSP_ENSANUT-ECU_06-10-2014.pdf (accessed on 31 January 2023).
13. Ministerio de Salud Pública (MSP). Normas y Protocolos de Alimentación Para Niños y Niñas Menores de 2 Años. Available online: https://www.salud.gob.ec/wp-content/uploads/2019/07/4_alimentacion_ni%C3%B1o_menor_2a%C3%B1os.pdf (accessed on 31 January 2023).
14. D'Auria, E.; Bergamini, M.; Staiano, A.; Banderali, G.; Pendezza, E.; Penagini, F.; Zuccotti, G.V.; Peroni, D.G. Baby-Led Weaning: What a Systematic Review of the Literature Adds On. *Ital. J. Pediatr.* **2018**, *44*, 49. [CrossRef]
15. Rapley, G. Baby-Led Weaning: Transitioning to Solid Foods at the Baby's Own Pace. *Community Pract.* **2011**, *84*, 20–23.
16. Ministry of Health (MOH). Baby-Led Weaning—Te Whatu Ora Position Statement. Available online: https://www.tewhatuora.govt.nz/health-services-and-programmes/nutrition/baby-led-weaning-te-whatu-ora-position-statement (accessed on 26 April 2024).
17. Daniels, L.; Heath, A.-L.M.; Williams, S.M.; Cameron, S.L.; Fleming, E.A.; Barry, J.T.; Wheeler, B.J.; Gibson, R.S.; Taylor, R.W. Baby-Led Introduction to SolidS (BLISS) Study: A Randomised Controlled Trial of a Baby-Led Approach to Complementary Feeding. *BMC Pediatr.* **2015**, *15*, 179. [CrossRef]
18. Núñez-Ramos, R.; Moreno-Villares, J.M. Los Cereales en la Alimentación del Lactante y el Niño Pequeño. *Acta Pediatr. Esp.* **2019**, *77*, 83–89.
19. Fernández-Palacios, L.; Ros, G.; Frontela, C. Nutrientes Clave en la Alimentación Complementaria: El Hierro en Fórmulas y Cereales. *Acta Pediatr. Esp.* **2015**, *73*, 269–276.

20. Gil Hernández, Á.; Martín-Lagos, R.A.; Ruiz López, M.D. *Tratado de Nutrición Composición y Calidad Nutritiva de los Alimentos*, 3rd ed.; Editorial Médica Panamericana, Ed.; Editorial Médica Panamericana: Madrid, Spain, 2017; pp. 54–111.
21. Latham, M.C. *Nutrición Humana en el Mundo en Desarrollo*; FAO, Ed.; FAO: Roma, Italy, 2002; Volume 29.
22. Sakashita, R.; Inoue, N.; Tatsuki, T. Selection of Reference Foods for a Scale of Standards for Use in Assessing the Transitional Process from Milk to Solid Food in Infants and Pre-School Children. *Eur. J. Clin. Nutr.* **2003**, *57*, 803–809. [CrossRef]
23. Fernández-Artigas, P.; Guerra Hernández, E.; García-Villanova, B. Changes in Sugar Profile during Infant Cereal Manufacture. *Food Chem.* **2001**, *74*, 499–505. [CrossRef]
24. Klerks, M.; Bernal, M.J.; Roman, S.; Bodenstab, S.; Gil, A.; Sanchez-Siles, L.M. Infant Cereals: Current Status, Challenges, and Future Opportunities for Whole Grains. *Nutrients* **2019**, *11*, 473. [CrossRef]
25. Theurich, M.A.; Zaragoza-Jordana, M.; Luque, V.; Gruszfeld, D.; Gradowska, K.; Xhonneux, A.; Riva, E.; Verduci, E.; Poncelet, P.; Damianidi, L.; et al. Commercial Complementary Food Use amongst European Infants and Children: Results from the EU Childhood Obesity Project. *Eur. J. Nutr.* **2020**, *59*, 1679–1692. [CrossRef]
26. Agencia Española de Consumo, Seguridad Alimentaria y Nutrición (AECOSAN). Plan de Colaboración la Mejora de la composición de los Alimentos y Bebidas Otras Medidas. Available online: https://www.aesan.gob.es/AECOSAN/docs/documentos/nutricion/PLAN_COLABORACION_2020.pdf (accessed on 13 November 2023).
27. Agencia Española de Seguridad Alimentaria y Nutrición (AESAN). Tabla Declaraciones Nutricionales Autorizadas 2019. Available online: https://www.aesan.gob.es/AECOSAN/docs/documentos/seguridad_alimentaria/gestion_ries-gos/Tabla_declaraciones_NUTRICIONALES_autorizadas.pdf (accessed on 13 November 2023).
28. Diario Oficial de la Unión Europea. Comunicación de La Comisión. Sobre Preguntas y Respuestas Relativas a la Aplicación del Reglamento (UE) n.o 1169/2011 del Parlamento Europeo y del Consejo Sobre la Información Alimentaria Facilitada al Consumidor. Available online: https://eur-lex.europa.eu/legal-content/ES/TXT/PDF/?uri=CELEX:52018XC0608(01) (accessed on 13 November 2023).
29. Calleja, C.A.; Hurtado, C.; Daschner, Á.; Fernández Escámez, P.; Manuel, C.; Abuín, F.-C.; María, R.; Pons, G.; Fandos, E.G.; José González Muñoz, M.; et al. Informe del Comité Científico de la Agencia Española de Seguridad Alimentaria y Nutrición (AESAN) Sobre Ingestas Nutricionales de Referencia para la Población Española. Available online: https://www.aesan.gob.es/AECOSAN/docs/documentos/seguridad_alimentaria/evaluacion_riesgos/informes_comite/INFORME_RECOMENDACIONES_DIETETICAS.pdf (accessed on 12 June 2023).
30. Quintiliano-Scarpelli, D.; Lehmann, N.; Castillo, B.; Blanco, E. Infant Feeding and Information Sources in Chilean Families Who Reported Baby-Led Weaning as a Complementary Feeding Method. *Nutrients* **2021**, *13*, 2707. [CrossRef]
31. Ladino, L.; Vázquez-Frias, R.; Montealegre, L.; Bagés-Mesa, M.C.; Ochoa-Ortiz, E.; Medina-Bravo, P.G. E-1500: Survey on Feeding Practices in the First 1,500 Days of Life, Recommended by Healthcare Professionals in Latin America. *Rev. Gastroenterol. Mex.* **2022**, *87*, 439–446. [CrossRef]
32. Zamanillo-Campos, R.; Rovira-Boixadera, L.; Rendo-Urteaga, T. Common Practices and Beliefs in the Preparation of Complementary Infant Feeding in a Spanish Sample: A Cross-Sectional Study. *Nutr. Hosp.* **2021**, *38*, 919–934. [CrossRef]
33. Grupo de Gastroenterología Pediátrica Zona sur Oeste de Madrid. Alimentación del Lactante y del Niño de Corta Edad. Available online: https://www.ampap.es/wp-content/uploads/2019/04/Alimentacion-del-lactante-y-del-ni%C3%B1o-de-corta-edad.pdf (accessed on 16 April 2024).
34. Jana, L.A.; Shu, J. Cereal in a Bottle: Solid Food Shortcuts to Avoid. Available online: https://www.healthychildren.org/English/ages-stages/baby/feeding-nutrition/Pages/Cereal-in-a-Bottle-Solid-Food-Shortcuts-to-Avoid.aspx (accessed on 10 April 2024).
35. Secretaria de Gobernación. NORMA Oficial Mexicana NOM-043-SSA2-2012, Servicios Básicos de Salud. Promoción y Educación para la Salud en Materia Alimentaria. Criterios para Brindar Orientación. Available online: https://www.dof.gob.mx/nota_detalle.php?codigo=5285372&fecha=22/01/2013#gsc.tab=0 (accessed on 10 April 2024).
36. Jiménez Ortega, A.I.; Martínez García, R.M.; Velasco Rodríguez-Belvis, M.; Ruiz Herrero, J. From Infant to Child. *Nutr. Hosp.* **2017**, *34*, 1699–5198.
37. Parlamento Europeo y del Consejo. Reglamento (UE) No 1169/2011 del Parlamento Europeo y Del Consejo. Available online: https://www.boe.es/doue/2011/304/L00018-00063.pdf (accessed on 12 June 2023).
38. *NTE INEN 2618:2013*; Elaborados a Base de Cereales para Lactantes y Niños Pequeños. Requisitos. Instituto Ecuatoriano de Normalización: Quito, Ecuador, 2013; pp. 1–9.
39. *NTE INEN 1334-2: 2011*; Rotulado de Productos Alimenticios para Consumo Humano. Parte 2. Rotulado Nutricional. Requisitos. Instituto Ecuatoriano de Normalización: Quito, Ecuador, 2011; pp. 3–5.
40. Ribes-Koninckx, C.; Dalmau-Serra, J.; Moreno Villares, J.M.; Diaz Martín, J.J.; Castillejo de Villasante, G.; Polanco Allue, I. La Introducción Del Gluten En La Dieta Del Lactante. Recomendaciones de Un Grupo de Expertos. *An. Pediatría* **2015**, *83*, 355. [CrossRef]
41. Perkin, M.R.; Logan, K.; Bahnson, H.T.; Marrs, T.; Radulovic, S.; Craven, J.; Flohr, C.; Mills, E.N.; Versteeg, S.A.; van Ree, R.; et al. Efficacy of the Enquiring About Tolerance (EAT) study among infants at high risk of developing food allergy. *J. Allergy Clin. Immunol.* **2019**, *144*, 1606–1614. [CrossRef]

42. European Commission. *Feeding Infants and Young Children*; European Commission: Brussels, Belgium, 2019; pp. 13–47.
43. Khosravi, A.; Bassetti, E.; Yuen-Esco, K.; Sy, N.Y.; Kane, R.; Sweet, L.; Zehner, E.; Pries, A.M. Nutrient Profiles of Commercially Produced Complementary Foods Available in Burkina Faso, Cameroon, Ghana, Nigeria and Senegal. *Nutrients* **2023**, *15*, 2279. [CrossRef]
44. Fidler Mis, N.; Braegger, C.; Bronsky, J.; Campoy, C.; Domellöf, M.; Embleton, N.D.; Hojsak, I.; Hulst, J.; Indrio, F.; Lapillonne, A.; et al. Sugar in Infants, Children and Adolescents: A Position Paper of the European Society for Paediatric Gastroenterology, Hepatology and Nutrition Committee on Nutrition. *J. Pediatr. Gastroenterol. Nutr.* **2017**, *65*, 681–696. [CrossRef]
45. Lin, A.H.M.; Nichols, B.L. The Digestion of Complementary Feeding Starches in the Young Child. *Starch-Stärke* **2017**, *69*, 1700012. [CrossRef]
46. Edson Bustos, A.; Alexis Medina, P. Recommendations and Effects of Dietary Fiber for Children. *Rev. Chil. Nutr.* **2020**, *47*, 457–462.
47. Fundación Iberoamericána de Nutrición. *International Life Sciences Institute Papel de los Cereales de Grano Entero en la Salud*; Fundación Iberoamericána de Nutrición: Granada, Spain, 2020; pp. 87–96.
48. Aparicio, A.; Salas-González, M.D.; Lorenzo-Mora, A.M.; Bermejo, L.M. Nutritional and Health Benefits of Whole Grains Cereals. *Nutr. Hosp.* **2022**, *39*, 3–7.
49. Organización de las Naciones Unidas para la Alimentación y la Agricultura (FAO); Organización Mundial de la Salud (OMS). Directrices sobre Preparados Alimenticios Complementarios para Lactantes de Más Edad y Niños Pequeños. Available online: https://www.fao.org/fao-who-codexalimentarius/sh-proxy/pt/?lnk=1&url=https%253A%252F%252Fworkspace.fao.org%252Fsites%252Fcodex%252FStandards%252FCXG+8-1991%252FCXG_008s.pdf (accessed on 8 January 2024).
50. Organización Panamericana de la Salud (OPS); Organización Mundial de la Salud (OMS). Modelo de Perfil de Nutrientes de la Organización Panamericana de la Salud. Available online: www.paho.org/permissions (accessed on 23 May 2023).
51. Gasol Foundation; Gómez, S.; Lorenzo, L.; Ribes, C.; Homs, C. Resultados principales del estudio PASOS 2019 sobre la actividad física, los estilos de vida y la obesidad de la población española de 8 a 16 años. In *Estudio PASOS*; Gasol Foundation: Barcelona, Spain, 2019; pp. 8–11.
52. Instituto Nacional de Estadística y Censos. Encuesta ENSANUT. Available online: https://www.ecuadorencifras.gob.ec/documentos/web-inec/Estadisticas_Sociales/ENSANUT/ENSANUT_2018/Principales%20resultados%20ENSANUT_2018.pdf (accessed on 2 June 2023).
53. Instituto Nacional de Estadística y Censos (INEC). Principales Resultados Nacional sobre Desnutrición Infantil—ENDI. Available online: https://www.ecuadorencifras.gob.ec/documentos/web-inec/ENDI/Presentacion_de_Resultados_ENDI_R1.pdf (accessed on 2 June 2023).
54. Vitoria Miñana, I. Current Content of Infant Cereals and Possible Alternatives: Not Everything Counts in Childhood Nutrition. In *Anales de Pediatria*; Elsevier: Barcelona, Spain, 2021; Volume 95, pp. 366–367.
55. Gómez-Álvarez Salinas, P. *Papillas de Cereales. Recomendaciones*; Elsevier: Barcelona, Spain, 2002; Volume 16, pp. 56–65.
56. Organización Mundial de la Salud (OMS). Alimentación Del Lactante y Del Niño Pequeño. Available online: https://www.who.int/es/news-room/fact-sheets/detail/infant-and-young-child-feeding (accessed on 1 September 2023).
57. Asociación Española de Pediatría. Vitaminas. Available online: https://enfamilia.aeped.es/vida-sana/vitaminas (accessed on 14 June 2024).
58. Ministerio de Salud Publica (MSP). *Normas, Protocolos y Consejería para la Suplementación con Micronutrientes*; Ministerio de Salud Publica (MSP): Quito, Ecuador, 2011; pp. 26–31.
59. Tello, B.; Rivadeneira, M.F.; Rubio-Codina, M.; Parra, J.; Medina, D. Reportes de la ENSANUT 2018. Available online: https://www.ecuadorencifras.gob.ec/documentos/web-inec/Bibliotecas/Libros/Reportes/Reportes_ENSANUT_Vol1_Salud_de_la_Ninez.pdf (accessed on 24 August 2023).
60. World Health Organization (WHO). *Guideline: Vitamin A Supplementation in Infants and Children 6–59 Months of Age*; World Health Organization: Geneva, Switzerland, 2011; pp. 1–5.
61. Bassetti, E.; Zehner, E.; Mayhew, S.H.; Nasser, N.; Mulder, A.; Badham, J.; Sweet, L.; Crossley, R.; Pries, A.M. Nutrient Profiles of Commercially Produced Complementary Foods Available in Cambodia, Indonesia and the Philippines. *Public Health Nutr.* **2022**, *25*, 2720–2730. [CrossRef]
62. Carbajal Azcona, Á. Manual de Nutrición y Dietética. Available online: https://www.ucm.es/data/cont/docs/458-2018-01-10-cap-14-alimentos-2018.pdf (accessed on 15 September 2023).
63. Organización Mundial de la Salud (OMS); Organización de las Naciones Unidas para la Alimentación y la Agricultura (FAO). Norma para Alimentos Elaborados a Base de Cereales para Lactantes y Niños Pequeños. Available online: https://www.fao.org/fao-who-codexalimentarius/sh-proxy/en/?lnk=1&url=https%253A%252F%252Fworkspace.fao.org%252Fsites%252Fcodex%252FStandards%252FCXS+74-1981%252FCXS_074s.pdf (accessed on 24 August 2023).
64. Mir-Marqués, A.; González-Masó, A.; Cervera, M.L.; De La Guardia, M. Mineral Profile of Spanish Commercial Baby Food. *Food Chem.* **2015**, *172*, 238–244. [CrossRef]
65. Fernández-Palacios, L.; Ros-Berruezo, G.; Barrientos-Augustinus, E.; Jirón de Caballero, E.; Frontela-Saseta, C. Aporte de Hierro y Zinc Bioaccesible a la Dieta de Niños Hondureños Menores de 24 Meses. *Nutr. Hosp.* **2017**, *34*, 290–300. [CrossRef]
66. Organización Panamericana de la Salud (OPS); Organización Mundial de la Salud (OMS). La Importancia del Hierro un Desarrollo Saludable. Available online: https://www3.paho.org/hq/dmdocuments/2011/Iron_Nutrition%20SPA.pdf (accessed on 2 December 2023).

67. Theurich, M.A.; Koletzko, B.; Grote, V. Nutritional Adequacy of Commercial Complementary Cereals in Germany. *Nutrients* **2020**, *12*, 1590. [CrossRef]
68. National Institutes of Health. Datos sobre El Zinc. Available online: https://ods.od.nih.gov/pdf/factsheets/Zinc-DatosEnEspanol.pdf (accessed on 26 June 2023).

nutrients

MDPI

Article

Safety and Suitability of Infant Formula Manufactured from Extensively Hydrolyzed Whey Protein Compared to Intact Protein: A Combined Analysis of Two Randomized Controlled Studies

Manja Fleddermann [1], Anette Knoll [2] and Berthold Koletzko [3,*]

1 HiPP GmbH & Co. Vertrieb KG, Georg-Hipp-Str. 7, 85276 Pfaffenhofen an der Ilm, Germany; manja.fleddermann@hipp.de
2 AK Statistics, Kreppe 2, 85276 Pfaffenhofen an der Ilm, Germany; office@anetteknoll.de
3 Division of Metabolic and Nutritional Medicine, Dr. von Hauner Children's Hospital, University of Munich Medical Center, Ludwig-Maximilians-Universität München, Lindwurmstr. 4, 80337 Muenchen, Germany
* Correspondence: berthold.koletzko@med.uni-muenchen.de; Tel.: +49-(0)89-4400-52826

Abstract: Our aim was to assess the nutritional safety and suitability of an infant formula manufactured from extensively hydrolyzed protein in comparison to infant formula manufactured from intact protein (both with low and standard protein content). We performed a combined analysis of raw data from two randomized infant feeding studies. An analysis of covariance (ANCOVA) model was used to determine the non-inferiority of daily weight gain (primary outcome; margin −3 g/day), with the intervention group as a fixed factor and geographic region, sex, and baseline weight as covariates (main model). The data of 346 infants exposed to the formula were included in the analysis. The sample size of the per-protocol analysis with 184 infants was too small to achieve sufficient statistical power. The lower limit of the 97.5% confidence interval (−0.807) of the mean group difference in daily weight gain (i.e., 2.22 g/day) was above the −3 g/day margin (full analysis set). Further anthropometric parameters did not differ between the infant formula groups throughout the study. Growth was comparable to breastfed infants. We conclude that the infant formula manufactured from extensively hydrolyzed protein meets infant requirements for adequate growth and does not raise any safety concerns.

Keywords: extensively hydrolyzed whey protein; protein hydrolysate; infant formula; infant nutrition; growth; formula fed; breastfed

1. Introduction

An adequate dietary protein supply is essential for healthy growth and development in infancy [1,2].

Human milk is recognized as the optimal source of nutrients for infants throughout at least the first 6 months of life [3]. However, if breastfeeding is not possible, available, or adequate, infant formulae are the only advisable breast milk substitutes. Infant formulae that are manufactured from cow's milk protein or other protein sources have been successfully used for many decades.

Next to infant formulae manufactured from intact proteins, infant formulae manufactured from hydrolyzed proteins are available for infants with an increased risk of developing allergies. Hydrolyzed proteins are smaller, easier to digest, and considered to be less allergenic when compared to intact proteins. However, the bioavailability of proteins, amino acids (AAs), and other nutritional components may be different between infant formulae manufactured from hydrolyzed protein (HP) formulae and intact protein (IP) formulae [4]. Based on the degree of hydrolysis and the proportion of small peptides, hydrolysates are classified as partially or extensively hydrolyzed.

Several studies evaluating HP formulae with standard or low protein content and using extensively or partially hydrolyzed whey or casein proteins indicate that HP formulae are safe in terms of growth when compared to human milk, intact cow's milk protein formulae, or growth standards [4–14].

Although the use of protein hydrolysates has been permitted for many years and the use of protein hydrolysates in the manufacturing of infant formulae is widespread in the market, the level of hydrolysis, the protein source, and other components may affect the safety and tolerance of different HP formulae; thus, the extrapolation of results from one HP formula to another is not accepted by regulators [15].

The growth effects and safety of infant formulae marketed by HiPP (Pfaffenhofen, Germany) compared to human milk have been evaluated in two studies: the HA study [16] evaluated different HP formulae with standard and low protein content, whereas the BeMIM study [17] compared IP formulae with standard and low protein content. In both studies, the standard and low-protein formulae manufactured from either protein hydrolysate or intact protein were considered safe and suitable for infants up to the age of 4 months.

To further explore the nutritional safety and suitability of these HP formulae comparatively, we compiled measures of growth between the HP formula and IP formula by performing a combined analysis of the HA and BeMIM studies.

2. Materials and Methods

2.1. Analysis Approach and Individual Studies

The HA and BeMIM studies were randomized, controlled, and double-blinded and investigated the non-inferiority of low-protein infant formulae to conventionally used infant formulae with standard protein content. While the HA study [16] evaluated infant formulae manufactured from hydrolyzed proteins, the BeMIM study [17] focused on IP formulae. Both studies used a non-randomized breastfed group as a reference. The intervention period of study formula feeding for each participant lasted from birth (starting, at the latest, from 1 month of life) until 4 months of life and included monthly study visits.

The combined data analysis was performed based on raw data from the two studies. The inclusion criteria differed slightly between studies and were aligned post-hoc to allow for comparable data. Healthy term newborns $\leq$ 28 days of life with a gestational age of $\geq$37 weeks and a birth weight between 2500 and 4500 g were included in the combined analysis.

2.2. Diet

The HP and IP formulae compared had similar protein content at the respective protein level (i.e., standard versus vs. low protein). HP formulae were whey-based, extensively hydrolyzed, and included 1.9 g protein/100 kcal (LP) or 2.3 g protein/100 kcal with or without synbiotics. For the synbiotics, *Limosilactobacillus fermentum* CECT5716 was used as a probiotic and galacto-oligosaccharides (GOS) as prebiotics. IP formulae were based on a whey:casein ratio of 60:40 and protein content of either 1.9 g/100 kcal (LP) or 2.2 g/100 kcal.

Both the HP and IP formulae were supplemented with individual AAs to meet regulatory requirements. Except for the IP formula containing 2.2 g/100 kcal, all formulae contained arachidonic and docosahexaenoic acid in a ratio of 1:1. For more information on the infant formulae compositions, see Supplementary Table S1.

Five intervention groups were investigated. From the HA study, eHF—infant formula manufactured from extensively hydrolyzed whey protein and LPeHF + Syn—low-protein infant formula manufactured from extensively hydrolyzed whey protein with synbiotics; from the BeMIM study, iPF—infant formula manufactured from intact protein and LPiPF—low-protein infant formula manufactured from intact protein; and, as a reference in both studies, BF—breastfeeding.

Infant formulae were administered orally ad libitum. Infant formula intake, as well as the number of breastfeeding meals and intake of other food or drinks, e.g., energy-containing liquids (sweetened tea or juice) or non-energy-containing liquids (tea and water), were documented using 3-day protocols.

2.3. *Primary and Secondary Outcome Assessments*

The primary outcome was the average daily weight gain in grams per day (g/day) between 1 and 4 months of life, to estimate adequate growth. Secondary outcomes included measurements of body length and head circumference, including respective z-scores as further growth indices, and nutrient intake, adverse events, stool characteristics, and biochemical markers (blood urea, albumin, AAs).

The aim of the combined analysis was to compare HP with the IP formula using formulae with standard protein content (i.e., eHF vs. iPF) and formulae with low protein content (i.e., LPeHF + Syn vs. LPiPF).

2.4. *Statistics and Power Estimation*

Retrospective sample size estimation scenarios were used to determine if sufficient infants were available in a confirmatory setting. Between 43 and 94 participants per group for LPeHF + Syn vs. LPiPF and eHF vs. iPF, respectively, were required to demonstrate non-inferiority. The power simulations were based on the means and standard deviations (SD) of the groups used in the HA and BeMIM studies, using both a per-protocol set (PPS) and full analysis set (FAS), a non-inferiority margin of −3.0 g/day at a one-sided significance level of 2.5%, and a power of 80% (Supplementary Table S2).

The FAS comprised all enrolled participants who participated at least in the month 1 visit and had received study formula. In PPS, only data from participants complying with the predefined conditions, such as completion of the intervention period up to 4 months of life, no intake of other infant formulae besides the study intervention, and breastfeeding at a maximum of once daily, were included. According to local practice, in the study countries, some infants receive liquids, like tea or water, in addition to breastmilk or infant formula, during the first 4 months of life, which was limited to a maximum amount of 50mL per day to still be included in the PPS. The main conclusions on the primary outcome measure were based on PPS; FAS served as a sensitivity analysis.

For the analysis of the daily weight gain, an analysis of covariance (ANCOVA) model was used to show non-inferiority, with the intervention group as a fixed factor and region, sex, and baseline weight as covariates (main model). An ANCOVA with only the intervention group as a fixed factor was used as a sensitivity analysis. Furthermore, additional covariates (maternal age at infant's birth, maternal body mass index (BMI), gestational age, smoking status of mother before and during pregnancy, weight at birth, maternal education, socioeconomic status) were included in the model. However, these additional covariates did not reveal any plausible and consistent relations with daily weight gain over all populations and group comparisons (LPeHF + Syn vs. LPiPF; eHF vs. iPF) in the ANCOVA model; thus, the results are not described.

The lower limit of the 97.5% confidence interval (CI) of the difference between formula groups was compared to the non-inferiority margin of −3.0 g/day. A hierarchical test design was assumed with ordered hypotheses (Step 1: eHF vs. iPF, Step 2: LPeHF + Syn vs. LPiPF), which was the only analysis that took multiple testing into account.

The European Food Safety Authority (EFSA) Guidance [18] stipulates an alternative way to analyze adequate growth, i.e., the equivalence in growth between intervention groups. Thus, this was also tested using an ANCOVA model, with the region and baseline value as covariates and weight-for-age z-scores at the age of 4 months. Equivalence was concluded if the calculated two-sided 90% CI of the estimated mean difference in the weight-for-age z-score was within the predefined margin of ± 0.5 SD, a bandwidth considered to be indicative for adequate growth.

Secondary outcome analyses were carried out in the PPS and FAS. Daily length and head circumference gains were compared between intervention groups using ANCOVA models similar to the model used for the primary outcome, with respective baseline characteristics included as covariates, but with a focus on superiority.

z-scores were calculated based on the World Health Organization (WHO) growth standards for breastfed children [19]. Comparisons between intervention groups for z-scores were done using a mixed model of repeated measurements (MMRM), with the region, visit, intervention group, and intervention group-by-visit interaction as fixed factors and participant as a random factor, as well as additional covariates (Supplementary Table S5).

Nutritional parameters (intake of study infant formula, other infant formula, energy-containing liquids, complementary feeding, and additional breastfeeding) as well as biochemical markers were evaluated using the van Elteren test adjusted for region. A Cochran–Mantel–Haenszel test, adjusted for region, was used to analyze gastrointestinal tolerance. The analysis of adverse events evaluated the number and frequency of intervention-emergent events by system organ class and preferred terms (according to the Medical Dictionary for Regulatory Activities (MedDRA) coding version 23.1). Amino acids and laboratory parameters were descriptively assessed and two-sided superiority tests on a significance level of 5% were applied.

Linear regression models were used to examine the dependencies between average liquid intake per day and weight gain, or infant formula intake between month 1 and month 4.

Statistical analyses were performed with the WPS Workbench version 4.3 (© Copyright World Programming Limited 2002–2022) using the SAS language code.

2.5. Study Population

The HA study was conducted between 2010 and 2013 as a multicenter study in Germany, Austria, and Serbia, and the BeMIM study between 2010 and 2011 as a single-center study in Serbia. Overall data from 1008 participants were available, of which 589 participants were included in the combined analysis (385 randomized formula-fed participants and 204 breastfed participants). The main reasons for the exclusion of 419 infants from the analysis were receiving infant formulae from a different protein source (see study design of Ahrens et al. (2018) [16], a missing visit at month 1, or screening failures.

To evaluate HP vs. IP formulae, the data of 385 randomized formula-fed participants were considered, of which 353 participants took part in the 1-month visit, had documented data, and received at least one bottle of study formula, and 307 completed the 4-month follow-up visit (Figure 1). The FAS comprised 346 participants (86 eHF, 89 iPF, 83 LPeHF + Syn, 88 LPiPF). For PPS, data were limited to 184 participants (39 eHF, 42 iPF, 54 LPeHF + Syn, 49 LPiPF). The predominant reasons for exclusion from PPS in the formula groups were the violation of the feeding regimen and an age outside the visit or enrolment window; not being allowed concomitant medication; early withdrawal; and the violation of the eligibility criteria. Data from 204 breastfed participants (203 FAS, 115 PPS) served as an external reference.

Baseline characteristics including sex, first-born status, maternal and paternal age and BMI, maternal smoking, age at randomization, mode of delivery, and anthropometry at birth were similar between the eHF and iPF groups and between the LPeHF + Syn and LPiPF groups for FAS (Supplementary Table S3) and PPS, except for education, where mothers in the iPF group had higher education levels compared to those in the eHF group (FAS). Due to the different study designs (multicenter vs. single center), all participants in the iPF and LPiPF groups were form Serbia, while over 66% of participants in the eHF and LPeHF + Syn groups were from Serbia and 33% from Germany and Austria.

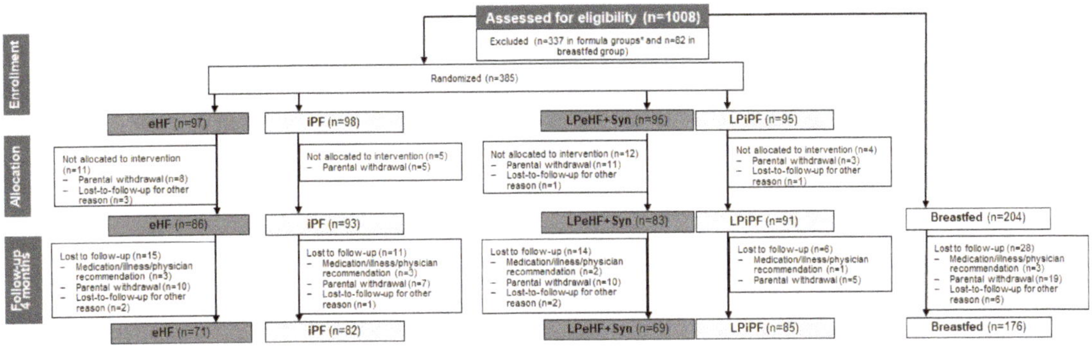

Figure 1. Participant disposition, randomization, and follow-up for infant formula groups compared in this analysis, and for the BF group. eHF = infant formula manufactured from extensively hydrolyzed whey protein, iPF = infant formula manufactured from intact protein, Syn = synbiotics, LP = low protein, BF = breastfeeding, * n = 210 infants received formulae from a different protein source.

3. Results

3.1. Weight Gain and Growth

The mean difference in daily weight gain in participants receiving eHF compared to participants fed iPF was 0.73 g/day (CI [−3.029, inf.]) for PPS, with the lower limit of the 97.5% CI narrowly missing the predefined non-inferiority margin of -3 g/day (Figure 2, Supplementary Table S4).

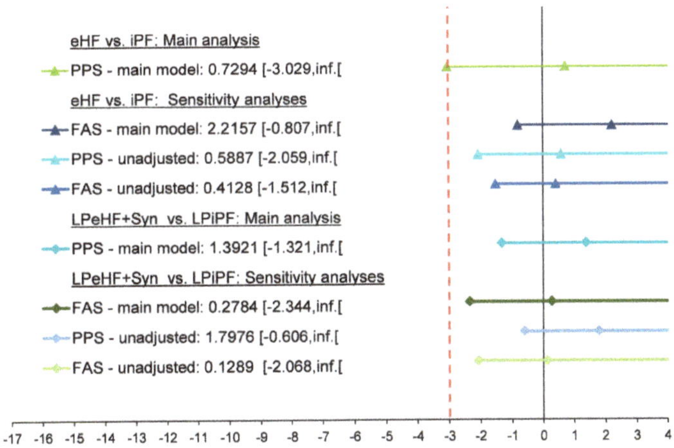

Figure 2. Weight gain/day differences [g/day] between infant formula manufactured from extensively hydrolyzed whey protein versus intact protein for PPS and FAS. Least square means and one-sided 97.5% confidence intervals are depicted. Main model = ANCOVA adjusted for sex, region, and baseline value. Unadjusted = ANCOVA with only the intervention group as fixed factor. The dotted line resembles the non-inferiority margin.

In a sensitivity analysis using FAS, the lower limit of the 97.5% CI (−0.807) of the mean group difference in daily weight gain (i.e., 2.22 g/day) was well above the −3 g/day margin (Figure 2, Supplementary Table S4). Similar results were seen in a further sensitivity analysis using an ANCOVA model without adjustments, yielding lower limits of the 97.5% CI above the −3 g/day margin (PPS: −2.059; FAS: −1.512, Figure 2).

The difference in daily weight gain between the LPeHF + Syn and LPiPF groups was 1.39 g/day (CI [−1.321, inf.[) in PPS, and 0.28 g/day (CI [−2.344, inf.[) in FAS (Figure 2, Supplementary Table S4). Similar results were obtained using an ANCOVA without adjustments (lower limit of the 97.5% CI, PPS: −0.606; FAS: −2.068, Figure 2). According to the hierarchical test scheme, the procedure stopped at the inferiority testing of eHF vs. iPF and no further inferential conclusions could be made when testing the LPeHF + Syn vs. LPiPF groups.

The length gain from months 1 to 4 did not differ between the HP and IP formula groups in PPS. Head growth was greater with LPeHF than LPiPF ($p = 0.0192$), but similar between eHF and iPF (PPS). The FAS analyses showed comparable results except for a significant difference in length gain between the eHF and iPF groups ($p = 0.0325$) (Supplementary Table S4). In BF participants, the gains in weight, length, and head circumference were smaller or similar to those observed in the formula groups (Supplementary Table S4).

Anthropometric measurements, expressed as z-scores (Figure 3 for PPS, Supplementary Figure S1 for FAS), were within -1 to 1 from months 1 to 4 of life, confirming age-appropriate development in all formula groups. No differences were observed between HP and IP formulae at any time between 1 and 4 months of life. For both PPS and FAS, an MMRM analysis confirmed that there were no differences between intervention groups (Supplementary Table S5).

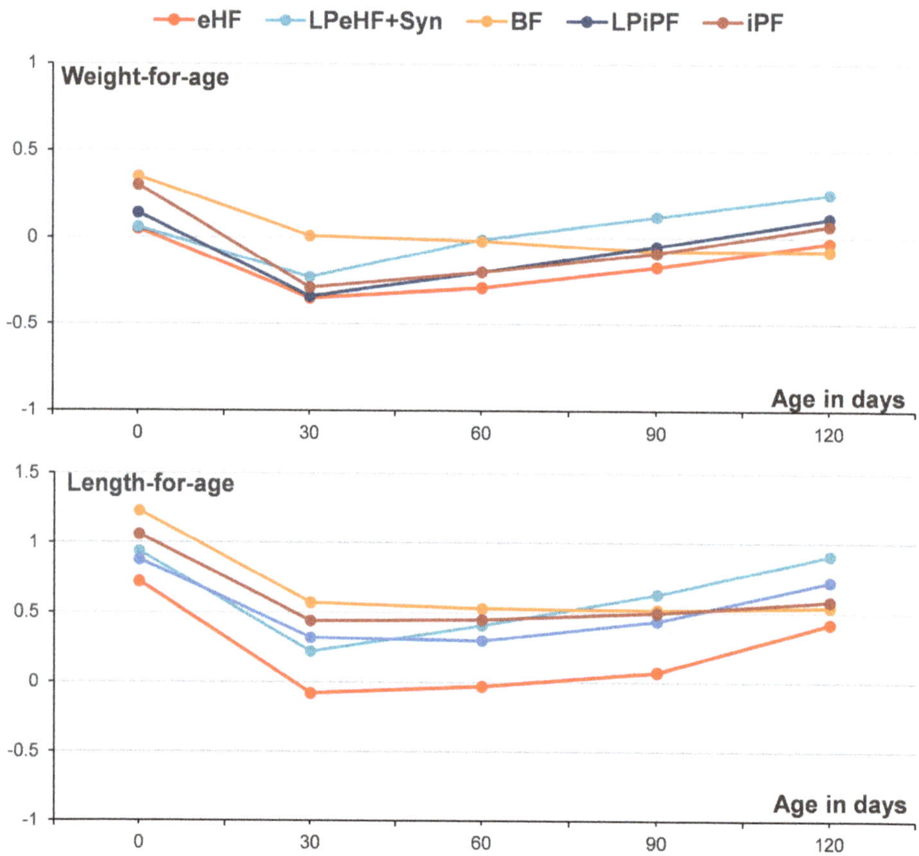

Figure 3. *Cont.*

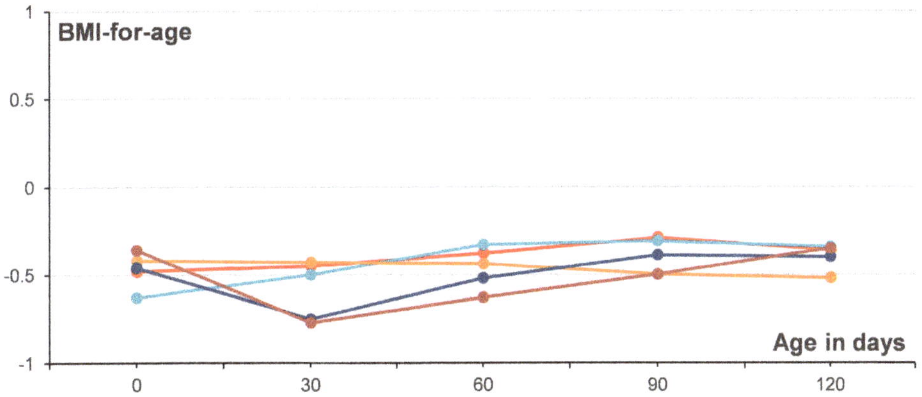

Figure 3. Anthropometric measurements (weight-for-age, length-for-age, and BMI-for-age) expressed as z-scores (growth standards of the WHO) (PPS). z-scores within −1 to 1 indicate age-appropriate development. BMI = body mass index, WHO = World Health Organization.

An ANCOVA at the age of 4 months confirmed equivalent growth with HP and IP formulae, i.e., the two-sided 90% CI of the mean difference in the weight-for-age z-score was contained within the pre-defined equivalence margin of ± 0.5 SD, in both FAS (eHF vs. iPF: [−0.140; 0.413]; LPeHF + Syn vs. LPiPF: [−0.346, 0.132]) and PPS (eHF vs. iPF: [−0.357, 0.327]; LPeHF + Syn vs. LPiPF: [−0.207, 0.280]).

3.2. Nutrient Intake

No differences in energy intake of the study infant formula between eHF and iPF were found throughout the observation period (PPS and FAS). The average energy intake in the LPeHF + Syn and LPiPF formula groups was comparable at months 2 and 3, but significantly higher in the LPeHF + Syn group at month 1 (FAS) and month 4 (FAS and PPS, Supplementary Tables S6 and S7).

The number of infants with documented additional breastfeeding was lower in infants fed the HP formula (Supplementary Tables S6 and S7). The same applied for energy-containing liquid intake (Supplementary Tables S6 and S7).

The number of infants in both the HP and IP groups who consumed other formulae and/or complementary food was too low (at a maximum of six infants) for a meaningful comparison (for FAS and PPS). Complementary feeding, generally, did not start before 4 months of life.

3.3. Impact of Liquid Intake on Growth and Formula Intake

Energy-containing liquids were consumed by 42.2% of infants in the formula-fed groups (FAS) and 28.6% of breastfed participants. No measurable effects of energy-containing liquid intake on participant weight gain were observed, as evidenced by a broad scatterplot and a Spearman's correlation coefficient near zero (Figure 4A). There was also no correlation between the intake of liquid and study formula for energy in kcal/days (Supplementary Figure S2), as well as for the amount of intake in mL/day (Supplementary Figure S3). In line with this, the weight-for-age z-scores did not correlate with energy-containing liquid intake at months 1, 2, 3, or 4 (Figure 4B). In addition, the influence of mean energy-containing liquid intake on the amount of infant formula intake from month 1 to month 4 could not be confirmed. Spearman's correlation coefficients were around zero (Supplementary Figure S4). Most infants consumed less than 50 mL/day of energy-containing liquids. As for the overall population, there was no obvious influence of energy-containing liquid intake on weight gain in infants consuming less than 50 mL/day of energy-containing liquids (Figure 4).

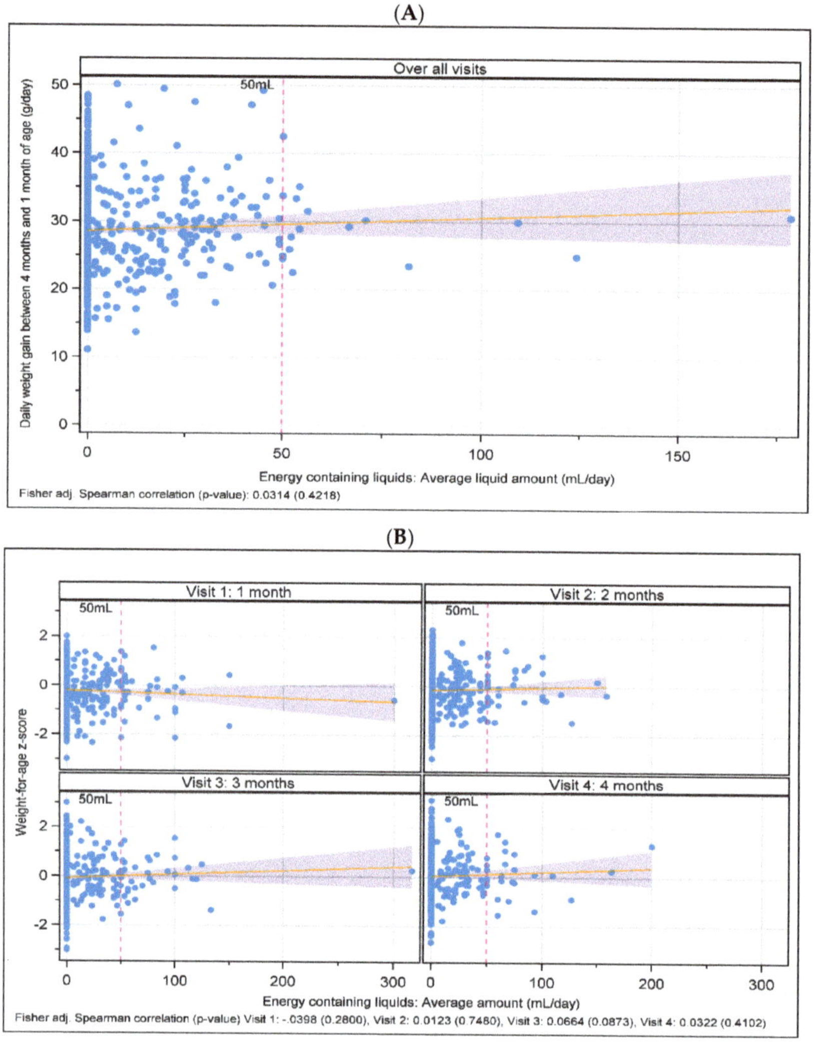

Figure 4. Scatterplots to correlate liquid intake and growth (FAS). (**A**) Impact of energy-containing liquid intake on weight gain between 1 and 4 months of life. (**B**) Impact of energy-containing liquid intake on weight-for-age z-scores at 1, 2, 3, and 4 months of life. Dotted line shows 50 mL cut-off.

3.4. Suitability

3.4.1. Adverse Events

The percentage of infants affected by adverse events was comparable in each intervention group and the BF group and no formula-related risks were observed (Supplementary Table S8). The incidence of serious adverse events was between 2.3% (iPF) and 6.8% (LPiPF), but none of the serious adverse events was related to infant formula intake. Adverse events associated with infections were more frequent in IP than in HP formula-fed participants, while pyrexia appeared to be more common in the HP formulae group. Overweight, which was documented in more detail in the HP study, was observed in HP formula-fed participants (Supplementary Table S8). An MMRM analysis, however, did not indicate any differences in growth (weight-for-age and BMI-for-age z-scores) between the HP and IP groups from 1 to 4 months of life (Supplementary Table S5).

3.4.2. Stool Characteristics

Stool characteristics were documented over a period of three days prior to each visit. For FAS, significantly more HP-fed infants showed a lower stool frequency than IP-fed infants at 1, 3, and 4 months ($p \leq 0.001$, eHF vs. iPF) and at 2, 3, and 4 months ($p < 0.001$, LPeHF + Syn vs. LPiPF, Supplementary Figure S4, Supplementary Table S10).

"Green" colored stools were reported more frequently in the HP formula groups (with increasing frequencies over the observation period; eHF: from 15.4% at month 1 to 34.2% at month 4 of life; LPeHF + Syn: from 27.8% at month 1 to 60.0% at month 4; FAS) compared to IP formula groups (iPF: 2.0% to 7.8% with the highest value at month 3, LPiPF: 4.9% to 7.5%, highest value at month 2; FAS). Statistically significant different stool color patterns were reached between the low-protein groups (LPeHF + Syn vs. LPiPF) at all timepoints in FAS (Supplementary Table S10). The stool color patterns between the standard protein groups (eHF vs. iPF) were only statistically different at month 1 in FAS. In the BF group, green stools were reported at a similar frequency as in the IP groups (3.6% to 9.9% (at month 2) of infants). In the BF and IP groups, most infants (>90%) reported stools ranging from yellow and brown to mustard-like during the entire observation period, while, in the HP groups, infants presenting these stool colors decreased over time (eHF: from 84.6% at month 1 to 64.7% at month 4 of life; LPeHF + Syn: from 71.8% at month 1 to 38.8% at month 4; FAS). Black/grey stools were hardly seen in any group (generally <1.5%, except for the eHF group at month 3 with 3.1%, FAS).

No significant differences between groups were observed for stool consistency in FAS (except for LPeHF + Syn vs. LPiPF at month 3 in FAS, $p = 0.019$). The stools of HP-fed participants were more frequently described as "watery" (eHF: 9.4% to 14.6% and LPeHF + Syn: 5.2% to 10.6% across observation period; FAS) compared to the stools of IP formula-fed participants (iPF 0.4% to 3.9%, LPiPF 0.8% to 3.5%; FAS), but most infants (85% to 95%, FAS) had a stool consistency ranging from soft, formed, sausage, and soft sausage to mushy stools (Supplementary Table S10). "Watery" refers only to the stool consistency and does not include diarrhea. The proportion of infants with "watery" stools tended to increase from month 1 to month 4 in all formula groups. Infants with hard stools were rare in the eHP and iPF groups (below 1%, except for the iPF group at month 1, 3.9%; FAS) but slightly more common in the LPiPF group (2.3% to 7.4%, FAS). Compared to the formula groups, BF infants reported more frequently watery stools (21.2% to 31.4%); stool consistencies ranging from soft, formed, sausage, and soft sausage to mushy were presented by 68.6% to 78.6% of BF infants and hard stools were rarely seen (≤0.2%).

3.4.3. Biochemical Markers

The values for plasma albumin and blood urea nitrogen (BUN) were within normal ranges (3.0–5.2 g/dL for albumin, 2.0–7.2 mmol/L for blood urea nitrogen [20]) for most participants in all intervention groups at month 4 in PPS and FAS (Table 1). While the BUN values did not differ significantly between the HP and IP formula groups, HP formula-fed participants had significantly higher plasma albumin values compared to respective IP participants (van Elteren test adjusted for region) in both PPS and FAS. BUN tended to be higher in the formula groups than in the BF group. While 5% (eHF) to 21% (LPeHF + Syn) of formula-fed infants had BUN concentrations below the reference range reported by Oster [20], more, i.e., 52%, of breast-fed infants had BUN concentrations below the reference range.

Amino acid plasma levels were evaluated at month 4. Although the AA profile appeared to be similar in all groups (Supplementary Table S9), the plasma concentrations of most AAs were significantly lower in the IP compared to the respective HP formula-fed participants. Exceptions were glutamic acid, ornithine, and phenylalanine, which were comparable between eHF and iPF, and aspargic acid, proline, and valine, which were comparable between LPeHF + Syn and LPiPF (FAS, Supplementary Table S9).

Table 1. Blood albumin and urea nitrogen at month 4. Reference ranges based on Oster 2007 [20].

FAS	Standard Protein Group				Low Protein Group					
	eHF		iPF		LPeHF + Syn		LPiPF		BF	
Albumin										
n	65		78		59		83		167	
Median (Q1, Q3) [g/dL]	4.1 *	(3.88,4.31)	3.7 *	(3.60, 3.90)	4.2 *	(4.04, 4.34)	3.8 *	(3.60, 3.90)	3.9	(3.70, 4.10)
n (%) of infants with values										
Within reference range	65	(100.0)	78	(100.0)	59	(100.0)	83	(100.0)	167	(100.0)
Above reference range	-		-		-		-		-	
Below reference range	-		-		-		-		-	
Blood urea nitrogen										
N	65		78		58		83		166	
Median (Q1, Q3) [mmol/L]	3.7	(3.16, 4.16)	2.8	(2.40, 3.10)	2.6	(2.16, 3.00)	2.5	(2.10, 3.00)	2.0	(1.50, 2.33)
n (%) of infants with values										
Within reference range	62	(95.4)	69	(88.5)	46	(79.3)	73	(88.0)	80	(48.2)
Above reference range	-		-		-		2	(2.4)	-	
Below reference range	3	(4.6)	9	(11.5)	12	(20.7)	8	(9.6)	86	(51.8)

* $p < 0.0001$ (two-sided, van Elteren test adjusted for region) for difference eHF vs. iPF and for difference LPeHF + Syn vs. LPIPF.

4. Discussion

We conducted a combined analysis of two randomized studies in healthy term infants to compare the effects of an HP formula to an IP formula on growth parameters during the first 4 months of life. The results indicated non-inferior weight gain between infants consuming formulae manufactured from extensively hydrolyzed whey protein at standard or low protein levels and infants receiving formulae manufactured from intact cow's milk with comparable protein content. The non-inferiority margin (−3 g/day for the lower limit of the 97.5% CI) for daily weight gain was reached, when comparing eHF vs. iPF (FAS) and LPeHF + Syn vs. LPiPF (PPS, FAS). For the eHF vs. iPF (PPS) comparison, the non-inferiority margin was narrowly missed (lower 95% CI: −3.029), presumably due to the low number of infants and inadequate sample size in PPS (39 eHF and 42 iPF vs. 94 per group required). Secondary endpoints of growth indices, i.e., weight, length, and head circumference, were generally similar between HP and IP formulae at both protein levels, except for greater monthly head circumference growth (low-protein infant formula, PPS and FAS) and length gains (standard protein level, FAS) in the HP compared to IP formula. However, compared to the WHO growth standards, the mean z-score values of all intervention groups were within ±1 SD during the intervention (Figure 3, in both PPS and FAS and at both low and standard protein levels), indicating comparable and adequate growth with all interventions. In addition, no significant differences between intervention groups were observed for all other z-score values assessed in this study, suggesting that the few observed differences were not clinically relevant.

The findings of this study are consistent with observations reported in other publications. Karaglani et al. (2020) [9], Picaud et al. (2020) [4], and Otten et al. (2023) [21] demonstrated in three randomized controlled studies comparable growth between infants fed a partially or extensively hydrolyzed whey-based formula and infants fed an intact cow's milk protein formula during the first 4 to 5 months of life. Similar results with no difference in growth characteristics between HP and IP formulae were observed by Wu et al. (2017) [22] in healthy term infants from enrolment to 7 and 13 weeks of life. A pooled analysis of seven clinical studies compared intact cow's milk infant formulae to a partially hydrolyzed whey infant formula from a single manufacturer on growth at 2 weeks and 1, 2, 3, and 4 months of life [23]. There were no differences in weight gain between infant formula groups. In contrast, in a rather small study (56 infants) performed by Mennella at al. (2011) [10], infants fed an HP formula had significantly lower weight-for-length z-scores compared to IP formula-fed infants across ages 2.5 to 7.5 months. As discussed by others [9], this difference may be due to the lower food consumption observed in this study in the HP formula group. HP formulae contain peptides that can display a bitter taste [24] and might also lead to more rapid satiation [25,26].

Despite recent improvements in infant formulae composition, formulae still contain slightly higher levels of protein than human milk, associated with increased rates of weight gain [27]. Consistent with other findings [28–30], we observed an increase in weight-for-age or BMI-for-age z-scores during the first 4 months of life in all formula intervention groups, while no increase was seen in BF infants.

The LPeHF + Syn that was compared with the LPiPF formula in our analysis contained additional synbiotics (combination of L. fermentum and GOS), making a direct comparison difficult. Results from other studies and meta-analyses do not indicate an impact of synbiotic-supplemented formulae on growth [31,32].

Generally, there were no differences in energy intake from the study infant formula between HP and IP formulae, except for significantly lower total energy intake in the IP formula group at the low protein level at months 1 and 4. However, this difference may be due to the higher breastfeeding rates in the IP formula groups, which is an additional energy source for the infant. Other studies did also not see a consistent difference in infant formula intake between HP and IP formulae. Karaglani et al. (2020) [9] observed higher weekly infant formula consumption (~+10.5%) in IP compared to HP formulae-fed infants but this difference disappeared when daily infant formula intake was corrected for body weight. Czerkies et al. (2018) [23] reported a more pronounced increase in infant formula intake over time in the HP than in the IP formula group, a difference that, however, was only evident among girls.

The number of infants consuming additional formulae and/or complementary food was low in all intervention groups, with no apparent differences. The consumption of energy-containing liquids was higher in the IP than HP formulae groups, but this, however, had no impact on growth or study formula intake. One factor that may have contributed to the differences in energy-containing liquid intake may be their more common use in Eastern European countries, as previously reported by Schiess et al. (2010) for Poland [33]. In our analysis, data for the IP groups were derived from the BeMIM study and thus solely from Serbia, whereas the HP formulae study was performed in Serbia, Germany, and Austria. Infants fed an IP formula (low or standard protein) received also more additional breastfeeding than HP-fed infants. Energy intake from breastfeeding could, however, not be quantified because the amount of breastmilk per meal and its composition were not recorded and analyzed.

In general, any additional intake of energy-containing liquids is considered a protocol deviation in infant growth studies. We therefore conducted a correlation analysis on the impact of energy-containing liquid intake on infant formula intake and weight-for-age z-scores. In contrast to Schiess et al. (2010) [33], who reported that infants receiving energy-containing liquids had an approximately 30 kcal lower infant formula intake based on data from a multicenter European study, the intake of liquids up to 50 mL/day did not correlate with the amount of or energy intake from the infant formula in our analysis. In the Schiess study, an inverse relationship between liquid/tea intake and energy intake from infant formulae was observed. Reasons for these inconsistent results are unclear, but they may arise in part from the different analysis approaches used: while Schiess et al. (2010) compared groups with and without energy-containing liquid intake with a Wilcoxon rank-sum test, we used a linear regression model/correlation measures to investigate the connection between growth, formula intake, and energy-containing liquid intake for all infants. The average energy intake in kcal/day from liquids was comparable between our analysis and the Schiess study. In the latter, the impact of energy-containing liquid consumption on growth was not evaluated, but, in our analysis, liquid intake (up to 50 mL/day) had no visible positive or negative effect on infant weight gain during the observation period. No conclusion can be drawn for liquid intake of more than 50 mL/day, as the number of participants who consumed more than 50 mL liquid/day was very low. The proportions of infant formula-fed infants consuming energy-containing liquids were comparable in our analyses and the Schiess study (about 42%), but differed for BF infants (29% in our analysis vs. 10% in the Schiess study).

Concerning adverse events, around a quarter of infants experienced adverse events, with no differences between intervention groups. No serious, formula-related adverse events occurred. A higher incidence of adverse events related to the study formula was reported for the HP formula groups versus their IP counterparts, but given the transient nature and mild severity, this was not considered a safety concern.

There were also no consistent differences in tolerance parameters between the HP and IP formula groups, in line with findings from other studies [5]. The reduced stool frequency observed for the HP formula was unexpected and contrasts with previous findings that report an equal or increased stool frequency [5,22]. HP formulae are supposed to shorten the gastrointestinal transit time [34,35], generally associated with an increased stool frequency. The trend towards more watery stools in the HP formula groups than in their IP formula counterparts aligns with a shorter transit time and is compatible with other findings [4,23]. The higher prevalence of "green" stools in the HP formula in our analysis is commonly seen in infants consuming HP formulae [36], which might be explained by the hydrolyzed proteins, which are absorbed and metabolized differently from intact proteins [37].

The plasma AA levels observed in our analysis generally reflected the composition of the different infant formulae tested, with lower AA levels in the IP than in the HP formula. The IP compared to the HP formula groups reached plasma concentrations closer to the BF reference, reflecting a more balanced AA intake typical for IP formulae due to a whey:casein ratio close to human milk. Glutamine and cysteine plasma concentrations were below the BF reference in both IP groups. Following the EU guidance on infant formula compositions, the amount of cysteine present in infant formulae can be summed up with methionine (if the ratio of the two amino acids is less than 2); thus, cysteine values must always be evaluated in light of methionine intake. While the plasma cysteine concentrations were below those of the BF reference group in the IP groups, the median methionine concentrations were above those of BF infants. The methionine concentrations in formulae were adequate and thus the sum of both AAs was in line with the EU guidance. Glutamine and glutamic acid and serine levels in infant formulae are not regulated by EU law. However, human milk contains significant amounts of glutamate, which has been suggested to be important for intestinal development in infants [38–42].

BUN values did not differ between the HP and IP formula-fed groups. Our results showed that a much larger proportion of breastfed infants had BUN values below the reference values than formula-fed infants. It appears that the reference ranges should be redefined based on the levels observed in healthy, growing breastfed infants.

Albumin levels were greater in the HP than in the IP formula group, which was unexpected. Previous studies with HP formulae indicated the lower protein quality of HP vs. IP formulae, which is generally associated with lower albumin serum levels and consistent with findings by Florendo et al. (2009) [43]. The unexpected difference in albumin levels in our study may be due, at least in part, to the use of different laboratories to evaluate serum albumin for the HP formula groups and IP formula groups, thus generating slightly different results. However, the serum levels for all intervention groups were well within normal reference limits [20]. In addition, no relevant differences were observed in growth indices between groups, suggesting that the observed differences in albumin levels may not be clinically important.

The unexpected results for serum albumin levels and the additional intake of energy-containing liquids highlight one limitation of this analysis: the intervention groups compared were from two different studies and geographical regions, i.e., all data from HP formula-fed infants were from the HA study conducted in Serbia, Austria, and Germany, while IP formula-fed participants were from the BeMIM study conducted solely in Serbia. Although the statistical tests were adjusted for region, differences in cultural feeding patterns and the differences in studies may have still impacted the results. Looking at our post-hoc sample size estimation, the number of infants in one PPS group comparison (eHF vs. iPF) is probably too low to draw robust conclusions. A further limitation of the study is that more than one component differed between HP and IP. Thereby, besides the protein source, the macro- and micronutrient composition, as well as the content of long-chain polyunsaturated fatty acids, differed slightly between formulae.

The strength of this analysis lies in the similarity of the study designs: both studies were randomized, controlled studies; data were collected at almost identical timepoints; anthropometric measurements and assessments for stool characteristics were done similarly; and diets were isocaloric and comparable for protein content on the respective protein levels (standard vs. low protein). The synbiotics that were included only in the low-protein HP formula were shown to not impact infant growth [31,32] and thus are unlikely to have biased the results. Another key strength of our analysis is the use of individual-level data, allowing the harmonization of covariates, definitions, and analytical approaches.

5. Conclusions

The analysis demonstrated that infant formulae manufactured from extensively hydrolyzed whey protein meet infant requirements for adequate growth with similar gains in weight and z-scores, compared to infant formulae manufactured from intact protein and a reference group of breastfed infants. Based on these results, it can be concluded that infant formulae manufactured from extensively hydrolyzed whey protein are suitable and safe for infants during the first 4 months of life. Local practices in some countries, providing small amounts of energy-containing liquids (up to 50 mL) during the first 4 months of life, do not impact infant growth.

Supplementary Materials: The following supporting information can be downloaded at: https://www.mdpi.com/article/10.3390/nu16020245/s1, Table S1. Nutritional characteristics of the formulas, Table S2. Retrospective sample size calculation, Table S3. Baseline characteristics of study participants (FAS), Table S4. Average weight gain, length, and head circumference between month 1 and month 4 (FAS and PPS), Table S5. Weight-for-age and BMI-for-age z-scores—MMRM (FAS and PPS), Table S6. Intake of study formula, other infant formula, energy-containing liquids, and complementary food between month 1 and month 4 (FAS), Table S7. Intake of study formula, other infant formula, energy-containing liquids, and complementary food between month 1 and month 4 (PPS), Table S8. Adverse events (FAS), Table S9. Plasma amino acid profile at month 4 (FAS), Table S10. Stool frequency, color, and consistency (FAS). Figure S1. Anthropometric measurements (weight-for-age, length-for-age, and BMI-for-age) expressed as z-scores (growth standards of the WHO) (FAS), Figure S2. Scatterplots to correlate the impact of average study formula intake/day at 1, 2, 3, and 4 month(s) of life on average energy intake from liquids (FAS), Figure S3. Scatterplots to correlate the impact of average amount of study formula intake/day at 1, 2, 3, and 4 month(s) of life on average amount of energy-containing liquid intake (FAS), Figure S4. Stool frequency at 1, 2, 3, and 4 month(s) of life (FAS).

Author Contributions: Conceptualization, M.F., A.K. and B.K.; methodology, M.F., A.K. and B.K.; formal analysis, A.K.; writing—original draft preparation, M.F., A.K. and B.K.; writing—review and editing, M.F., A.K. and B.K.; visualization, M.F. and A.K.; project administration, M.F. All authors have read and agreed to the published version of the manuscript.

Funding: The combined analysis and the therein included studies were sponsored by HiPP GmbH & Co. Vertrieb KG, which also provided the infant formulae and financial support to the participating centers to conduct the two studies. The employer of B.K., LMU University Hospitals, received funding from HiPP GmbH & Co. Vertrieb KG for research contributions to the BEMIM study. B.K. is the Else Kröner Seniorprofessor of Paediatrics at LMU—University of Munich, financially supported by the charitable Else Kröner-Fresenius Foundation, LMU Medical Faculty, and LMU University Hospitals.

Institutional Review Board Statement: Both studies included in the analysis were conducted in accordance with the Declaration of Helsinki and the International Council for Harmonisation Guidelines on Good Clinical Practice and were approved by respective ethics committees. HA safety I: Berlin (Ethikkommission Charité Ethikausschuss 1 am Campus Charité—Mitte, Charitéplatz 1, 10117 Berlin): EA1/240/09 (1 February 2010), Vienna (Ethikkommission der Med. Universität Wien, Boschekgasse 8b/E06, 1090 Wien): 362/2011 (31 August 2011), Rostock (Ethikkommission an der Medizinischen Fakultät der Universität Rostock, St.-Georg-Straße 108, 18055 Rostock): A 2011 27 (14 April 2011), Bochum (Ethik-Kommission der Medizinischen Fakultät der Ruhr-Universität Bochum Geschäftsstelle BG-Universitätskliniken Bermannsheil, Bürkle-da-la-Camp-Platz 1, 44789 Bochum): 4013-11 (3 May 2011), Belgrade (KBC "Dr Dragiša Mišović—Dedinje" Belgrade, Ethical Committee, KBC "Dr Dragiša Mišović-Dedinje", ETIČKI ODBOR, NAUČNI SAVET, Vladislav Diligenski): 18-1472/18 (6 February 2012); BeMIM study: Belgrade (KBC "Dr Dragiša Mišović—Dedinje" Belgrade, Ethical Committee, KBC "Dr Dragiša Mišović-Dedinje", ETIČKI ODBOR, NAUČNI SAVET, Vladislav Diligenski): 1734/12 (17 December 2009).

Informed Consent Statement: Informed consent was obtained from the caregivers of all participants involved in the studies.

Data Availability Statement: The data presented here are available upon request from the corresponding author due to intellectual property limitations.

Acknowledgments: The authors would like to thank all the families who participated in the study. We also thank, in addition to the authors of this article, for their contribution to this analysis, Kristin L. Ritzenthaler (HiPP GmbH & Co. Vertrieb KG) and Annette Rempel (FGK Clinical Research GmbH).

Conflicts of Interest: A.K. and B.K. declare no conflicts of interest. M.F. is employed by HiPP GmbH & Co. Vertrieb KG, which provided the product and financially sponsored the two studies. M.F. was involved in the design of the combined analysis, the interpretation of the data, and the writing of the manuscript.

References

1. EFSA NDA Panel (EFSA Panel on Dietetic Products, Nutrition and Allergies). Scientific Opinion on nutrient requirements and dietary intakes of infants and young children in the European Union. *EFSA J.* **2013**, *11*, 3408.
2. Yon, B.A.; Johnson, R.K. US and Canadian Dietary Reference Intakes (DRIs) for the macronutrients, energy and physical activity. *Nutr. Bull.* **2005**, *30*, 176–181. [CrossRef]
3. Insitute of Medicine. *Nutrition during Lactation*; The National Academies Press: Washington, DC, USA, 1991. [CrossRef]
4. Picaud, J.-C.; Pajek, B.; Arciszewska, M.; Tarczón, I.; Escribano, J.; Porcel, R.; Adelt, T.; Hassink, E.; Rijnierse, A.; Abrahamse-Berkeveld, M.; et al. An Infant Formula with Partially Hydrolyzed Whey Protein Supports Adequate Growth and Is Safe and Well-Tolerated in Healthy, Term Infants: A Randomized, Double-Blind, Equivalence Trial. *Nutrients* **2020**, *12*, 2072. [CrossRef]
5. Berseth, C.L.; Mitmesser, S.H.; Ziegler, E.E.; Marunycz, J.D.; Vanderhoof, J. Tolerance of a standard intact protein formula versus a partially hydrolyzed formula in healthy, term infants. *Nutr. J.* **2009**, *8*, 27. [CrossRef]
6. Exl, B.M.; Deland, U.; Secretin, M.C.; Preysch, U.; Wall, M.; Shmerling, D.H. Improved general health status in an unselected infant population following an allergen reduced dietary intervention programme. The ZUFF-study-programme. Part I: Study design and 6-month nutritional behaviour. *Eur. J. Nutr.* **2000**, *39*, 89–102. [CrossRef] [PubMed]
7. Hernell, O.; Lönnerdal, B. Nutritional evaluation of protein hydrolysate formulas in healthy term infants: Plasma amino acids, hematology, and trace elements. *Am. J. Clin. Nutr.* **2003**, *78*, 296–301. [CrossRef] [PubMed]
8. Isolauri, E.; Sütas, Y.; Mäkinen-Kiljunen, S.; Oja, S.S.; Isosomppi, R.; Turjanmaa, K. Efficacy and safety of hydrolyzed cow milk and amino acid-derived formulas in infants with cow milk allergy. *J. Pediatr.* **1995**, *127*, 550–557. [CrossRef] [PubMed]
9. Karaglani, E.; Thijs-Verhoeven, I.; Gros, M.; Chairistanidou, C.; Zervas, G.; Filoilia, C.; Kampani, T.M.; Miligkos, V.; Matiatou, M.; Valaveri, S.; et al. A Partially Hydrolyzed Whey Infant Formula Supports Appropriate Growth: A Randomized Controlled Non-Inferiority Trial. *Nutrients* **2020**, *12*, 3056. [CrossRef]
10. Mennella, J.A.; Inamdar, L.; Pressman, N.; Schall, J.I.; Papas, M.A.; Schoeller, D.; Stallings, V.A.; Trabulsi, J.C. Type of infant formula increases early weight gain and impacts energy balance: A randomized controlled trial. *Am. J. Clin. Nutr.* **2018**, *108*, 1015–1025. [CrossRef]
11. Nentwich, I.; Pazdírková, A.; Lokaj, J.; Szepfalusi, Z.; Hrstková, H. Early feeding in infancy and atopic dermatitis—A prospective observational study. *Klin. Padiatr.* **2009**, *221*, 78–82. [CrossRef]
12. Rigo, J.; Schoen, S.; Verghote, M.; van Overmeire, B.; Marion, W.; Abrahamse-Berkeveld, M.; Alliet, P. Partially Hydrolysed Whey-Based Formulae with Reduced Protein Content Support Adequate Infant Growth and Are Well Tolerated: Results of a Randomised Controlled Trial in Healthy Term Infants. *Nutrients* **2019**, *11*, 1654. [CrossRef]
13. Vandenplas, Y.; Hauser, B.; Blecker, U.; Suys, B.; Peeters, S.; Keymolen, K.; Loeb, H. The nutritional value of a whey hydrolysate formula compared with a whey-predominant formula in healthy infants. *J. Pediatr. Gastroenterol. Nutr.* **1993**, *17*, 92–96. [CrossRef] [PubMed]
14. Ziegler, E.E.; Jeter, J.M.; Drulis, J.M.; Nelson, S.E.; Haschke, F.; Steenhout, P.; Brown, C.; Maire, J.-C.; Hager, C. Formula with reduced content of improved, partially hydrolyzed protein and probiotics: Infant growth and health. *Monatsschrift Kinderheilkd.* **2003**, *151*, 65–71. [CrossRef]
15. Commission Delegated Regulation. (EU) 2016/127 of 25 September 2015 supplementing Regulation (EU) No. 609/2013 of the European Parliament and of the Council as regards the specific compositional and information requirements for infant formula and follow-on formula and as regards requirements on information relating to infant and young child feeding. *OJEU* **2016**, *59*, L25/1–L25/29.
16. Ahrens, B.; Hellmuth, C.; Haiden, N.; Olbertz, D.; Hamelmann, E.; Vusurovic, M.; Fleddermann, M.; Roehle, R.; Knoll, A.; Koletzko, B.; et al. Hydrolyzed Formula With Reduced Protein Content Supports Adequate Growth: A Randomized Controlled Noninferiority Trial. *J. Pediatr. Gastroenterol. Nutr.* **2018**, *66*, 822–830. [CrossRef]
17. Fleddermann, M.; Demmelmair, H.; Grote, V.; Nikolic, T.; Trisic, B.; Koletzko, B. Infant formula composition affects energetic efficiency for growth: The BeMIM study, a randomized controlled trial. *Clin. Nutr.* **2014**, *33*, 588–595. [CrossRef]
18. EFSA Panel on Dietetic Products, Nutrition and Allergies (NDA); Turck, D.; Bresson, J.-L.; Burlingame, B.; Dean, T.; Fairweather-Tait, S.; Heinonen, M.; Hirsch-Ernst, K.I.; Mangelsdorf, I.; McArdle, H.J.; et al. Scientific and technical guidance for the preparation and presentation of an application for authorisation of an infant and/or follow-on formula manufactured from protein hydrolysates. *EFSA J.* **2017**, *15*, e04779. [CrossRef]
19. WHO Multicentre Growth Reference Study Group. *WHO Child Growth Standards: Length/Height-for-Age, Weight-for-Age, Weight-for-Length, Weight-for-Height and Body Mass Index-for-Age: Methods and Development*; World Health Organization: Geneva, Sweitzerland, 2006.
20. Oster, O. Pädiatrisch Relevante Referenzwerte: Klinische Chemie. Available online: https://www.springermedizin.de/emedpedia/paediatrie/paediatrisch-relevante-referenzwerte-klinische-chemie?epediaDoi=10.1007/978-3-642-54671-6_352 (accessed on 3 September 2021).
21. Otten, L.; Schelker, E.; Petersen, H.; Nomayo, A.; Fleddermann, M.; Arendt, B.M.; Britzl, T.; Haberl, E.M.; Jochum, F. Safety and Suitability of an Infant Formula Manufactured from Extensively Hydrolysed Protein in Healthy Term Infants. *Nutrients* **2023**, *15*, 1901. [CrossRef]

22. Wu, S.L.; Ding, D.; Fang, A.P.; Chen, P.Y.; Chen, S.; Jing, L.P.; Chen, Y.M.; Zhu, H.L. Growth, Gastrointestinal Tolerance and Stool Characteristics of Healthy Term Infants Fed an Infant Formula Containing Hydrolyzed Whey Protein (63%) and Intact Casein (37%): A Randomized Clinical Trial. *Nutrients* **2017**, *9*, 1254. [CrossRef]
23. Czerkies, L.A.; Kineman, B.D.; Cohen, S.S.; Reichert, H.; Carvalho, R.S. A Pooled Analysis of Growth and Tolerance of Infants Exclusively Fed Partially Hydrolyzed Whey or Intact Protein-Based Infant Formulas. *Int. J. Pediatr.* **2018**, *2018*, 4969576. [CrossRef]
24. Mennella, J.A.; Forestell, C.A.; Morgan, L.K.; Beauchamp, G.K. Early milk feeding influences taste acceptance and liking during infancy. *Am. J. Clin. Nutr.* **2009**, *90*, 780s–788s. [CrossRef]
25. Diepvens, K.; Häberer, D.; Westerterp-Plantenga, M. Different proteins and biopeptides differently affect satiety and anorexigenic/orexigenic hormones in healthy humans. *Int. J. Obes.* **2008**, *32*, 510–518. [CrossRef] [PubMed]
26. Foltz, M.; Ansems, P.; Schwarz, J.; Tasker, M.C.; Lourbakos, A.; Gerhardt, C.C. Protein Hydrolysates Induce CCK Release from Enteroendocrine Cells and Act as Partial Agonists of the CCK1 Receptor. *J. Agric. Food Chem.* **2008**, *56*, 837–843. [CrossRef] [PubMed]
27. Koletzko, B.; von Kries, R.; Closa, R.; Escribano, J.; Scaglioni, S.; Giovannini, M.; Beyer, J.; Demmelmair, H.; Gruszfeld, D.; Dobrzanska, A.; et al. Lower protein in infant formula is associated with lower weight up to age 2 y: A randomized clinical trial. *Am. J. Clin. Nutr.* **2009**, *89*, 1836–1845. [CrossRef]
28. Dewey, K.G. Growth Characteristics of Breast-Fed Compared to Formula-Fed Infants. *Biol. Neonate* **1998**, *74*, 94–105. [CrossRef] [PubMed]
29. Kramer, M.S.; Guo, T.; Platt, R.W.; Vanilovich, I.; Sevkovskaya, Z.; Dzikovich, I.; Michaelsen, K.F.; Dewey, K. Feeding effects on growth during infancy. *J. Pediatr.* **2004**, *145*, 600–605. [CrossRef]
30. Victora, C.G.; Morris, S.S.; Barros, F.C.; Horta, B.L.; Weiderpass, E.; Tomasi, E. Breast-feeding and growth in Brazilian infants. *Am. J. Clin. Nutr.* **1998**, *67*, 452–458. [CrossRef] [PubMed]
31. Gil-Campos, M.; López, M.Á.; Rodriguez-Benítez, M.V.; Romero, J.; Roncero, I.; Linares, M.D.; Maldonado, J.; López-Huertas, E.; Berwind, R.; Ritzenthaler, K.L.; et al. Lactobacillus fermentum CECT 5716 is safe and well tolerated in infants of 1-6 months of age: A randomized controlled trial. *Pharmacol. Res.* **2012**, *65*, 231–238. [CrossRef]
32. Janmohammadi, P.; Nourmohammadi, Z.; Fazelian, S.; Mirzababaei, A.; Alizadeh, S.; Zarei, M.; Daneshzad, E.; Djafarian, K. Does infant formula containing synbiotics support adequate growth in infants? A meta-analysis and systematic review of randomized controlled trials. *Crit. Rev. Food Sci. Nutr.* **2021**, *63*, 707–718. [CrossRef] [PubMed]
33. Schiess, S.A.; Grote, V.; Scaglioni, S.; Luque, V.; Martin, F.; Stolarczyk, A.; Vecchi, F.; Koletzko, B. Intake of energy providing liquids during the first year of life in five European countries. *Clin. Nutr.* **2010**, *29*, 726–732. [CrossRef] [PubMed]
34. Mihatsch, W.A.; Högel, J.; Pohlandt, F. Hydrolysed protein accelerates the gastrointestinal transport of formula in preterm infants. *Acta Paediatr.* **2001**, *90*, 196–198. [CrossRef]
35. Picaud, J.C.; Rigo, J.; Normand, S.; Lapillonne, A.; Reygrobellet, B.; Claris, O.; Salle, B.L. Nutritional efficacy of preterm formula with a partially hydrolyzed protein source: A randomized pilot study. *J. Pediatr. Gastroenterol. Nutr.* **2001**, *32*, 555–561. [CrossRef]
36. Borschel, M.W.; Baggs, G.E. A New Hydrolyzed Formula is Well Tolerated in Infants with Suspected Food Protein Allergy or Intolerance. *Open Nutr. J.* **2015**, *9*, 1–4. [CrossRef]
37. Worsøe, P.S.; Sangild, P.T.; van Goudoever, J.B.; Koletzko, B.; van der Beek, E.M.; Abrahamse-Berkeveld, M.; Burrin, D.G.; van de Heijning, B.J.M.; Thymann, T. Growth and Clinical Variables in Nitrogen-Restricted Piglets Fed an Adjusted Essential Amino Acid Mix: Effects of Partially Intact Protein-Based Diets. *J. Nutr.* **2018**, *148*, 1118–1125. [CrossRef]
38. Blachier, F.; Boutry, C.; Bos, C.; Tomé, D. Metabolism and functions of L-glutamate in the epithelial cells of the small and large intestines. *Am. J. Clin. Nutr.* **2009**, *90*, 814s–821s. [CrossRef] [PubMed]
39. Rao, R.; Samak, G. Role of Glutamine in Protection of Intestinal Epithelial Tight Junctions. *J. Epithel. Biol. Pharmacol.* **2012**, *5*, 47–54. [CrossRef] [PubMed]
40. Rook, D.; Te Braake, F.W.; Schierbeek, H.; Longini, M.; Buonocore, G.; Van Goudoever, J.B. Glutathione synthesis rates in early postnatal life. *Pediatr. Res.* **2010**, *67*, 407–411. [CrossRef]
41. Ruth, M.R.; Field, C.J. The immune modifying effects of amino acids on gut-associated lymphoid tissue. *J. Anim. Sci. Biotechnol.* **2013**, *4*, 27. [CrossRef]
42. van Sadelhoff, J.H.J.; van de Heijning, B.J.M.; Stahl, B.; Amodio, S.; Rings, E.; Mearin, M.L.; Garssen, J.; Hartog, A. Longitudinal Variation of Amino Acid Levels in Human Milk and Their Associations with Infant Gender. *Nutrients* **2018**, *10*, 1233. [CrossRef]
43. Florendo, K.N.; Bellflower, B.; van Zwol, A.; Cooke, R.J. Growth in preterm infants fed either a partially hydrolyzed whey or an intact casein/whey preterm infant formula. *J. Perinatol.* **2009**, *29*, 106–111. [CrossRef] [PubMed]

nutrients

MDPI

Article

Impact of Maternal Fish Consumption on Serum Docosahexaenoic Acid (DHA) Levels in Breastfed Infants: A Cross-Sectional Study of a Randomized Clinical Trial in Japan

Ayu Kasamatsu [1], Hiroshi Tachimoto [2] and Mitsuyoshi Urashima [1,2,*]

[1] Division of Molecular Epidemiology, The Jikei University School of Medicine, 3-25-8 Nishi-Shimbashi, Minato-Ku, Tokyo 105-8461, Japan; ayu.kasamatsu@gmail.com

[2] Department of Pediatrics, The Jikei University School of Medicine, 3-25-8 Nishi-Shimbashi, Minato-Ku, Tokyo 105-8461, Japan; hiroshitachimoto@gmail.com

* Correspondence: urashima@jikei.ac.jp; Tel.: +81-3-3433-1111 (ext. 2405)

Abstract: Docosahexaenoic acid (DHA), an essential n-3 long-chain polyunsaturated fatty acid (LCPUFA) abundant in fish, is crucial for infant brain development. We investigated the associations between maternal dietary habits, infant feeding patterns, and serum levels of DHA and other LCPUFAs in infants aged 5–6 months in Japan, where fish consumption is high. This cross-sectional study used serum samples from 268 infants enrolled in a randomized clinical trial. The frequency of mothers' consumption of 38 food items and infant feeding patterns were prospectively surveyed. Cow's milk formula (CMF) supplemented with 15.9% linolenic acid, 1.6% α-linolenic acid, 0.40% DHA, and 0.27% arachidonic acid was used. Significant positive associations with infants' serum DHA levels were found for "Blue-back fish" (rho = 0.24; $p = 0.0001$) and "White fish" (rho = 0.25, $p = 0.0001$). The combined variable "Blue-White fish" was found to be significantly associated with higher serum DHA levels in infants (rho = 0.29, $p < 0.0001$). Predominantly breastfed infants had significantly higher serum DHA levels than those fed more CMF (rho = 0.32, $p < 0.0001$). After multivariate analysis, "Blue-White fish" and "Feeding patterns" remained significantly and independently associated with serum DHA levels. These findings suggest that frequent consumption of "Blue-back fish" and/or "White fish" by lactating mothers, along with prioritizing breastfeeding over DHA-supplemented CMF, might effectively increase infants' serum DHA levels.

Keywords: infants; Japanese; seafood; breast feeding; docosahexaenoic acid; eicosapentaenoic acid; fatty acids; milk; omega-3; omega-6

1. Introduction

Exclusive breastfeeding is recommended for the first 6 months after birth [1,2] due to its numerous benefits for infants [3], one of which is the potential to enhance intelligence via unknown mechanisms [3–5]. Breastfed infants exhibit higher plasma levels of docosahexaenoic acid (DHA) than those fed DHA-unsupplemented infant formula [6–8]. DHA is an n-3 fatty acid belonging to the group of long-chain polyunsaturated fatty acids (LCPUFAs) and is essential for infant brain development [9], aiding myelination and improving the speed of electrical impulses in neurons [10]. Indeed, higher serum DHA levels are linked to increased brain volumes in neonates [11]. The process of incorporating DHA into the brain membrane structure in early life relies on its maternal transfer and dietary intake, as well as endogenous LCPUFA synthesis, as there is no de novo LCPUFA synthesis [12]. Thus, efforts have been made to maintain the DHA levels of formula-fed infants at levels comparable to those of breastfed infants using DHA supplementation. Recently, evidence of the clinical benefits of DHA supplementation has been accumulating. Multiple randomized controlled trials (RCTs) have suggested the possible effect of DHA supplementation on the development of visual acuity and cognitive outcomes in both preterm and full-term infants, although they have shown inconsistent results due to variations in outcome measurements and in DHA supplementation dosages among studies [13–15]. Some RCTs have also shown improvements in cognitive outcomes in very low birth weight infants with DHA supplementation [16,17]. Furthermore, DHA supplementation not only offers short-term advantages but also long-term benefits, enhancing brain structure and function and improving neurochemical outcomes in children aged 5 years and older [16,18,19].

To promote such favorable effects, it is recommended that lactating mothers consume seafood, which is rich in DHA [20]. This recommendation is based on the evidence that maternal dietary choices can affect breast milk fatty acid composition [21]. However, it remains unknown whether lactating mothers' diets affect their infants' fatty acid levels. Moreover, blood DHA levels were reported to be equivalent between breastfed infants and LCPUFA-supplemented formula-fed infants during the first several months of life in previous studies, although those studies were mostly from Western countries [22–25].

Japanese dietary habits are characterized by the consumption of considerable amounts of seafood. In fact, Japanese people consume more fish, with an average intake of 31.2–52.5 g/day, than Caucasian Americans, who consume 8.9 g/day [26]. The high consumption of fish in Japan makes it an ideal location to examine the effects of maternal fish consumption on serum DHA levels in breastfed infants. Thus, this study aimed to investigate the association between the dietary habits of lactating mothers and serum DHA and other LCPUFA levels in Japanese term infants before they start eating solid foods. We hypothesized that, in contrast to studies from Western countries, Japanese breastfed infants might have higher serum DHA levels than those fed cow's milk formula (CMF) supplemented with LCPUFAs. Hence, this study also aimed to elucidate the association between infant feeding patterns and their serum DHA levels.

2. Materials and Methods

2.1. Study Design

This study was designed as a pre-specified cross-sectional study conducted as a supplemental analysis of the Atopy Induced by Breastfeeding or Cow's Milk Formula (ABC) trial [27]. Since the effects of allergen avoidance in neonates on reducing the risk of food allergy are not well established, the trial aimed to determine if avoiding or introducing CMF for at least the first three days of life might decrease the risk of sensitization to cow's milk protein and clinical food allergies. Details of the background and methods of the ABC trial are described elsewhere [27]. Briefly, in the ABC trial, newborn infants were randomized to breastfeeding (BF) with or without amino acid–based elemental formula (EF) for at least the first 3 days of life group (BF/EF group) or a BF supplemented with CMF ($\geq$5 mL/day) from the first day of life to 5 months of age group (BF + CMF group) and were followed up until their second birthday. Enrollment began on 1 October 2013, and follow-up was completed on 31 May 2018 at a single university hospital in Tokyo, Japan. Written, informed consent was obtained from the parents of all the enrolled infants. The trial protocol was approved by the ethics committee of Jikei University School of Medicine and the institutional review board of Jikei University Hospital (25-057(7192)). The trial was registered with the UMIN Clinical Trials Registry (UMIN000011577). This cross-sectional study used information from a maternal dietary questionnaire and serum fatty acid levels in blood samples from infants aged 5 months that were specifically collected for this trial in order to analyze their association at this single time point.

2.2. Study Population

The ABC trial included infants at risk of atopy due to at least one of their parents or siblings having current and/or past atopic diseases (e.g., asthma). Infants whose parents intended to exclusively provide breastfeeding or CMF before birth, or infants who were born at less than 36 weeks' gestational age, had a birth weight of less than 2000 g, or had serious congenital anomalies (e.g., cleft palate) were excluded.

2.3. Infant Formula and Intervention

To evaluate sensitization to cow's milk protein, this trial incorporated both CMF (Meiji Hohoemi®, Meiji Holdings Co., Ltd., Tokyo, Japan) and EF (Meiji Elemental® formula, Meiji Holdings Co., Ltd.) alongside breast milk; EF does not contain cow's milk protein, but it does contain fundamental nutrients in approximately equivalent proportions to CMF. The CMF was supplemented with α-linolenic acid (ALA) = 1.6%, DHA = 0.40%, linolenic acid (LA) = 15.9%, and arachidonic acid (AA) = 0.27% per total fatty acid weight, but not with eicosapentaenoic acid (EPA). The EF was supplemented with ALA = 12.4% and LA = 60.2%. Details of the fatty acid composition and other nutritional components of the infant formulas are provided in the Supplementary Materials (Tables S1–S3). Newborns were centrally assigned in a 1:1 ratio to the BF/EF and BF + CMF groups using permuted blocks of 4 by computer randomization. Infants in the BF/EF group were to avoid CMF for at least the first 3 days of life but were allowed to receive EF when mothers believed that the amount of breast milk was not enough. If they added more than 150 mL/day of EF to breastfeeding for three consecutive days, the EF was switched to CMF after the fourth day. Infants in the BF + CMF group were to receive at least 5 mL/day of CMF from the first day of life and at least 40 mL/day after 1 month of age until the first blood test at 5–6 months of age or before starting solid foods to supplement breastfeeding.

2.4. Sample Size

The primary outcome of the ABC trial was defined as a CM-IgE level of 0.35 UA/mL or greater at 24 months of age. For sample size calculation, it was assumed that this outcome would be achieved in 10% of one group and 25% of the other, with a bilateral type I error of 5%, 90% power, and an estimated 3% loss to follow-up. Therefore, we calculated that a sample size of 300 participants in a 1:1 ratio would be required to detect this difference.

2.5. Data Collection

Data on maternal age, maternal body mass index, gestational weeks, birth weight, and neonatal sex were obtained from the neonatal summary record at birth. Participating parents were prospectively interviewed regarding their child's daily amount of CMF intake during follow-up visits to the outpatient clinic when their child was 5–6 months old. The feeding patterns were prospectively classified into the following four grades based on the pre-specified cutoff points of CMF intake: BF with CMF > 100 mL/day, BF with CMF 40–100 mL/day, BF with CMF 5–40 mL/day, and exclusive BF. If the feeding patterns were not recorded at 5–6 months of age, data on their feeding patterns at 3 months of age were used instead. Moreover, during a previous visit, mothers were given a self-administered questionnaire regarding their diet, which included 38 food items. The completed answers were to be brought to the visit when the child was 5–6 months old. In the questionnaire, mothers were asked to check the most applicable box on a 6-point scale, ranging from "rarely" to "three times a day", for the frequency of consumption of each listed food item over the previous month.

2.6. Serum Fatty Acid Measurements and Primary/Secondary Outcomes

Blood was collected from the infants at 5–6 months of age, prior to the introduction of solid foods. In the ABC trial, 25-hydroxyvitamin D, total IgE, and antigen-specific IgE levels were measured. If sufficient residual serum samples were available, they were utilized to measure the composition of 24 serum fatty acids. The serum samples were stored at −80 °C and sent to Standard Reference Laboratory Inc. (Tokyo, Japan) for analysis. The concentration of each fatty acid was measured by gas chromatography-mass spectrometry using a calibration curve method and expressed as the weight percentage of total fatty acids [28]. The primary outcome was set as the infant serum DHA level. The secondary outcomes were infant serum EPA, AA, ALA, and LA levels. Moreover, n-3 LCPUFA, which includes the sum of ALA, EPA, docosapentaenoic acid (DPA), and DHA, as well as n-6 LCPUFA, which includes the sum of LA, γ-linolenic acid, eicosadienoic acid, dihomo-γ-linolenic acid (DGLA), AA, and docosatetraenoic acid (DTA), were also evaluated as secondary outcomes.

2.7. Statistical Analysis

Spearman's rank correlation (rho) was employed to assess the associations between the frequency of maternal food intake of the 38 listed items or grades of feeding patterns and seven outcomes, and among n-3 LCPUFAs and n-6 LCPUFAs to quantify the strength of correlations a rho value of $\geq$0.9 was considered a very strong correlation, 0.9 > rho $\geq$ 0.7 was strong, 0.7 > rho $\geq$ 0.4 was moderate, 0.4 > rho $\geq$ 0.1 was weak, and rho < 0.1 was a negligible correlation [29]. Univariate and multivariate regression analyses were also conducted to explore factors associated with serum DHA levels in infants. The Bonferroni correction was applied to account for multiple comparisons (e.g., 300 times), and a two-sided p value of <0.00016 was considered statistically significant. All data were analyzed using Stata, version 17.0 (StataCorp, College Station, TX, USA).

3. Results

3.1. Study Population

The ABC trial included 312 pregnant women who were randomly assigned to either the BF/EF group or the BF + CMF group from the first day of their infant's life in a 1:1 ratio (Figure 1); there was no loss to follow-up until 5–6 months of age. Blood samples were collected from 309 out of 312 infants at 5–6 months of age. A total of 268 residual serum samples from the infants were available for measurement of the 24 different types of fatty acids (Cohort I). In addition, food intake frequency questionnaires were prospectively collected from 254 participants (Cohort II), and 223 participants were prospectively interviewed regarding their infant's feeding patterns (Cohort III). The number of participants in each grade of feeding patterns was as follows: (1) CMF >100 mL/day (n = 121); (2) CMF 40–100 mL/ day (n = 10); (3) CMF 5–40 mL/day (n = 23); and (4) exclusive BF (n = 69). None of the infants were receiving EF at the time of blood sampling. The participants' characteristics are shown in Table 1.

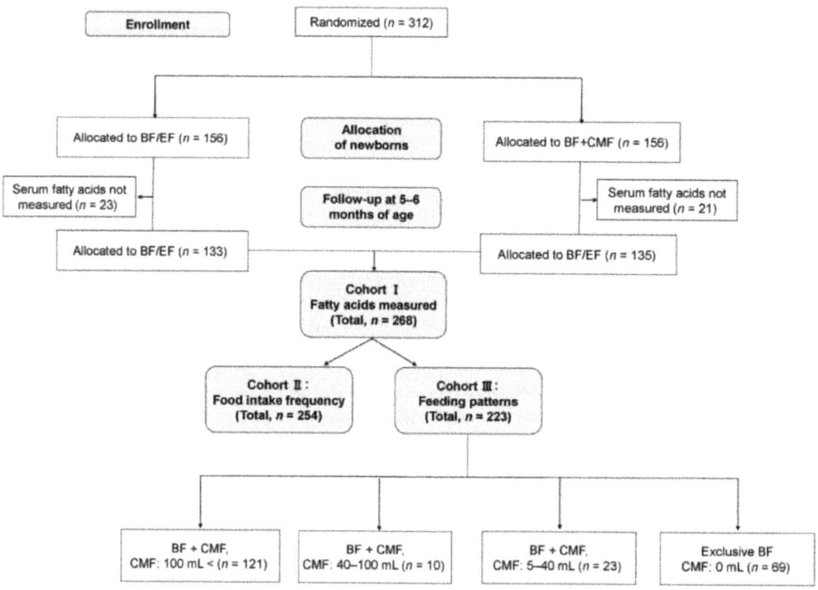

Figure 1. Participant flow through the ABC trial. BF + CMF, breastfeeding, and cow's milk formula; BF/EF, breastfeeding and/or elemental formula; CMF, cow's milk formula.

Table 1. Participants' characteristics.

	Fatty Acid Measured n = 268	Fatty Acid Unmeasured n = 42
Maternal age, mean (SD)—years	35.1 (4.3)	35.4 (4.8)
Maternal body mass index, mean (SD)—kg/m^2	20.6 (4.3)	20.9 (2.8)
Gestational weeks, median (IQR)—weeks	39 (38–39)	39 (38–39)
Birth weight, mean (SD)—g	2993 (314)	2983 (309)
Female, no. (%)	69 (53.9)	65 (50.0)

3.2. Serum Fatty Acid Compositions at 5–6 Months of Age

The present study first investigated fatty acid compositions in 268 infants (Cohort I), analyzing 24 different types of fatty acids (Table 2). For n-3 LCPUFA, strong positive associations were observed between serum levels of EPA, DPA, and DHA, while a moderate negative association was found between ALA and DHA (Figure 2A). Additionally, moderate associations were found between DGLA, AA, and DTA levels among the n-6 LCPUFAs, but negligible associations were found between LA and other fatty acids (Figure 2B). Interestingly, strong negative associations were observed between monounsaturated fatty acids (MUFA) and n-6 LCPUFA, and moderate negative associations were found between saturated fatty acids (SFA) and n-6 LCPUFA, as well as between MUFA and n-3 LCPUFA. Conversely, negligible associations were observed between n-3 and n-6 LCPUFA (Figure 2C).

Table 2. Values of 24 types of serum fatty acids measured at 5–6 months of age (n = 268).

No.	Fatty Acids		µg/mL	Weight %
			Measured Value	Measured Value
			Median (IQR) Min–Max	Median (IQR) Min–Max
1	Lauric acid	12:0	25.5 (16.0–41.9) 2.9–206	0.76 (0.50–1.11) 0.11–2.96
2	Myristic acid	14:0	45.6 (31.4–67.4) 16.3–298	1.32 (1.04–1.75) 0.57–4.50
3	Myristoleic acid	14:1n-5	1.4 (1.0–2.0) 0.30–10.2	0.04 (0.03–0.05) 0.01–0.14
4	Palmitic acid	16:0	723 (654–934) 434–2280	22.3 (21.6–22.9) 19.5–26.0
5	Palmitoleic acid	16:1n-7	43.4 (32.3–55.4) 18.8–153	1.24 (1.11–1.43) 0.77–2.56
6	Stearic acid	18:0	300 (264–348) 180–846	8.67 (8.23–9.14) 6.82–10.2
7	Oleic acid	18:1n-9	719 (594–925) 327–2758	21.1 (19.5–23.1) 14.6–32.8
8	Linoleic acid	18:2n-6	931 (818–1072) 540–1840	26.9 (24.6–28.8) 18.2–31.8
9	γ-linolenic acid	18:3n-6	4.70 (3.85–5.80) 1.50–15.8	0.13 (0.11–0.16) 0.05–0.53
10	α-linolenic acid	18:3n-3	22.5 (17.0–31.4) 9.7–87.4	0.65 (0.53–0.77) 0.31–1.48
11	Arachidic acid	20:0	12.9 (11.6–14.6) 6.90–29.4	0.36 (0.34–0.40) 0.27–0.55
12	Eicosenoic acid	20:1n-9	6.60 (5.00–9.15) 2.50–28.8	0.19 (0.16–0.23) 0.10–0.48
13	Eicosadienoic acid	20:2n-6	8.90 (7.60–22.1) 4.90–22.1	0.26 (0.24–0.27) 0.18–0.35
14	5,8,11-eicosatrienoic acid	20:3n-9	2.1 (1.7–2.6) 0.7–6.1	0.06 (0.05–0.07) 0.005–0.17

Table 2. *Cont.*

No.	Fatty Acids		μg/mL	Weight %
			Measured Value	Measured Value
			Median (IQR) Min–Max	Median (IQR) Min–Max
15	Dihomo-γ-linolenic acid	20:3n-6	30.4 (24.3–37.1) 14.0–79.0	0.84 (0.72–1.01) 0.30–1.82
16	Arachidonic acid	20:4n-6	221 (191–257) 103–437	6.22 (5.41–7.15) 2.45–10.3
17	Eicosapentaenoic acid	20:5n-3	24.3 (17.2–39.5) 3.9–165	0.66 (0.51–1.07) 0.15–4.58
18	Behenic acid	22:0	23.1 (20.6–25.6) 13.4–41.0	0.66 (0.57–0.75) 0.35–0.99
19	Erucic acid	22:1n-9	1.6 (1.2–2.0) 0.5–4.2	0.05 (0.04–0.05) 0.005–0.09
20	Docosatetraenoic acid	22:4n-6	6.5 (5.7–7.6) 2.8–14.2	0.19 (0.16–0.21) 0.10–0.30
21	Docosapentaenoic acid	22:5n-3	16.0 (12.6–19.0) 4.6–46.1	0.44 (0.36–0.53) 0.22–0.76
22	Lignoceric acid	24:0	19.5 (17.4–22.0) 10.3–32.6	0.56 (0.48–0.65) 0.26–0.91
23	Docosahexaenoic acid	22:6n-3	150.0 (127.4–178.3) 42.8–368.6	4.17 (3.69–4.90) 1.63–7.75
24	Nervonic acid	24:1n-9	41.7 (35.0–46.8) 24.2–85.0	1.19 (0.96–1.41) 0.52–1.98

IQR, interquartile range.

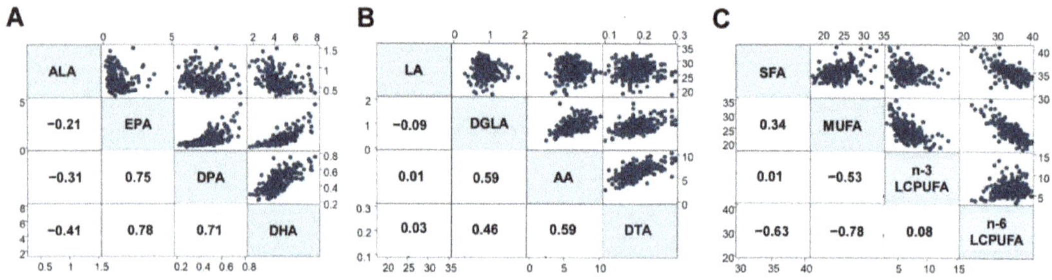

Figure 2. Associations between different fatty acids (%), including (**A**) n-3 LCPUFA, (**B**) n-6 LCPUFA, and (**C**) the relationship between SFA, MUFA, n-3 LCPUFA, and n-6 LCPUFA. DGLA, dihomo-γ-linolenic acid; DTA, docosatetraenoic acid; LCPUFA, long-chain polyunsaturated fatty acid. Numbers in squares represent Spearman's rho. Blue dots represent the corresponding fatty acid levels (%).

3.3. *Frequency of Maternal Intake of the Listed Items and Serum DHA Levels in Infants*

This study next examined the association between the frequency of consumption of 38 food items by lactating mothers and serum DHA levels in their infants (Table 3). Of the 38 food items, only two types of fish, "Blue-back fish" (rho = 0.24, p = 0.0001) (Figure 3A) and "White fish" (rho = 0.25, p = 0.0001) (Figure 3B), were found to have significant positive associations with serum DHA levels in infants. In contrast, other types of fish, such as salmon, tuna, and swordfish, as well as food categories such as nuts, dairy products, eggs, vegetable oil, fried foods, meat, and beans, did not have any significant associations with DHA levels. A new variable, "Blue-White fish", created by combining the frequency of consumption of these two fish types, was found to be significantly associated with higher levels of serum DHA in infants (rho = 0.29, $p < 0.0001$) (Figure 3C). When stratified by infant sex, the relationship between frequency of "Blue-White fish" intake and serum DHA levels persisted in both males (rho = 0.40, $p < 0.0001$) and females (rho = 0.39, $p < 0.0001$), showing no evident interaction of sex (p for interaction = 0.112) (Figure S1A,B).

Table 3. Associations between frequency of maternal intake of specific foods and infant serum DHA levels.

No.	Food Item	*n*	rho	*p* Value
	Fish			
1	Blue-back fish: Mackerel, sardine, horse mackerel, Pacific saury (including canned)	252	0.24	0.0001
2	White fish (sea bream, snapper, flounder, eel, cod, trout, etc.)	249	0.25	0.0001
3	Salmon (including canned salmon)	250	0.03	0.64
4	Tuna (canned tuna, sashimi, etc.)	252	−0.02	0.78
5	Swordfish	249	0.01	0.82
	Nuts			
6	Peanuts (including peanut butter)	249	−0.06	0.36
7	Walnuts	250	−0.01	0.92
8	Almonds	251	0.04	0.49
9	Cashew nuts	250	0.06	0.32
10	Macadamia nuts	251	0.04	0.50
11	Hazelnuts	249	−0.00	0.98
12	Coconut (including that in processed foods)	244	−0.02	0.78
	Dairy products			
13	Cow's milk	254	0.11	0.07
14	Cheese	252	−0.05	0.45
15	Cream (including cream for coffee)	254	−0.11	0.07
16	Ice cream	253	0.05	0.44
17	Butter	249	0.01	0.90
	Egg			
18	Heated eggs	252	−0.03	0.62
19	Raw eggs	221	0.02	0.79
20	Mayonnaise	251	−0.06	0.33
21	Fish eggs (salmon roe, flying fish roe, sea urchin, dried mullet roe, caviar, etc.)	250	−0.02	0.81
	Vegetable oil			
22	Unspecified vegetable oil	247	−0.04	0.55
23	Olive oil	250	0.03	0.61
24	Rapeseed oil	268	−0.05	0.45
25	Sesame oil	268	−0.08	0.21
26	Safflower oil	268	−0.09	0.16
27	Other	268	−0.01	0.92
28	Margarine	248	−0.07	0.25

Table 3. *Cont.*

No.	Food Item	*n*	rho	*p* Value
	Fried food			
29	Junk food (potato chips, etc.)	253	−0.11	0.08
30	Instant noodles	250	−0.12	0.06
31	Fried food at home (tempura, fried chicken, fried potatoes, etc.)	254	0.03	0.59
32	Fried food from outside (tempura, fried chicken, fried potatoes, etc.)	254	−0.11	0.09
	Meat			
33	Beef	246	0.05	0.43
34	Pork	252	0.05	0.46
35	Chicken	251	0.08	0.23
36	Processed meat (sausage, salami, hotdogs, bacon, etc.)	253	−0.05	0.40
37	Hamburger at fast-food restaurant	248	−0.08	0.22
	Beans			
38	Soybean (natto, tofu, miso, green soybeans, soy milk) and sweet red (adzuki) beans	252	0.14	0.02

A *p* value of <0.00016 was considered statistically significant. "*n*" denotes the number of respondents to the questionnaire.

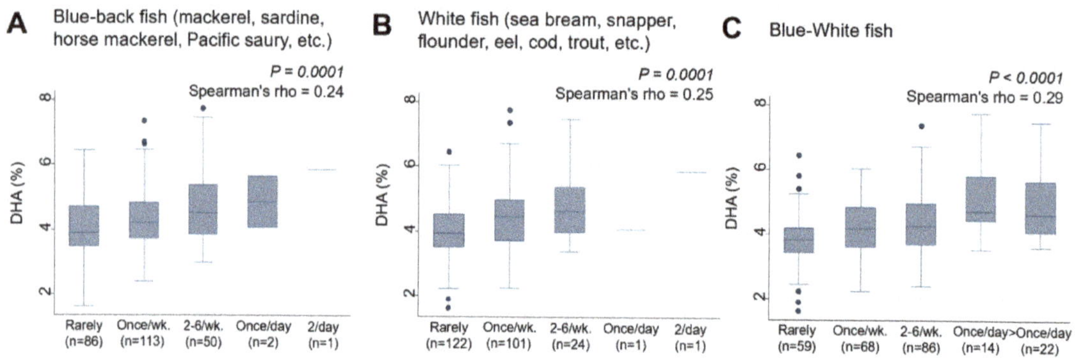

Figure 3. Frequency of (**A**) Blue-back fish, (**B**) White fish, and (**C**) Blue-White fish consumption by lactating mothers and the levels of serum DHA (%) in their infants. Number of non-respondents: (**A**) 2, (**B**) 5, (**C**) 5. Box presents interquartile range (IQR) from 25% to 75%. Middle line of the box means the median. The upper and lower whiskers represent minimum within 25% − 1.5*IQR and maximum within 75% + 1.5*IQR. Outliers that differ significantly from the rest of the dataset are plotted as individual points outside of the whiskers on the box-plot. A *p* value of <0.00016 was considered statistically significant.

3.4. *Frequency of Maternal Intake of the Listed Items and Serum EPA and Other LCPUFA Levels in Infants*

The study also examined the associations between the frequency of maternal intake of certain foods and the levels of serum EPA and other LCPUFAs in their infants. "Blue-back fish" and "White fish", which were found to be associated with DHA levels, also showed significant positive associations with EPA levels in the infants (rho = 0.32, $p < 0.0001$ for both) (Figure 4A,B). The combined intake of "Blue-White fish" was also significantly and positively associated with EPA levels (rho = 0.40, $p < 0.0001$) (Figure 4C). Weak negative and positive trends were observed between "Junk food" (rho = −0.19, $p = 0.003$) (Figure 4D) and "Beans" (rho = 0.17, $p = 0.008$) (Figure 4E), respectively, and EPA levels, although their p values did not reach statistical significance using the cutoff point of $p = 0.00016$.

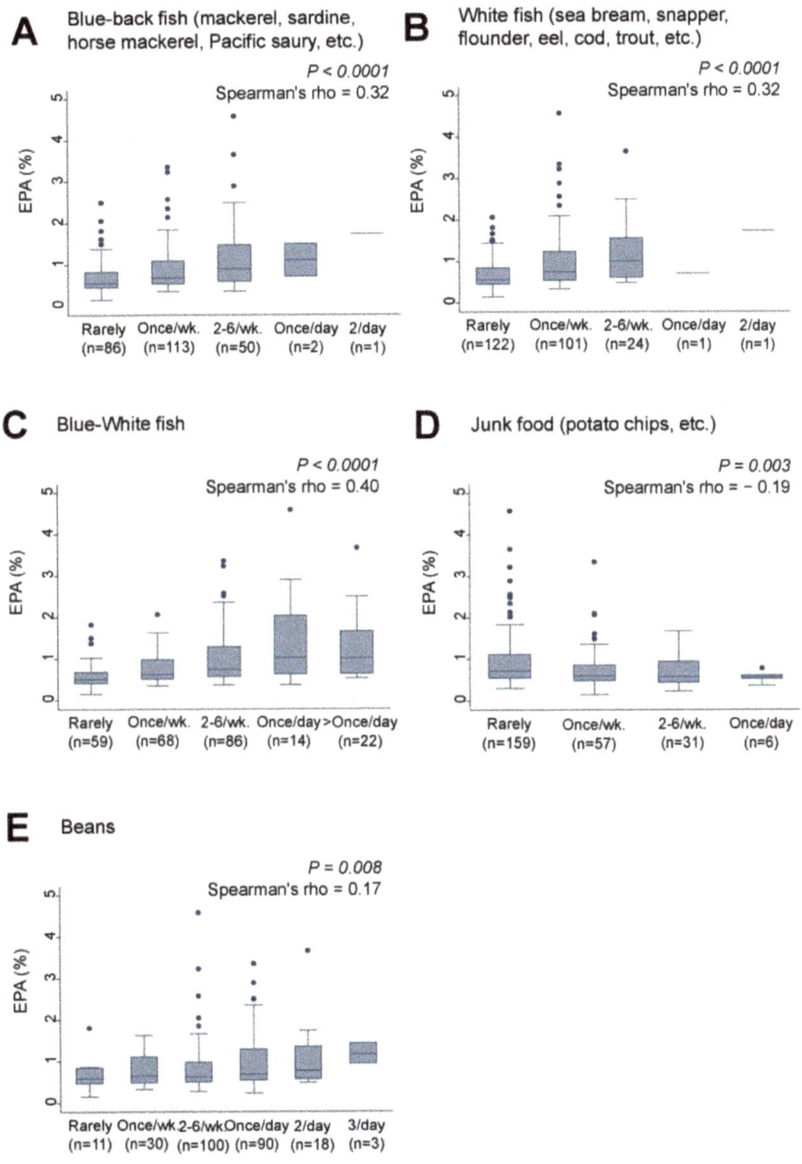

Figure 4. Frequency of (**A**) Blue-back fish, (**B**) White fish, (**C**) Blue-White fish, (**D**) Junk food, and (**E**) Bean consumption by lactating mothers and levels of serum EPA (%) in their infants. Number of non-respondents: (**A**) 2, (**B**) 5, (**C**) 5, (**D**) 1, (**E**) 2. Box presents interquartile range (IQR) from 25% to 75%. Middle line of the box means the median. The upper and lower whiskers represent minimum within 25% − 1.5*IQR and maximum within 75% + 1.5*IQR. Outliers that differ significantly from the rest of the dataset are plotted as individual points outside of the whiskers on the box-plot. A p value of <0.00016 was considered statistically significant.

Similarly, the intake of 'Blue-back fish' (rho = 0.29, $p < 0.0001$) (Figure 5A), "White fish" (rho = 0.31, $p < 0.0001$) (Figure 5B), and the combined intake of "Blue-White fish" (rho = 0.37, $p < 0.0001$) (Figure 5C) were significantly and positively associated with n-3 LCPUFA levels. Weak positive and negative trends were also observed between "Junk food" (rho = −0.16, $p = 0.009$) (Figure 5D) and "Beans" (rho = 0.18, $p = 0.004$) (Figure 5E) and n-3 LCPUFA levels, respectively. However, none of the 38 food items analyzed showed significant associations with serum levels of AA, LA, ALA, or n-6 LCPUFA.

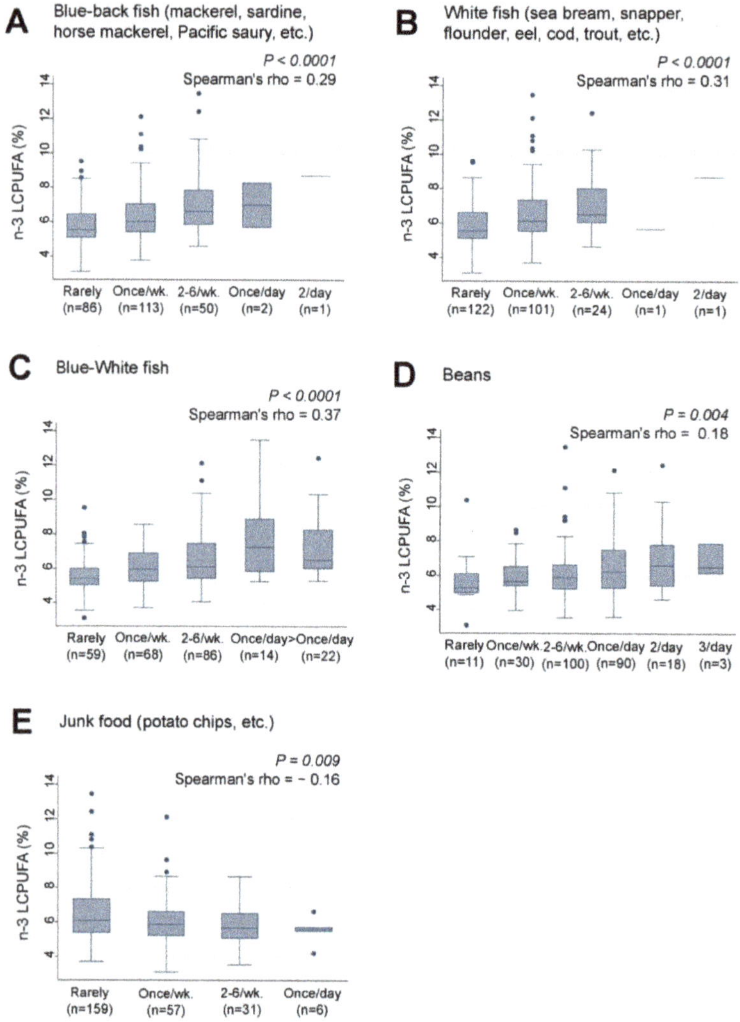

Figure 5. Frequency of (**A**) Blue-back fish, (**B**) White fish, (**C**) Blue-White fish, (**D**) Beans, and (**E**) Junk food consumption by lactating mothers and levels of serum n-3 LCPUFA (%) in their infants. LCPUFA, long-chain polyunsaturated fatty acid. Number of non-respondents: (**A**) 2, (**B**) 5, (**C**) 5, (**D**) 2, (**E**) 5. Box presents interquartile range (IQR) from 25% to 75%. Middle line of the box means the median. The upper and lower whiskers represent minimum within 25% − 1.5*IQR and maximum within 75% + 1.5*IQR. Outliers that differ significantly from the rest of the dataset are plotted as individual points outside of the whiskers on the box-plot. A p value of <0.00016 was considered statistically significant.

3.5. Feeding Patterns and Serum DHA and Other n-3 LCPUFA Levels in Infants

Examination of the association between the infants' feeding patterns and their serum n-3 LCPUFA levels revealed that infants who were predominantly breastfed had significantly higher levels of serum DHA (rho = 0.32, $p < 0.0001$) (Figure 6A), EPA (rho = 0.35, $p < 0.0001$) (Figure 6B), AA (rho = 0.30, $p < 0.0001$) (Figure 6C), and n-3 LCPUFA (rho = 0.36, $p < 0.0001$) (Figure 6D) compared to those who received larger amounts of CMF to supplement breastfeeding. Conversely, infants who were fed less CMF had significantly lower levels of serum LA (rho = −0.33, $p < 0.0001$) (Figure 6E) compared to those who were predominantly breastfed. No significant associations were found between feeding patterns and serum ALA (Figure 6F) or n-6 LCPUFA levels (Figure 6G).

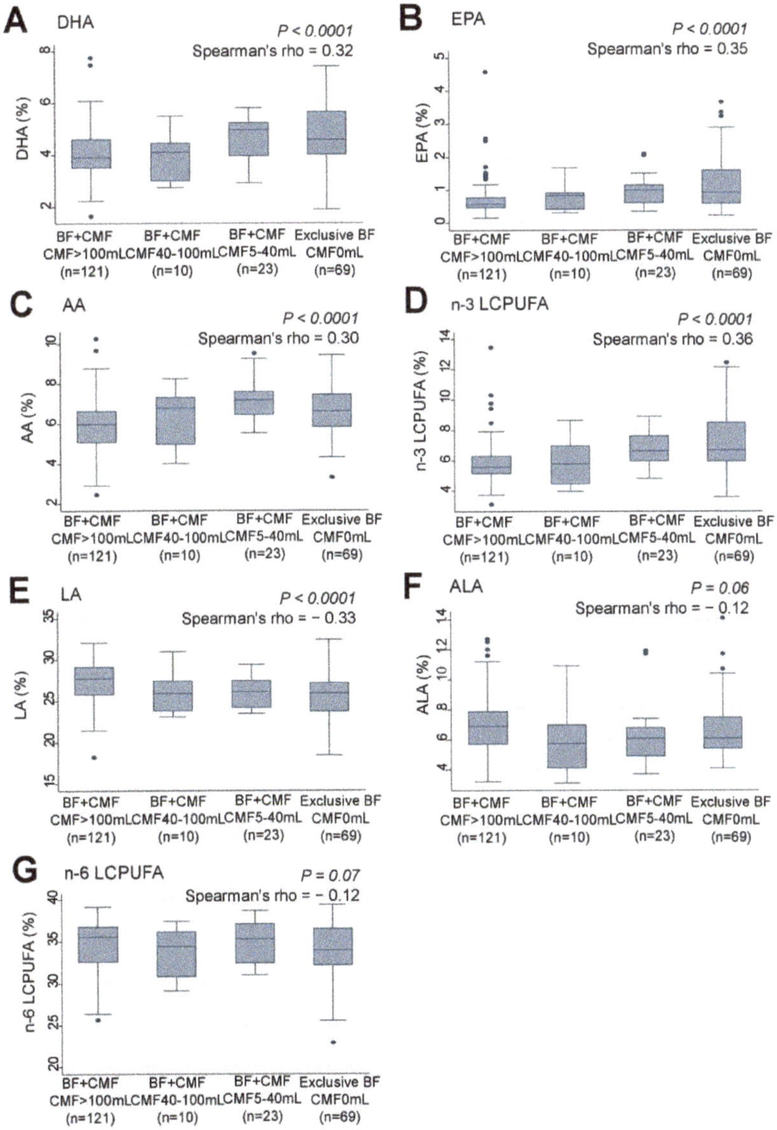

Figure 6. Correlations between feeding pattern grades and serum levels (%) of (**A**) DHA, (**B**) EPA, (**C**) AA, (**D**) n-3 LCPUFA, (**E**) LA, (**F**) ALA, and (**G**) n-6 LCPUFA in infants. LCPUFA, long-chain

polyunsaturated fatty acid. Box presents interquartile range (IQR) from 25% to 75%. Middle line of the box means the median. The upper and lower whiskers represent minimum within 25% − 1.5*IQR and maximum within 75% + 1.5*IQR. Outliers that differ significantly from the rest of the dataset are plotted as individual points outside of the whiskers on the box-plot A p value of <0.00016 was considered statistically significant.

3.6. Factors Associated with Serum DHA Levels in Infants: Univariate and Multivariate Regression Analyses

We assessed the infants' serum DHA levels in relation to six variables: "Blue-White fish" consumption, feeding patterns, group allocation in the ABC trial, maternal age, maternal body mass index, gestational weeks, birth weight, and infant sex (Table 4). Univariate analysis revealed that both "Blue-White fish" consumption and "feeding patterns" were significantly associated with serum DHA levels, while there was no significant association for the other factors (Model I). In the subsequent multivariate analysis (Model II), including the two significant factors identified in univariate analyses, "Blue-White fish" consumption and "feeding patterns" remained significant variables. After adjusting for all six variables, both "Blue-White fish" consumption and "feeding patterns" remained significant variables (Model III). Notably, when infant sex was included in the univariate analysis for "Blue-White fish" and serum DHA levels, the coefficient for "Blue-White fish" remained virtually unchanged (coefficient = 0.29 for both), showing no evidence of a confounding effect of sex.

Table 4. Univariate and multivariate regression analysis of factors associated with serum DHA levels in infants.

	Univariate Analysis			Multivariate Analysis					
	Model I			Model II			Model III		
	CE	95% CI	p Value	CE	95% CI	p Value	CE	95% CI	p Value
Blue-White fish	0.29	0.19–0.39	<0.001	0.29	0.18–0.41	<0.001	0.24	0.11–0.38	0.001
Feeding patterns	0.25	0.15–0.35	<0.001	0.18	0.09–0.28	<0.001	0.17	0.05–0.29	0.006
Allocated group in ABC trial	0.18	−0.07–0.44	0.15				0.07	−0.23–0.37	0.64
Maternal age	−0.02	−0.05–0.01	0.27				0.01	−0.02–0.04	0.54
Maternal body mass index	0.01	−0.03–0.04	0.74				0.00	−0.03–0.03	0.94
Gestational weeks	0.05	−0.01–0.11	0.13				0.05	−0.10–0.19	0.54
Birth weight	0.00	−0.00–0.00	0.20				0.31	−0.00–0.00	0.72
Female	0.19	−0.06–0.44	0.13				0.31	0.00–0.63	0.05

CE, coefficient; 95% CI, 95% confidence interval. Model I presents the results of univariate regression analysis evaluating the association of infant serum DHA levels with six variables: "Blue-White fish" intake, feeding pattern, allocation group in the ABC trial, maternal age, maternal body mass index, gestational age in weeks, birth weight, and infant sex; Model II presents the results of multivariate regression analysis, including the factors of "Blue-White fish" consumption and feeding pattern, both of which showed significant associations in Model I; and Model III presents the results of multivariate regression analysis including all six variables. A p value of <0.00016 was considered statistically significant.

4. Discussion

To the best of our knowledge, this is the first study to explore the association between maternal diet and serum LCPUFA levels in infants who have not yet started solid foods. The results indicated that the infants of lactating mothers who frequently consumed "Blue-back fish" and/or "White fish" from the list of 38 food items had higher levels of serum DHA than infants whose mothers did not consume these fish regularly. The study also found that infants who were predominantly breastfed had higher levels of serum DHA compared to those who were formula-fed. Even following multivariate analysis, frequent intake of

"Blue-White fish" by lactating mothers and "feeding patterns" remained significant factors related to infant DHA levels, indicating that both factors were independently associated with higher serum DHA levels in infants. These results suggest that higher serum DHA levels might be more effectively achieved by frequent maternal consumption of "Blue-back fish" and/or "White fish", or by prioritizing breastfeeding rather than relying on CMF supplemented with DHA.

A previous meta-analysis revealed that the concentration of DHA in breast milk varies considerably by country and is generally higher in coastal populations with a higher consumption of seafood [30]. A large Canadian birth cohort study showed that maternal intake of fish oil supplements and cold-water fish (such as salmon, mackerel, and bluefish) was positively associated with DHA and n-3 LCPUFA levels in breast milk but not with AA and n-6 LCPUFA levels [31]. Similarly, the Japanese Human Milk Study reported that maternal consumption of grilled fish was associated with increased DHA levels in breast milk [32]. These previous reports support the finding of this study that serum DHA levels are higher in infants fed by mothers who frequently consume "Blue-White fish" as compared to those who only infrequently consume such fish. Hence, our findings imply that mothers can potentially enhance their infants' DHA levels by frequently consuming "Blue-back fish" and/or "White fish," even when breastfeeding is limited due to milk supply or maternal lifestyle. In Japan, these types of fish are affordable and readily available, often as convenient, ready-to-eat options, such as canned or convenience store offerings. This accessibility makes it feasible for even busy mothers to incorporate these fish into their daily diets. It should be cautioned, however, that causality was not determined in this study due to the nature of the study design. Additionally, the study did not assess LCPUFA levels in breast milk or maternal serum, necessitating further longitudinal investigations to comprehensively evaluate the relationship between maternal dietary intake of these fish, LCPUFA levels in maternal serum and breast milk, and infant DHA levels.

No interaction of sex was evident in the association between maternal "Blue-White fish" intake frequency and infant serum DHA levels in this study. As demonstrated in a systematic review predominantly involving adults, females have higher plasma DHA levels (%) compared to males. This could be attributed to differences in n-3 LCPUFA synthesis from ALA, dietary patterns, and age [33]. However, only limited data on children are available, with studies showing no sex differences in plasma or erythrocyte membrane LCPUFA composition among individuals from infancy to young adulthood [34]. These previous findings are consistent with our observations. On the other hand, DHA levels in breast milk are suggested to be higher when the infant is female [35]. Thus, further studies are warranted to elucidate the effects of sex on the association between maternal diet, LCPUFA levels in breast milk, and the levels in infant serum.

The present study also revealed that serum DHA levels were higher in breastfed infants compared to those fed CMF, even when it was supplemented with DHA. Contrary to our findings, most studies from Western countries indicated similar [22–25] or lower [36,37] blood DHA levels in 3–9-month-old, full-term, breastfed infants compared to those fed LCPUFA-supplemented formula. This discrepancy might be due to the comparable or lower DHA levels observed in breast milk versus formula in these studies. Conversely, Japanese mothers in previous studies exhibited higher DHA levels in breast milk (ranging from 0.53% to 1.10%) [38–40], exceeding the 0.4% DHA supplementation in CMF used in our study. Indeed, a previous Japanese study involving 6-month-old infants showed a similar trend in mean erythrocyte membrane DHA as that in our present findings [41]. Data from our Japanese study thus offer insights into the potential influence of relative DHA levels in breast milk and infant formula on the relationship between feeding patterns and infant blood DHA levels.

In addition to DHA, AA is also crucial for infant growth, brain development, and overall health [42]. Thus, 0.27% AA was added to the CMF used in this study. However, contrary to expectations, the results showed that breastfed infants had higher serum AA levels compared to those fed CMF, even when it was supplemented with AA. Interestingly, unlike DHA, maternal consumption of specific foods, such as fish, did not appear to affect serum AA levels in infants. AA is found in small amounts in a variety of animal-derived foods, such as meat, poultry, eggs, fish, and dairy products [43]. This contrasts with DHA and EPA, which are primarily found in seafood. As such, EPA and DHA were associated with the consumption of "Blue-back fish" and/or "White fish", while AA was not associated with the consumption of any specific food items. It is noteworthy that AA is exclusively found in animal-derived foods because plants cannot synthesize C-20 LCPUFAs, including AA. In fact, compared with omnivorous women, vegetarian women had lower blood concentrations of AA during pregnancy [44]. Several decades ago, the Japanese diet consisted mainly of rice, fish, beans, and vegetables. However, recent dietary changes towards a more westernized diet, which includes more animal-derived foods, might have resulted in higher serum AA levels in breastfed infants compared to those fed CMF, even when it was supplemented with LCPUFA, including AA.

Infants predominantly fed CMF had significantly higher levels of LA in their serum than breastfed infants. Moreover, the levels of ALA did not appear to be affected by feeding patterns. The CMF used in this study was supplemented with a higher percentage of LA (15.9%) than ALA (1.6%), both of which are found in high percentages in Japanese breast milk [40]. The findings indicate that the LA content in CMF was sufficient to increase serum LA levels in infants, but the ALA content was insufficient. Since infants' bodies can convert ALA and LA into DHA and AA, respectively [45], it was expected that infants fed CMF supplemented with ALA and LA would have higher serum DHA and AA levels. However, infants predominantly fed CMF supplemented with higher ALA and LA levels than breast milk had significantly lower levels of DHA and AA in their serum than breastfed infants. In addition, a previous RCT showed that blood DHA and AA levels were higher in infants fed CMF supplemented with higher amounts of DHA and AA than those supplemented with more ALA and LA [46]. These findings suggest that directly supplementing CMF with DHA and AA might more effectively increase their levels in infants, as compared to supplementing CMF with their precursors, ALA and LA.

One of the strengths of this study is that it used blood samples collected from 268 infants to measure 24 different types of fatty acids, despite the challenge of performing venous blood sampling in infants aged 5 to 6 months. This unique approach sets this study apart from most other studies on LCPUFA, which have relied on measuring their concentrations in breast milk.

The results of this study should be considered in light of several limitations. First, due to a lack of information on the amount of breast milk intake, evaluation of the ratio of CMF to breast milk could not be accurately assessed despite the study being prospective. Infants exclusively fed with CMF were grouped together with those fed a mixture of breast milk and CMF in the CMF >100 mL/day category. Second, the exposure to CMF might not have been adequately classified, as the exact amount of CMF and the frequency of intake were not recorded, and data on the feeding patterns for 15% (31/207) of the participants had to be substituted with their feeding patterns at 3 months of age. Further, the amount of breast milk consumed could not usually be measured. Third, there might have been residual confounding as CMF doses were not randomized. For example, mothers who exclusively breastfeed their infants might be more likely to have a healthy lifestyle, exercise habits, and high socioeconomic status. Fourth, the questionnaire survey on food intake only considered the frequency of the consumption of specific foods and did not record the amount or cooking method, both of which would affect the results. Moreover, the questionnaires utilized in this study have not undergone validation and reliability assessments for evaluating dietary intake. Fifth, the results of the interview and questionnaire survey on food patterns might have been affected by a recall bias. Sixth, the levels of DHA in infant serum might be different from those in plasma, red blood cells, or in the brain. Seventh, the study population consisted of infants at risk of atopy, and hence, generalization of our findings to healthy infants might not be appropriate. Eighth, the sample size was calculated for the ABC trial and might not be adequate for the objectives of this cross-sectional study.

Therefore, associations with food items other than "Blue-White fish" might have remained undetected. Lastly, the study was conducted in the center of Tokyo, and hence, the results might not be generalizable to populations in rural areas of Japan or to the populations of other countries.

5. Conclusions

The present results suggest that the infants of lactating mothers who frequently consume "Blue-back fish" and/or "White fish" and are predominantly breastfed might experience a more effective increase in serum DHA levels compared to the infants of mothers who rely on DHA-supplemented CMF alone.

Supplementary Materials: The following supporting information can be downloaded at: https://www.mdpi.com/article/10.3390/nu15204338/s1, Table S1: Fatty acid composition of cow's milk formula (CMF) (Hohoemi®); Table S2: Fatty acid composition of the elemental formula (EF) (Meiji Elemental® formula); Table S3: Nutritional composition of cow's milk formula (CMF) (Hohoemi®) and elemental formula (EF) (Meiji Elemental formula®); Figure S1: Frequency of Blue-White fish consumption by lactating mothers and the levels of serum DHA (%) in their infants. (A) Males, (B) Females.

Author Contributions: Conceptualization, A.K. and M.U.; methodology, A.K. and M.U.; validation, H.T. and M.U.; formal analysis, A.K. and M.U.; writing—original draft preparation, A.K. and M.U.; writing—review and editing, A.K. and M.U.; visualization, A.K. and M.U.; supervision, H.T. and M.U.; project administration, H.T. and M.U.; funding acquisition, H.T. and M.U. All authors have read and agreed to the published version of the manuscript.

Funding: This research was supported by (1) the Ministry of Education, Culture, Sports, Science and Technology in the Japan-Supported Program for the Strategic Research Foundation at Private Universities, (2) JSPS KAKENHI Grant Number JP16K09074, (3) the Practical Research Project for Allergic Diseases and Immunology of the Japan Agency for Medical Research and Development, AMED (15ek0410019h0101), (4) Dairy Products Health Science Council and Japan Dairy Association, and (5) The Jikei University School of Medicine. The funders of the study played no role in study design, collection, analysis, or interpretation of data, the writing of the report, or the placement of any restrictions regarding the submission of the report for publication.

Institutional Review Board Statement: The study was conducted in accordance with the Declaration of Helsinki and approved by the Institutional Review Board of the Jikei University School of Medicine (25-057(7192), 1 August 2013).

Informed Consent Statement: Informed consent was obtained from all subjects involved in the study.

Data Availability Statement: The data in the article for the clinical trials will not be made available because permission was not obtained from the study participants to share their data publicly. Other data, the code book, and analytic code will be made available on request.

Acknowledgments: The authors would like to thank Haruka Wada for data management and data monitoring at the Division of Molecular Epidemiology, Jikei University School of Medicine (Tokyo, Japan).

Conflicts of Interest: The authors declare no conflict of interest. The funders had no role in the design of the study; in the collection, analyses, or interpretation of data; in the writing of the manuscript; or in the decision to publish the results.

References

1. Meek, J.Y.; Noble, L.; Section on Breastfeeding. Policy statement: Breastfeeding and the use of human milk. *Pediatrics* **2022**, *150*, e2022057988. [CrossRef]
2. World Health Organization. *Breastfeeding*; World Health Organization: Geneva, Switzerland, 2018.
3. Victora, C.G.; Bahl, R.; Barros, A.J.; Franca, G.V.; Horton, S.; Krasevec, J.; Murch, S.; Sankar, M.J.; Walker, N.; Rollins, N.C.; et al. Breastfeeding in the 21st century: Epidemiology, mechanisms, and lifelong effect. *Lancet* **2016**, *387*, 475–490. [CrossRef] [PubMed]
4. Horwood, L.J.; Darlow, B.A.; Mogridge, N. Breast milk feeding and cognitive ability at 7–8 years. *Arch. Dis. Child. Fetal Neonatal Ed.* **2001**, *84*, F23–F27. [CrossRef] [PubMed]

5. Plunkett, B.A.; Mele, L.; Casey, B.M.; Varner, M.W.; Sorokin, Y.; Reddy, U.M.; Wapner, R.J.; Thorp, J.M., Jr.; Saade, G.R.; Tita, A.T.N.; et al. Association of breastfeeding and child IQ score at age 5 Years. *Obstet. Gynecol.* **2021**, *137*, 561–570. [CrossRef] [PubMed]
6. Decsi, T.; Thiel, I.; Koletzko, B. Essential fatty acids in full term infants fed breast milk or formula. *Arch. Dis. Child. Fetal Neonatal Ed.* **1995**, *72*, F23–F28. [CrossRef] [PubMed]
7. Boehm, G.; Borte, M.; Bohles, H.J.; Muller, H.; Kohn, G.; Moro, G. Docosahexaenoic and arachidonic acid content of serum and red blood cell membrane phospholipids of preterm infants fed breast milk, standard formula or formula supplemented with n-3 and n-6 long-chain polyunsaturated fatty acids. *Eur. J. Pediatr.* **1996**, *155*, 410–416. [CrossRef] [PubMed]
8. Foreman-van Drongelen, M.M.; van Houwelingen, A.C.; Kester, A.D.; Blanco, C.E.; Hasaart, T.H.; Hornstra, G. Influence of feeding artificial-formula milks containing docosahexaenoic and arachidonic acids on the postnatal long-chain polyunsaturated fatty acid status of healthy preterm infants. *Br. J. Nutr.* **1996**, *76*, 649–667. [CrossRef] [PubMed]
9. Bradbury, J. Docosahexaenoic acid (DHA): An ancient nutrient for the modern human brain. *Nutrients* **2011**, *3*, 529–554. [CrossRef] [PubMed]
10. Schneider, N.; Bruchhage, M.M.K.; O'Neill, B.V.; Hartweg, M.; Tanguy, J.; Steiner, P.; Mutungi, G.; O'Regan, J.; McSweeney, S.; D'Sa, V.; et al. A nutrient formulation affects developmental myelination in term infants: A randomized clinical trial. *Front Nutr.* **2022**, *9*, 823–893. [CrossRef] [PubMed]
11. Hortensius, L.M.; Hellstrom, W.; Savman, K.; Heckemann, R.A.; Bjorkman-Burtscher, I.M.; Groenendaal, F.; Andersson, M.X.; Nilsson, A.K.; Tataranno, M.L.; van Elburg, R.M.; et al. Serum docosahexaenoic acid levels are associated with brain volumes in extremely preterm born infants. *Pediatr. Res.* **2021**, *90*, 1177–1185. [CrossRef]
12. Lauritzen, L.; Brambilla, P.; Mazzocchi, A.; Harslof, L.B.; Ciappolino, V.; Agostoni, C. DHA effects in brain development and function. *Nutrients* **2016**, *8*, 6. [CrossRef] [PubMed]
13. Jasani, B.; Simmer, K.; Patole, S.K.; Rao, S.C. Long chain polyunsaturated fatty acid supplementation in infants born at term. *Cochrane Database Syst. Rev.* **2017**, *3*, CD000376. [CrossRef] [PubMed]
14. Moon, K.; Rao, S.C.; Schulzke, S.M.; Patole, S.K.; Simmer, K. Longchain polyunsaturated fatty acid supplementation in preterm infants. *Cochrane Database Syst. Rev.* **2016**, *12*, CD000375. [CrossRef] [PubMed]
15. Newberry, S.J.; Chung, M.; Booth, M.; Maglione, M.A.; Tang, A.M.; O'Hanlon, C.E.; Wang, D.D.; Okunogbe, A.; Huang, C.; Motala, A.; et al. Omega-3 fatty acids and maternal and child health: An updated systematic review. *Evid. Rep. Technol. Assess.* **2016**, *224*, 1–826.
16. Gould, J.F.; Makrides, M.; Gibson, R.A.; Sullivan, T.R.; McPhee, A.J.; Anderson, P.J.; Best, K.P.; Sharp, M.; Cheong, J.L.Y.; Opie, G.F.; et al. Neonatal docosahexaenoic acid in preterm infants and intelligence at 5 years. *N. Engl. J. Med.* **2022**, *387*, 1579–1588. [CrossRef]
17. Henriksen, C.; Haugholt, K.; Lindgren, M.; Aurvag, A.K.; Ronnestad, A.; Gronn, M.; Solberg, R.; Moen, A.; Nakstad, B.; Berge, R.K.; et al. Improved cognitive development among preterm infants attributable to early supplementation of human milk with docosahexaenoic acid and arachidonic acid. *Pediatrics* **2008**, *121*, 1137–1145. [CrossRef] [PubMed]
18. Lepping, R.J.; Honea, R.A.; Martin, L.E.; Liao, K.; Choi, I.Y.; Lee, P.; Papa, V.B.; Brooks, W.M.; Shaddy, D.J.; Carlson, S.E.; et al. Long-chain polyunsaturated fatty acid supplementation in the first year of life affects brain function, structure, and metabolism at age nine years. *Dev. Psychobiol.* **2019**, *61*, 5–16. [CrossRef] [PubMed]
19. Liao, K.; McCandliss, B.D.; Carlson, S.E.; Colombo, J.; Shaddy, D.J.; Kerling, E.H.; Lepping, R.J.; Sittiprapaporn, W.; Cheatham, C.L.; Gustafson, K.M. Event-related potential differences in children supplemented with long-chain polyunsaturated fatty acids during infancy. *Dev. Sci.* **2017**, *20*, e12455. [CrossRef]
20. U.S. Department of Agriculture; U.S. Department of Health and Human Services. *The Dietary Guidelines for Americans, 2020–2025*, 9th ed.; U.S. Department of Agriculture: Washington, DC, USA, 2020.
21. Bravi, F.; Wiens, F.; Decarli, A.; Dal Pont, A.; Agostoni, C.; Ferraroni, M. Impact of maternal nutrition on breast-milk composition: A systematic review. *Am. J. Clin. Nutr.* **2016**, *104*, 646–662. [CrossRef]
22. Bondia-Martinez, E.; Lopez-Sabater, M.C.; Castellote-Bargallo, A.I.; Rodriguez-Palmero, M.; Gonzalez-Corbella, M.J.; Rivero-Urgell, M.; Campoy-Folgoso, C.; Bayes-Garcia, R. Fatty acid composition of plasma and erythrocytes in term infants fed human milk and formulae with and without docosahexaenoic and arachidonic acids from egg yolk lecithin. *Early Hum. Dev.* **1998**, *53* (Suppl. 1), S109–S119. [CrossRef]
23. Schwartz, J.; Drossard, C.; Dube, K.; Kannenberg, F.; Kunz, C.; Kalhoff, H.; Kersting, M. Dietary intake and plasma concentrations of PUFA and LC-PUFA in breastfed and formula fed infants under real-life conditions. *Eur. J. Nutr.* **2010**, *49*, 189–195. [CrossRef] [PubMed]
24. Visentin, S.; Vicentin, D.; Magrini, G.; Santandreu, F.; Disalvo, L.; Sala, M.; Fasano, V.; Gonzalez, H.F. Red blood cell membrane fatty acid composition in infants fed formulas with different lipid profiles. *Early Hum. Dev.* **2016**, *100*, 11–15. [CrossRef] [PubMed]
25. Uhl, O.; Fleddermann, M.; Hellmuth, C.; Demmelmair, H.; Koletzko, B. Phospholipid species in newborn and 4 month old infants after consumption of different formulas or breast milk. *PLoS ONE* **2016**, *11*, e0162040. [CrossRef]
26. Iso, H.; Sato, S.; Folsom, A.R.; Shimamoto, T.; Terao, A.; Munger, R.G.; Kitamura, A.; Konishi, M.; Iida, M.; Komachi, Y. Serum fatty acids and fish intake in rural Japanese, urban Japanese, Japanese American and Caucasian American men. *Int. J. Epidemiol.* **1989**, *18*, 374–381. [CrossRef] [PubMed]

27. Urashima, M.; Mezawa, H.; Okuyama, M.; Urashima, T.; Hirano, D.; Gocho, N.; Tachimoto, H. Primary prevention of cow's milk sensitization and food allergy by avoiding supplementation with cow's milk formula at birth: A randomized clinical trial. *JAMA Pediatr.* **2019**, *173*, 1137–1145. [CrossRef] [PubMed]
28. Ozawa, A.; Takayanagi, K.; Fujita, T.; Hirai, A.; Hamazaki, T.; Terano, T.; Tamura, Y.; Kumagai, A. Determination of long chain fatty acids in human total plasma lipids using gas chromatography. *Bunseki Kagaku.* **1982**, *31*, 87–91. [CrossRef]
29. Schober, P.; Boer, C.; Schwarte, L.A. Correlation coefficients: Appropriate use and interpretation. *Anesth. Analg.* **2018**, *126*, 1763–1768. [CrossRef] [PubMed]
30. Brenna, J.T.; Varamini, B.; Jensen, R.G.; Diersen-Schade, D.A.; Boettcher, J.A.; Arterburn, L.M. Docosahexaenoic and arachidonic acid concentrations in human breast milk worldwide. *Am. J. Clin. Nutr.* **2007**, *85*, 1457–1464. [CrossRef]
31. Miliku, K.; Duan, Q.L.; Moraes, T.J.; Becker, A.B.; Mandhane, P.J.; Turvey, S.E.; Lefebvre, D.L.; Sears, M.R.; Subbarao, P.; Field, C.J.; et al. Human milk fatty acid composition is associated with dietary, genetic, sociodemographic, and environmental factors in the CHILD Cohort Study. *Am. J. Clin. Nutr.* **2019**, *110*, 1370–1383. [CrossRef] [PubMed]
32. Ueno, H.M.; Higurashi, S.; Shimomura, Y.; Wakui, R.; Matsuura, H.; Shiota, M.; Kubouchi, H.; Yamamura, J.I.; Toba, Y.; Kobayashi, T. Association of DHA concentration in human breast milk with maternal diet and use of supplements: A cross-sectional analysis of data from the Japanese human milk study cohort. *Curr. Dev. Nutr.* **2020**, *4*, nzaa105. [CrossRef] [PubMed]
33. Lohner, S.; Fekete, K.; Marosvolgyi, T.; Decsi, T. Gender differences in the long-chain polyunsaturated fatty acid status: Systematic review of 51 publications. *Ann. Nutr. Metab.* **2013**, *62*, 98–112. [CrossRef] [PubMed]
34. Decsi, T.; Kennedy, K. Sex-specific differences in essential fatty acid metabolism. *Am. J. Clin. Nutr.* **2011**, *94*, 1914S–1919S. [CrossRef] [PubMed]
35. Ordnung, M.; Mank, M.; Stahl, B.; Kurz, D.; Marosvolgyi, T.; Decsi, T.; Rothenbacher, D.; Genuneit, J.; Siziba, L.P. Potential sex differences in human milk fatty acids and their association with atopic dermatitis: Results of the Ulm SPATZ health study. *Pediatr. Allergy Immunol.* **2023**, *34*, e13992. [CrossRef] [PubMed]
36. Makrides, M.; Neumann, M.A.; Simmer, K.; Gibson, R.A. Erythrocyte fatty acids of term infants fed either breast milk, standard formula, or formula supplemented with long-chain polyunsaturates. *Lipids* **1995**, *30*, 941–948. [CrossRef] [PubMed]
37. Miller, M.R.; Seifert, J.; Szabo, N.J.; Clare-Salzler, M.; Rewers, M.; Norris, J.M. Erythrocyte membrane fatty acid content in infants consuming formulas supplemented with docosahexaenoic acid (DHA) and arachidonic acid (ARA): An observational study. *Matern. Child Nutr.* **2010**, *6*, 338–346. [CrossRef]
38. Ogunleye, A.; Fakoya, A.T.; Niizeki, S.; Tojo, H.; Sasajima, I.; Kobayashi, M.; Tateishi, S.; Yamaguchi, K. Fatty acid composition of breast milk from Nigerian and Japanese women. *J. Nutr. Sci. Vitaminol.* **1991**, *37*, 435–442. [CrossRef]
39. Yuhas, R.; Pramuk, K.; Lien, E.L. Human milk fatty acid composition from nine countries varies most in DHA. *Lipids* **2006**, *41*, 851–858. [CrossRef]
40. Wang, L.; Shimizu, Y.; Kaneko, S.; Hanaka, S.; Abe, T.; Shimasaki, H.; Hisaki, H.; Nakajima, H. Comparison of the fatty acid composition of total lipids and phospholipids in breast milk from Japanese women. *Pediatr. Int.* **2000**, *42*, 14–20. [CrossRef]
41. Katoku, Y.; Yamada, M.; Yonekubo, A.; Kuwata, T.; Kobayashi, A.; Sawa, A. Effect of the cholesterol content of a formula on the lipid compositions of plasma lipoproteins and red blood cell membranes in early infancy. *Am. J. Clin. Nutr.* **1996**, *64*, 871–877. [CrossRef]
42. Hadley, K.B.; Ryan, A.S.; Forsyth, S.; Gautier, S.; Salem, N., Jr. The essentiality of arachidonic acid in infant development. *Nutrients* **2016**, *8*, 216. [CrossRef]
43. Kawashima, H. Intake of arachidonic acid-containing lipids in adult humans: Dietary surveys and clinical trials. *Lipids Health Dis.* **2019**, *18*, 101. [CrossRef]
44. Crozier, S.R.; Godfrey, K.M.; Calder, P.C.; Robinson, S.M.; Inskip, H.M.; Baird, J.; Gale, C.R.; Cooper, C.; Sibbons, C.M.; Fisk, H.L.; et al. Vegetarian diet during pregnancy is not associated with poorer cognitive performance in children at age 6–7 years. *Nutrients* **2019**, *11*, 3029. [CrossRef]
45. De Caterina, R. n-3 fatty acids in cardiovascular disease. *N. Engl. J. Med.* **2011**, *364*, 2439–2450. [CrossRef] [PubMed]
46. Hoffman, D.R.; Wheaton, D.K.; James, K.J.; Tuazon, M.; Diersen-Schade, D.A.; Harris, C.L.; Stolz, S.; Berseth, C.L. Docosahexaenoic acid in red blood cells of term infants receiving two levels of long-chain polyunsaturated fatty acids. *J. Pediatr. Gastroenterol. Nutr.* **2006**, *42*, 287–292. [CrossRef]

nutrients

MDPI

Article

Validation of the Scale on Parental Feeding Behaviors (ECOPAL) for Caregivers of Mexican Children

Marina Liliana González-Torres [1,*], Xochitl Garza-Olivares [2], Gabriela Navarro-Contreras [3] and Lidia Alejandra González-Orozco [1]

1 Department of Psychology, Autonomous University of Aguascalientes, Aguascalientes 20100, Mexico; lidia.gonzalez@edu.uaa.mx
2 Department of Clinical and Health Psychology, Tecnológico de Monterrey, Monterrey 64849, Mexico; xochitl.garza@tec.mx
3 Department of Psychology, University of Guanajuato, Guanajuato 37670, Mexico; g.navarro@ugto.mx
* Correspondence: liliana.gonzalez@edu.uaa.mx

Abstract: Parental feeding practices can be crucial to preventing childhood obesity. This study aimed to validate a self-applicable instrument for evaluating the diverse parental feeding behaviors of Mexican caregivers based on the theoretical constructs of coercive control, structure, and autonomy support. The scale's content validity achieved significant values when assessed by expert judges, with moderate intensity in congruence (Kendall's W = 0.462; $p = 0.000$) and clarity (Kendall's W = 0.369; $p = 0.001$). The participants were 1185 Mexican adults (32.7 ± 7.6 years of age, 97% women, and 90% mothers) responsible for the main meal of at least one child (4.8 ± 3 years old). The data were subdivided randomly for an exploratory factor analysis ($n = 581$) and a confirmatory factorial analysis (n = 604). The first analysis grouped the items into 11 factors, with an accumulated variance of 63.9%. In the confirmatory analysis, a 10-factor model showed a better fit (CMIN = 1531.5, $p < 0.001$, CMIN/df = 2.20, RSEA = 0.045, CFI = 0.92, TLI, 0.91, and NFI = 0.87). The factors in this model were (1) the disposition of non-recommended foods, (2) nutritional education, (3) pressure to eat, (4) praise for healthy eating, (5) monitoring of consumption, (6) structured offer of fruits and vegetables, (7) consumption conditioning, (8) overt restriction, (9) guided choices, and (10) covert restriction. The Cronbach's alpha value was 0.816. Therefore, this scale presents good psychometric properties with which to evaluate the frequency of child caregivers' feeding behaviors in the context of ten different feeding practices in Mexico's urban areas and contributes to the knowledge of current practices in the Mexican population. It also evaluates changes resulting from future interventions that promote eating practices that favor the formation of healthy eating habits.

Keywords: parental feeding behaviors; healthy feeding; prevention; childhood obesity; upbringing

1. Introduction

Globally, at least one in three children under the age of five is malnourished or overweight [1]. In Mexico, both problems are present. However, childhood obesity has the most significant impact, as Mexico is considered a country with one of the highest worldwide rates of obesity [2], which has aroused a growing interest in the study of obesity. It has been noted that a fundamental step in the search for a means of preventing childhood obesity is the analysis of parental feeding practices [3,4], which are a set of behaviors and actions that parents carry out to influence the eating behavior of their children [5]. This definition can be applied to many behaviors carried out by parents, but there needs to be more clarity about its operationalization and its consequences on child eating behavior [6].

The results of some studies suggest practices that can be beneficial for the development of healthy eating habits by promoting autonomy, stimulating self-regulation and self-control, such as providing nutritional education, involving children in the selection of foods, diet, motivation, modeling, reasoning, and negotiation, among others [5–7]. However, it has been found that parents receive little guidance on how to contribute to the development of their children's feeding autonomy from an early age and how to manage the problems of feeding children, for example, knowing how to face a refusal to consume food [8].

The family context determines lifestyle development, including activity and eating patterns [3]. Recently, an observational study of Mexican caregiver–child interactions in a natural feeding context, in which parental feeding behaviors were operationalized from previous theoretical proposals [5,6], revealed that the adults offered low proportions of fruits and vegetables to the children during their meals, and that eating together with the child, praising the child's intake, and highlighting the properties of foods were highly probable behaviors to appear with the acceptance of food. Still, these behaviors were infrequent in the caregivers [9]. However, this observational study evaluated a few parents (n = 10), and evaluating a larger sample would be very costly. A questionnaire for assessing family eating practices is a valuable research tool for nutritionists, psychologists, nurses, and other specialists seeking to understand and promote healthy eating habits in children [10].

Current measures only assess select parental feeding practices and conceptualize these practices differently [10], and fewer culturally appropriate instruments exist for the Latina population. In Mexico, two instruments have been adapted for the study of parental feeding practices, both with good psychometric properties. The Child Feeding Questionnaire [11], adapted and validated for Mexico [12], presents a Cronbach's alpha of 0.858, which was validated in a sample of mothers of children between 5 and 12 years of age, and the Comprehensive Feeding Practices Questionnaire [13], adapted for Mexico [14], obtained a Cronbach's alpha > 0.60; its validation process also occurred in a sample of mothers, but they had preschool-age children. In addition, these adaptations only consider one of each child's caregivers: the mother. These questionnaires have not been applied to other caregivers such as grandmothers, parents, or other individuals responsible for feeding children.

Although there are instruments for measuring parental feeding practices that have been validated in the Mexican population, these include items that do not directly reference behaviors but rather attitudes and beliefs about infant feeding. For example, the Child Feeding Questionnaire [11,12] presents item 30, which says, "If I did not guide or regulate their feeding, my child would eat less than he/she should", and item 28, "I have to be especially careful to make sure my daughter eats enough", both of which refer to beliefs and not necessarily to actions. Similarly, the Comprehensive Feeding Practices Questionnaire [13,14] presents items such as item 46, which indicates, "I try to eat healthy foods in front of my child even though I will not be my favorites", and item 47, "I try to show enthusiasm about healthy foods", which refer to behaviors, but lack precision when evaluating the attempt and not the performance of the behavior. In the study of parental eating practices, it is imperative to establish which behaviors are carried out and at what frequency.

For its part, the HomeSTEAD survey [10], which consists of three subscales and 86 items, assesses 24 parental feeding practices based on the authors' proposed theoretical classification [5], i.e., coercive control, structure, and autonomy support practices; the latter two represent positive constructs that promote healthy eating behaviors in children. Each of the subscales of the instrument proposed by the authors shows an acceptable internal consistency (Cronbach's alpha > 0.62). However, the sample with which this instrument was validated comprised inhabitants of the United States of America. Recently, a Portuguese version of the HomeSTEAD family food practices survey was validated in a sample of parents of children aged 3–12 years old and proved an acceptable level of internal consistency (Cronbach's alpha > 0.61) [15]. At present, the survey has undergone no validation in the Spanish-speaking population.

In addition, several items in this survey have the same lack of precision with respect to specific behaviors; for instance, "My child learns to eat healthy snacks from me" is an affirmation that does not describe how the parent achieves the result. The following is another example: "How often do you plan your family's meals to provide a variety of food groups?" This question does not specifical ask how often the participant includes a variety of food groups in their family's meals.

Therefore, this work aimed to develop and validate a self-applicable instrument that evaluates the frequency with which caregivers of children between the ages of 1 and 11 perform parental eating behaviors that can describe parental feeding practices according to the classification in Table 1 [5]. The items developed in this instrument are not a translation of the HomeSTEAD survey, since they were written with a focus on defining the constructs based on Mexican culture, and care was taken to ensure that each item refers to specific, observable behaviors.

Table 1. The theoretical basis of the instrument.

Category	Construct	Items
Coercive control: parental pressure and the domination of the child's feelings, thoughts, and behaviors.	Restriction: the caregiver places strict limitations on access to food, usually to control the consumption of unhealthy foods.	7, 16, 17, 40, 51, 66, 71, 78, 80
	Pressure to eat: the caregiver insists, verbally or through physical force, that the child consume more food.	6, 23, 25, 26, 35, 59, 73
	Determinants of consumption: the caregiver offers food that the child likes to encourage consumption or promises to carry out an activity in exchange for consuming a specific food.	13, 21, 33, 58, 69, 77
Structure in feeding: how the parents organize the environment to facilitate the development of skills in the child.	Food availability: the variety of foods the caregiver offers and has available for the child's consumption.	2, 15, 38, 42, 45, 47, 50, 54, 67, 69, 76, 79
	Modeling: the caregiver purposely shows their eating habits to encourage similar behaviors in the child or involuntarily displays unhealthy food consumption in front of the child.	8, 18, 19, 30, 37, 61, 65, 72
	Eating habits: the caregiver creates a consistent routine that is implemented during feeding time, considering the location, time, and presence of family members.	3, 9, 14, 39, 43, 44, 75
	Unstructured practices: the caregiver allows the child to have complete control during the feeding period, including the timing, frequency, and type of food.	10, 20, 34, 48, 52
	Guided choices: the caregiver allows the child to choose what to consume among options proposed by the caregiver.	12, 27, 36, 55
	Monitoring feeding: the caregiver actively tracks what and how much the child is eating, ensuring that the child eats enough healthy food and avoids unhealthy food.	22, 24, 46, 56, 57
Support and autonomy: allowing the child, according to their age, to make choices, allowing them to self-regulate in the future without their parents.	Motivation for food consumption and interaction: the caregiver praises the child for consuming new or healthy food.	5, 11, 32, 70
	Nutritional education and reasoning: the caregiver explains the nutritional qualities of food, the benefits of eating healthy foods, and the consequences of eating unhealthy foods.	28, 62, 64, 74

Table 1. *Cont.*

Category	Construct	Items
	The involvement of the child in eating: the caregiver actively includes the child in the choice of food when buying and preparing food, allows them to interact with the food, and is interested in knowing the child's perception of the food. Food for consumption.	1, 31, 49, 53, 63, 68
	Negotiation: the caregiver engages the child in reaching an acceptable compromise about what and how much the child will eat.	4, 29, 41

Note: operational definitions were based on Vaughn and colleagues, 2016 [5] and translated into Spanish in Mexico in 2018 [6].

2. Materials and Methods

The scale construction and validation process followed the steps shown in the diagram in Figure 1.

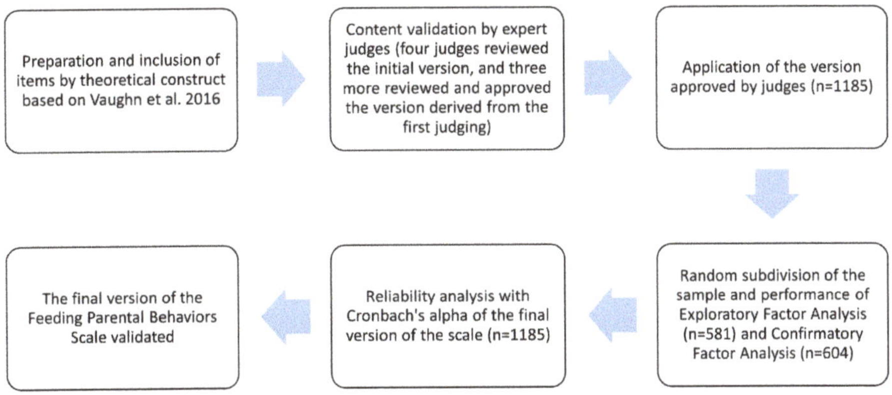

Figure 1. Diagram of the process of validating the Scale of Parental Feeding Behaviors.

2.1. *The Development of the Scale on Parental Feeding Behavior*

The objective of this instrument is to evaluate the weekly frequency with which caregivers utilize behavioral strategies when feeding children between 1 and 11 years of age. The items were developed by three experts (bilingual psychologists), considering the constructs [5] shown in Table 1. The operational definitions allowed the constructs to be included as instrument dimensions.

2.2. *Content Validation by Expert Judges*

The content validation method [16] provided an instrument for measuring the judges' verdicts on the items and the stages in the content validation process.

The experts were selected according to their knowledge and experience concerning parental feeding practices (two psychologists), psychometry (one psychologist), or both (two psychologists and one nurse). All are postgraduates in their fields (five Ph.D. degrees and one Master's degree). The six expert judges are from different states in the country's north, center, and south (Aguascalientes, Guanajuato, Jalisco, Nuevo León, and Veracruz).

In the first stage, four judges evaluated each item of the first version of the instrument in terms of its congruence (whether the item has a logical relationship with the dimension or indicator that measures) and clarity (whether the item is easily understood; if its syntax and semantics are adequate) on a scale from 1 to 4, according to a widely used instrument [16]. The mode and median of each item were obtained for the judges' evaluations, and the agreement between judges was calculated via Kendall's W to validate the content of the congruence criteria (Kendall's W = 0.462, X2= 118.24, and p = 0.000) and clarity (Kendall's W = 0.369, X2 = 94.518, and p = 0.008. Likewise, the judges were asked to provide comments, observations, or suggestions for each item's correction. Items that obtained a median score equal to or less than 3.5 were corrected, considering all of the judges' observations. In the second stage, the updated version was sent to three final expert judges (psychologist researchers with Ph.D. degrees in parental feeding practices and with experience in psychometry) who agreed to approve the final version, which contained 80 items.

The cultural adequacy of the instrument was assessed in a field test, as recommended by the literature [17], with 13 Mexican mothers of children 1–5 years of age. These participants indicated that the items were clear and understandable.

2.3. *The Application and Validation of the Instrument*

2.3.1. Participants

The participants comprised 1185 Mexican adults responsible for the main meal of at least one child in Mexico's urban zone. The participants were identified through non-probabilistic sampling via the initial dissemination of the publication in an essential educational institution, in addition to its promotion on social networks in November 2022, taking into account the following considerations about the public to which it was directed: men and women between 18 and 65 years of age from Mexico's urban areas, with children between 1 and 12 years of age, with interests in parenting, paternity, maternity, and fitness. In total, 1210 caregivers provided answers to the scale via a digital form, but we eliminated data from 25 caregivers with children whose ages fell outside of the age range. The final sample was subdivided into two random subsamples for the EFA (n = 581) and CFA (n = 604).

2.3.2. Materials and Instruments

Each participating caregiver provided their digital informed consent. The scale, which comprised 80 items regarding the frequency of parental behaviors exhibited while feeding a child in the last week, was distributed via Google Forms. The participants' response options were never (1), a few times (2), sometimes (3), many times (4), and always (5).

2.3.3. Data Analysis

Skewness and kurtosis values were used to analyze the normality assumption for each item's distribution. We excluded items with high skewness values and kurtosis > $|1.5|$. We confirmed the adequacy of the sampling using the Kaiser–Meyer–Olkin (KMO) measure ($\geq$0.6), and the factorability of the data was confirmed using Bartlett's test of sphericity ($p < 0.05$). We performed an exploratory factor analysis (EFA), according to recommendations [18,19], using the maximum likelihood extraction method and Kaiser's Oblimin rotation to study the scale's psychometric properties via SPSS v. 29. Modeling was carried out by eliminating the items with a factorial weight of less than 0.350 or those with a weight greater than 0.300 for more than one factor. A confirmatory factorial analysis (CFA) was then performed using AMOS v.29. For reliability, Cronbach's alpha value was calculated for the final version of the scale (40 items), and McDonald's omega value was calculated for each dimension.

3. Results

3.1. *Participants*

The caregivers were 32.7 (7.6) years old, with a mean BMI of 26.9 (9.3). Among the participants, 52.7% reported answering the scale while thinking about their behaviors when feeding a girl, while the rest did so while thinking about feeding a boy. The child's age was 4.8 (3) years. According to the regionalization reported in the Encuesta Nacional de

Salud y Nutrición, 35.4% of participants lived in the urban areas of the western region, 30.9% lived in the northern part, 24.5% lived in the central region, and 9.2% lived in the southern region [20]. Finally, 97% of the participants were women, 2.4% were men, and 0.6% preferred not to indicate their gender; 89.9% were mothers, 2.6% were fathers, 2.5% were aunts, 1.9% were grandparents, 0.6% were cousins, and 2.2% were unrelated to the child. Table 2 presents the economic income ranges and academic levels of the participants.

Table 2. Economic income ranges and academic levels of the participants.

	Elementary *f*	High School *f*	College *f*	Postgraduate *f*
MXN 4999 or less	36 (36%)	49 (17%)	29 (5%)	5 (3%)
MXN 5000 to MXN 9999	35 (35%)	109 (37%)	158 (27%)	10 (5%)
MXN 10,000 to MXN 14,999	10 (10%)	64 (22%)	132 (22%)	32 (16%)
MXN 15,000 to MXN 19,999	3 (3%)	29 (10%)	77 (13%)	26 (13%)
MXN 20,000 to MXN 24,999	2 (2%)	11 (4%)	55 (9%)	34 (17%)
MXN 25,000 to MXN 29,999	2 (2%)	2 (1%)	31 (5%)	29 (15%)
MXN 30,000 or more	1 (1%)	7 (7%)	42 (22%)	43 (22%)
I prefer not to answer	10 (10%)	24 (8%)	68 (11%)	20 (10%)

Note: Incomes are provided by month in Mexican pesos. n = 1185, *f* = Frecuencia.

3.2. Exploratory Factorial Analysis

The KMO (0.892) value and Bartlett's test of sphericity (X2 = 13,141.025, df = 1176, p = 0.000) indicated an adequate sample and the utility of the factorial analysis. The items were grouped into 11 factors in the EFA, which explained 63.9% of the accumulated variance.

As shown in Table 3, the eleven factors obtained from the rotation, given its coincidence with the theoretical construct, were named as follows: (1) disposition of non-recommended foods (DNR), (2) nutritional education (EN), (3) pressure to eat (P), (4) praise for healthy eating (El), (5) meal times (MT), (6) monitoring of consumption (Mn), (7) structured offer of fruits and vegetables (OFV), (8) consumption conditioning (Co), (9) overt restriction (RO), (10) guided choices (EG), and (11) covert restriction (RC). This version of the instrument comprised 49 items.

Table 3. Factorial rotation matrix of the EFA items and internal consistency with Cronbach's alpha and McDonald's omega.

Factor Names and Items in Spanish and English	DNR	EN	P	EI	MT	Mn	OFV	Co	RO	EG	RC
Disposición de alimentos no recomendables (DNR). ***Disposition of non-recommended foods.***	α = 0.847	**ω = 0.845**									
40. Ofrezco al niño(a), botanas, dulces, postres o cereales endulzados (por ejemplo: Zucaritas, Froot Loops, papas fritas, dulces, frituras, caramelos, chocolates, galletas, pastelitos, etc.). *I offer the child snacks, sweets, desserts, or sweetened cereals.*	−0.764										
47. Ofrezco al niño(a) alimentos procesados y comida rápida (por ejemplo: alimentos enlatados, embutidos como salchicha o jamón, hamburguesas, pizza, pollo frito, etc.). *I offer the child processed foods and fast food.*	−0.661										
39. Le doy al niño(a) botanas, dulces o postres a media mañana y media tarde. *I give the child snacks, sweets, or desserts in the mid-morning and mid-afternoon.*	−0.575										
45. Ofrezco al niño(a) bebidas endulzadas procesadas (por ejemplo: jugos procesados, refrescos, bebidas lácteas endulzadas como yogurt, Danonino, Yakult, etc.). *I offer the child processed sweetened beverages.*	−0.523										
72. Muestro mi agrado al comer botanas, dulces, postres o cereales endulzados, antojitos mexicanos o alimentos procesados frente al niño(a). *I show my pleasure by eating snacks, sweets, sweetened desserts or cereals, Mexican fried food, or processed foods in front of the child.*	−0.482										
* 37. Consumo frente al niño(a) botanas, dulces o postres, antojitos mexicanos o comida procesada (por ejemplo: papitas, dulces, chocolates, galletas, pastelitos, sopes, etc.). *I eat snacks, sweets or desserts, Mexican fried foods, or processed food in front of the child.*	−0.449										
Educación Nutricional (EN). ***Nutritional education.***				α = 0.856					ω = 0.869		
64. Cuando el niño(a) rechaza un alimento le digo los beneficios de consumirlo. *When the child rejects a food, I tell him/her the benefits of consuming it.*		0.822									
62. Le digo al niño(a) de los beneficios de consumir alimentos como frutas y verduras de forma cotidiana. *I tell the child about the benefits of consuming foods such as fruits and vegetables daily*		0.802									

Table 3. *Cont.*

Factor Names and Items in Spanish and English	DNR	EN	P	El	MT	Mn	OFV	Co	RO	EG	RC
28. Le digo al niño(a) las propiedades nutricionales de los alimentos que le ofrezco. *I tell the child about the nutritional properties of the food that I offer*		0.696									
74. Le digo al niño(a) de los efectos que tienen alimentos como botanas, dulces o postres si se consumieran de forma cotidiana. *I tell the child about the effects of foods such as snacks, sweets or desserts if consumed daily.*		0.663									
* 63. Involucro al niño(a) en la preparación de los alimentos. *I involve the child in the preparation of food.*		0.413									
Presión para comer (P). ***Pressure to eat.***			α = 0.818				**ω = 0.828**				
25. Durante la comida le insisto al niño(a) para que siga comiendo a pesar de que diga que ya está lleno. *During the meal, I insist that the child continue to eat even if he/she says he/she is full.*			0.745								
59. Le insisto al niño(a) para que se coma todo lo que le sirvo en cada comida. *I insist that the child eat everything I serve him/her at each meal.*			0.674								
26. Le insisto al niño(a) que se termine un alimento o porción específica de lo que le sirvo en cada comida. *I urge the child to finish a specific food or portion that I serve at each meal.*			0.667								
* 35. Insisto al niño(a) a que siga comiendo introduciendo alimento en su boca. *I urge the child to continue eating by introducing food into his/her mouth.*			0.554								
22. Permito que el niño(a) deje de comer cuando dice que ya está lleno (R). *I allow the child to stop eating when he/she says he/she is full (R).*			0.463								
73. Le digo al niño(a) que la comida no se desperdicia por lo que se la tiene que acabar. *I tell the child that food is not wasted, so he/she must finish it.*			0.388								
Elogios ante alimentación saludable (El). ***Praise for healthy eating.***		α = 0.857			ω = 0.861						
70. Felicito o elogio al niño(a) cuando prueba un nuevo alimento. *I congratulate or praise the child when trying a new food.*				0.927							

Table 3. *Cont.*

Factor Names and Items in Spanish and English	DNR	EN	P	El	MT	Mn	OFV	Co	RO	EG	RC
32. Felicito o elogio al niño(a) por haber probado un alimento que había rechazado. *I congratulate or praise the child for tasting a food that he/she had rejected.*				0.817							
5. Felicito o elogio al niño(a) cuando come alimentos como frutas o verduras. *I congratulate or praise the child when he/she eats fruits or vegetables.*				0.642							
Horarios de comida desestructurados (MT). ***Meal times.***		α = 0.684		ω = 0.746							
* 34. El niño(a) no tiene horario de comida y puede comer cuando quiera. *The child does not have a meal schedule, he/she can eat whenever he/she wants.*					0.858						
* 44. El niño(a) tiene horarios establecidos para cada una de las comidas del día(R). *The child has established times for each of the meals of the day(R)*					0.566						
* 20. Permito que el niño(a) decida cuándo quiere comer. *I allow the child to decide when he/she wants to eat.*					0.545						
Monitoreo del consumo (Mn). ***Monitoring of consumption***		α = 0.795		ω = 0.787							
56. Llevo la cuenta de las botanas, dulces y postres que consume el niño(a) durante el día (por ejemplo: Zucaritas, Froot Loops, papas fritas, dulces, frituras, caramelos, chocolates, galletas, pastelitos, etc.) *I keep track of the snacks, sweets and desserts that the child consumes during the day.*						0.841					
24. Llevo la cuenta de las bebidas endulzadas que toma el niño(a) durante el día (por ejemplo: jugos de fruta natural, jugos procesados, aguas frescas, refrescos, bebidas lácteas endulzadas como yogurt, Danonino, Yakult, etc.) *I keep track of the sweetened drinks the child drinks during the day*						0.686					
57. Llevo la cuenta de las frutas y verduras que come el niño(a) durante el día. *I keep track of the fruits and vegetables that the child eats during the day*						0.552					

Table 3. *Cont.*

Factor Names and Items in Spanish and English	DNR	EN	P	El	MT	Mn	OFV	Co	RO	EG	RC
46. Llevo la cuenta de la cantidad de agua natural que bebe el niño(a) durante el día. *I keep track of the amount of natural water the child drinks during the day*						0.393					
Oferta estructurada de Frutas y Verduras (OFV). ***Structured offer of fruits and vegetables***		α = 0.729			ω = 0.733						
43. Le doy al niño(a) frutas o verduras a media mañana y media tarde. *I give the child fruits or vegetables in the mid-morning and mid-afternoon*							0.837				
9. Le doy al niño(a) algún alimento de colación a media mañana y media tarde. *I give the child some snack food in the mid-morning and mid-afternoon*							0.658				
50. Ofrezco al niño(a) diferentes frutas o verduras en cada comida. *I offer the child different fruits or vegetables at each meal.*							0.513				
Restricción abierta o manifiesta (RO). ***Overt restriction.***			α = 0.785				ω = 0.786				
78. Le niego el consumo de comidas preparadas con aceite como antojitos mexicanos (por ejemplo: sopes, enchiladas, flautas, etc.). *I deny the intake of foods prepared with oil, such as Mexican fried food.*								0.870			
* 30. Evito tener al alcance del niño(a) antojitos mexicanos (por ejemplo: sopes, enchiladas, flautas, etc.). *I avoid having Mexican fried food within the reach of the child.*								0.605			
* 54. Ofrezco al niño(a) antojitos mexicanos (por ejemplo: sopes, enchiladas, flautas, etc.)(R) *I offer the child Mexican fried food.*								0.572			
51. Le niego el consumo de botanas, dulces, postres o cereales endulzados al niño(a) (por ejemplo: Zucaritas, Choco Krispis, papas fritas, frituras, dulces, chocolates, galletas, pastelitos, etc.). *I deny the intake of snacks, sweets, desserts or sweetened cereals to the child.*								0.417			
17. Le niego el consumo de alimentos procesados y comida rápida (por ejemplo: alimentos enlatados, embutidos como salchicha o jamón, hamburguesas, etc.). *I deny the intake of processed foods and fast food to the child.*								0.406			

Table 3. *Cont.*

Factor Names and Items in Spanish and English	DNR	EN	P	El	MT	Mn	OFV	Co	RO	EG	RC
Condicionamiento del consumo de alimentos (Co). ***Consumption conditioning.***			$\alpha = 0.828$				$\omega = 0.831$				
58. Cuando el niño(a) rechaza un alimento le digo que realizará alguna actividad a cambio de terminarse el alimento (por ejemplo: ver televisión, salir al parque, jugar videojuegos). *When the child rejects a food, I tell him/her that he/she will do some activity in exchange for finishing the food.*									0.725		
23. Le digo al niño(a) que termine todo lo que está en su plato a cambio de permitirle hacer cosas que le gustan (por ejemplo: ver TV, salir a jugar, etc.). *I tell the child to finish everything on his plate in exchange for allowing him to do things he likes.*									0.694		
33. Le digo al niño(a) que si se porta bien le daré un alimento de su agrado. *I tell the child that if he behaves well I will give him/her a food he likes.*									0.680		
* 13. Le ofrezco al niño(a) algún alimento de su agrado para celebrar algo que logró con éxito. *I offer the child some food they like to celebrate something they have successfully achieved.*									0.513		
60. Cuando el niño(a) rechaza un alimento le ofrezco otro de su agrado con la condición de que consuma el que rechazó. *When the child rejects a food, I offer him/her another to his/her liking on the condition that he eats the one he refused.*									0.432		
Elecciones Guiadas (EG). ***Guided choices.***			$\boldsymbol{\alpha = 0.742}$				$\boldsymbol{\omega = 0.743}$				
55. Le sirvo al niño(a) dos o más opciones del mismo grupo de alimentos para que al menos coma uno de ellos. *I serve the child two or more options from the same food group so that they eat at least one of them.*										0.732	
36. Cuando el niño(a) rechaza un alimento le ofrezco otro del mismo grupo de alimentos. *When the child rejects a food, I offer another from the same food group.*										0.554	
27. Pongo al centro de la mesa dos o más opciones del mismo grupo de alimentos para que el niño(a) coma lo que prefiera. *I put two or more options from the same food group in the center of the table so that the child can eat what he/she prefers.*										0.554	

Table 3. *Cont.*

Factor Names and Items in Spanish and English	DNR	EN	P	El	MT	Mn	OFV	Co	RO	EG	RC
12. Le muestro al niño(a) dos o más opciones del mismo grupo de alimento y le pregunto cuál prefiere comer. *I show the child two or more options from the same food group and ask him/her which he/she prefers to eat,*										0.504	
Restricción encubierta (RC). ***Covert restriction.***		$\alpha = 0.829$			$\omega = 0.831$						
2. Evito llevar a casa bebidas que considero no recomendables para consumo diario. *I avoid taking home drinks that I consider not recommended for daily consumption.*											0.552
16. Evito tener al alcance del niño(a) botanas, dulces, postres o cereales endulzados (por ejemplo, papitas, frituras, dulces, chocolates, galletas, pastelitos, etc.). *I avoid having snacks, sweets, desserts, or sweetened cereals within the child's reach.*											0.567
7. Evito tener al alcance del niño(a) alimentos procesados y comida rápida (por ejemplo: alimentos enlatados, embutidos como salchicha o jamón, hamburguesas, etc.). *I avoid having processed foods and fast food within the child's reach.*											0.500
66. Evito tener al alcance del niño(a) bebidas endulzadas procesadas (por ejemplo: jugos y néctares procesados, refrescos, bebidas lácteas endulzadas como yogurt, Danonino, Yakult, etc.). *I avoid having processed sweetened beverages within the child's reach.*											0.472
76. Evito llevar a casa alimentos que considero no recomendables para el consumo diario. *I avoid taking home foods that I consider not recommended for daily consumption*											0.432
Global						$\alpha = 0.795$					

Note: The extraction method was the maximum likelihood. The rotation method was Oblimin with Kaiser normalization. The factors are the result of the EFA. Items with * were eliminated for the final version of the instrument according to the confirmatory factor analysis, thus revealing better adjustment and better psychometric properties. The reliability of the total scale with 40 items was $\alpha = 0.816$.

3.3. Confirmatory Factor Analysis

Different models were used for the CFA, as indicated in Table 4. The proposal with ten factors and 40 items showed the best properties and fit (CMIN = 1531.5, $p < 0.001$, CMIN/df = 2.20, RSEA = 0.045, CFI = 0.92, TLI, 0.91, and NFI = 0.87). Among the eleven items that showed a weight of less than 0.490 were those belonging to the meal time (MT) factor, so this factor was eliminated in the final version of the instrument.

Table 4. Comparison of values of each confirmatory factor analysis model.

Models	Chi-Square	*p*	Chi-Normed Square	Root Mean Square Error of Approximation (RMSEA)	Comparative Fit Index (CFI)	Non-Normalized Index of Fit (NNFI o TLI)	Normalized Fit Index (NFI)	Parsimonious Comparative Fit (PCFI)	Parsimonious Normed Fit (PNFI)	Akaike's Information Criterion (AIC)
Expected		>0.05	<3/5	<0.05/0.08	0.9–1	0.9–1	0.9–1	0.9–1	Close to 1	Close to 0
11 factors and 49 items	2672.22	0	2.49	0.05	0.871	0.862	0.815	0.769	0.713	2897.89
10 factors and 40 items	1531.5	0	2.204	0.045	0.924	0.915	0.871	0.824	0.776	1861.53

Regarding the correlations between the ten factors, as shown in Figure 2, correlations were high among the factors of coercive control, specifically the correlation of the practice disposition of non-recommended foods (DNR) with overt (RO, −0.736) and covert restriction (RC, −0.791), as well as pressure to eat (P, 0.402) and the consumption conditioning (Co, 0.49). P correlated with Co (0.65). Factors of RC were correlated with RO (0.795) and negatively correlated with Co (−0.32). There were also correlations between the positive practices of autonomy or structure, specifically monitoring (Mn) with the structured offer of fruits and vegetables (OFV, 0.56), as well as with nutritional education (EN, 0.43) and guided choices (EG, 0.41). The EG correlated with OFV (0.48) and EN (0.33). The EN correlated with OFV (0.36) and praise behaviors (El, 0.41). In addition, positive correlations were observed between the practice of CR with OFV (0.61), with Mn (0.49), and with EG (0.32). The behaviors of RA correlated with Mn (0.41), OFV (0.44), and with EG (0.3). The practice of Co correlated with El (0.36). The practice of DNR was negatively correlated with Mn (−0.31), with OFV (−0.45), and with CR (−0.79).

3.4. Consistency Analysis

The final version with 40 items obtained a Cronbach's alpha value of 0.816, and a single-item consistency analysis showed a Cronbach's alpha greater than 0.8 in all cases (Table 5), indicating a reliable instrument. In addition, McDonald's omega was acceptable for each dimension (>0.7) (see Table 3).

Table 5. Consistency analysis, subtracting the unique elements.

	Mean Scale If the Element Has Been Suppressed	Scale Variance If the Element Has Been Suppressed	Total Item Correlation Corrected	Cronbach's Alpha If the Item Has Been Deleted
item_76	114.5620	257.111	0.294	0.812
item_66	114.6616	257.923	0.214	0.815
item_16	114.7806	258.856	0.198	0.815
item_7	114.8633	257.064	0.249	0.814
item_2	114.7865	256.700	0.255	0.813
item_27	115.9544	256.564	0.277	0.813

Table 5. *Cont.*

	Mean Scale If the Element Has Been Suppressed	Scale Variance If the Element Has Been Suppressed	Total Item Correlation Corrected	Cronbach's Alpha If the Item Has Been Deleted
item_12	115.4869	253.568	0.340	0.811
item_36	115.6481	255.541	0.309	0.812
item_55	115.6422	255.103	0.352	0.811
item_60	116.2844	255.580	0.329	0.811
item_23	116.1688	255.830	0.272	0.813
item_33	116.1426	257.658	0.227	0.814
item_58	116.3131	254.046	0.341	0.811
item_51	115.2641	258.632	0.199	0.815
item_17	115.2751	257.642	0.246	0.814
item_50	114.5308	254.835	0.351	0.811
item_78	115.5249	258.905	0.184	0.816
item_9	114.6101	257.103	0.265	0.813
item_43	114.4464	256.806	0.308	0.812
item_46	115.1139	247.142	0.406	0.808
item_57	114.9468	245.550	0.469	0.806
item_56	114.7511	245.739	0.431	0.807
item_24	114.7013	249.301	0.333	0.811
item_32	114.5316	248.908	0.424	0.808
item_5	114.6034	249.701	0.375	0.809
item_70	114.5080	246.946	0.470	0.806
item_73	115.9004	255.007	0.261	0.813
item_22	116.5595	263.691	0.093	0.817
item_25	116.5063	259.929	0.216	0.814
item_26	115.7418	254.661	0.299	0.812
item_59	115.7932	253.549	0.315	0.812
item_74	114.7806	245.759	0.470	0.806
item_28	115.3823	243.539	0.508	0.804
item_62	114.4481	245.822	0.486	0.806
item_64	115.0093	241.947	0.574	0.802
item_72	115.6810	269.412	−0.089	0.822
item_45	116.0700	270.036	−0.113	0.822
item_39	116.2692	267.771	−0.036	0.820
item_47	116.0219	270.445	−0.135	0.822
item_40	115.9443	268.786	−0.071	0.821

Note: the global Cronbach's alpha value is 0.816.

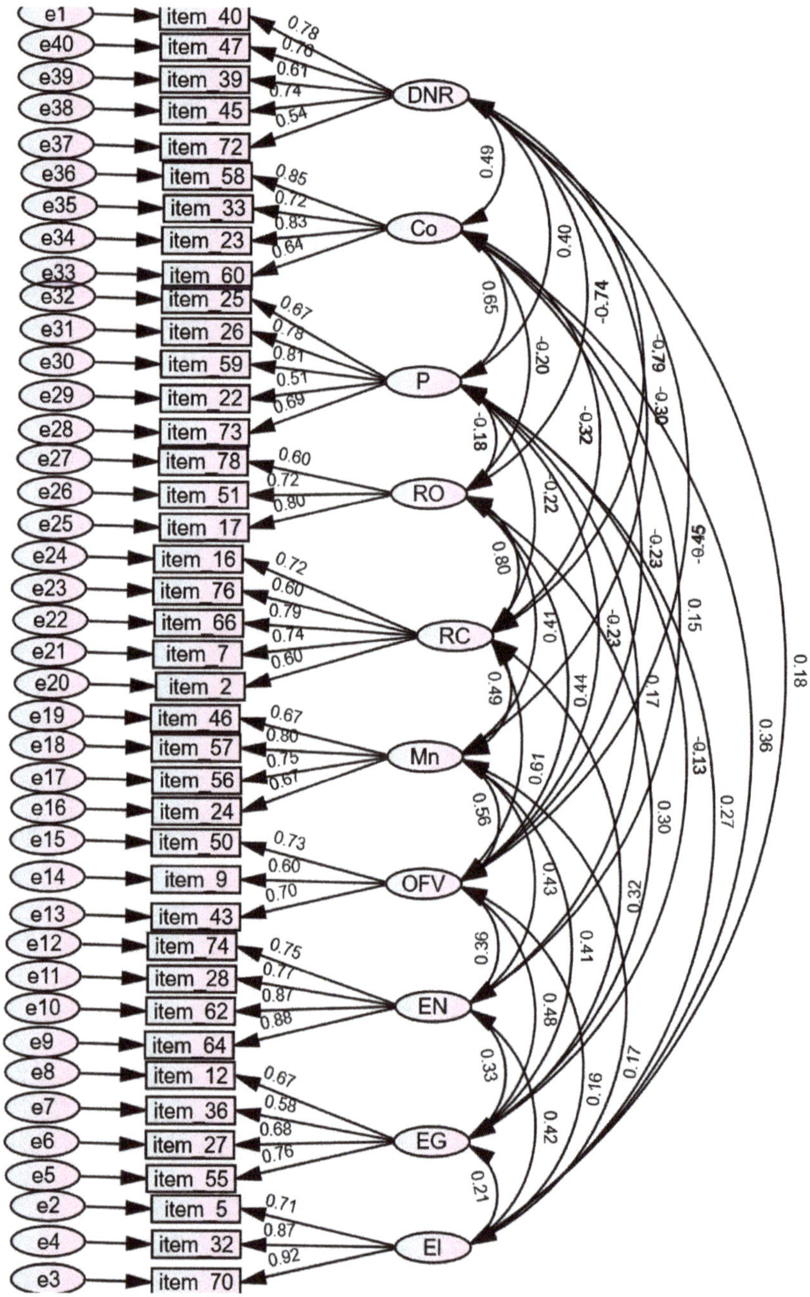

Figure 2. Confirmatory factor analysis diagram of the final model with ten factors and 40 items. Note: DNR = disposition of non-recommended foods; RO = overt restriction; RC =covert restriction; P = pressure to eat; Co = consumption conditioning; Mn = monitoring; OFV = structured offer of fruits and vegetables; EN = nutritional education; EG = guided choices; El = praise for healthy eating.

4. Discussion

The present work provides evidence of the construct validity and internal consistency of the self-applicable Scale on Parental Feeding Behaviors (ECOPAL). For this reason, it is considered suitable for evaluating the frequency with which caregivers or adults responsible for feeding children between 1 and 12 years of age perform positive and negative parental eating behaviors to promote healthy eating. The scale's internal consistency was analyzed, and evidence of its construct validity was provided. Similarly, the scale provides empirical evidence of the theoretical basis [6] with respect to the classification of parental feeding practices. The results were compared with the results of two other instruments with the same theoretical basis, the HomeSTEAD family food practices survey [10,15], which does not have a Spanish version, and the Comprehensive Feeding Practices Questionnaire in Spanish to Mexican Mothers [14], which changes the original construct of parental feeding practices to include attitudes and beliefs towards food.

The dimensions of the ECOPAL scale showed adequate consistency (>0.68); some were better than the original version of the HomeSTEAD survey (>0.62) and its Portuguese version (>0.61). Although the ECOPAL questionnaire evaluates fewer practices than the three subscales of the HomeSTEAD survey, it can determine them globally and comprehensively on the same scale. It can account for the frequency of behaviors of each practice and provide information regarding their relative frequency to other practices.

Compared with the Comprehensive Feeding Practices Questionnaire for Mexican Mothers (CIPA) [14], ECOPAL presented better consistency of global scale ($\alpha = 0.64$ vs. $\alpha = 0.816$, respectively). The CIPA remained the modeling's dimension with high consistency ($\alpha = 0.965$) but with items that evaluate beliefs on modeling more than actions.

The instrument resulting from the psychometric validation process shows adequate construct validity, since it presents nine of the thirteen theoretical constructs, namely restriction (overt and covert); pressure to eat; the consumption conditioning; food disposal (not recommended and fruits and vegetables); guided choices; unstructured practices (meal times); intake monitoring; nutritional education; and motivation for healthy eating (praise). In addition, some components were grouped by the type of food they offer, such as the structured offer of fruits and vegetables (OFV) and the disposition of non-recommended foods (DNR). This finding is particularly relevant because it accounts for the practice of food availability and is part of the structure construct [5].

The MT factor, which refers to a lack of structure at meal times, is obtained via the EFA. These items can account for unstructured eating practices. However, the MT factor was not maintained in the CFA; it is considered theoretically relevant, since meal times and accompanying the child and sharing food are indicated as part of the modeling climate for children's eating behaviors [21].

The constructs not maintained in the instrument from the EFA were modeling, eating habits, the involvement of the child in eating, and negotiation. It should be noted that these practices belong to categories of structure and autonomy support. Five items that presented significant biases were lost from the beginning, as evidenced by high kurtosis and asymmetry values (>1.5); these were structure practices such as modeling and eating habits. The values could have occurred since caregivers reported having performed these behaviors with extreme scores, such as never or always. The negotiation construct disappeared due to the low communality (<0.3) presented by the items from the extraction method and was affected by having only included three items in this factor since its creation. Reviewing the wording and including more items in future applications to evaluate this parental practice would be convenient. Although a minimum of three or four items per factor is recommended [22], if there is a minimum of 200 cases, which this study fulfills, having 581 cases for the EFA, current recommendations indicate that the more items there are that accurately measure a factor, the more determined this factor will be and the more stable the factorial solution will be [19]. Finally, the items regarding the child's involvement in feeding were lost for two reasons: two items had saturations lower than 0.3, and the rest presented saturations > 0.3 with more than one factor, which was shared with the nutritional education factor and with consumption motivation. After considering the reviewed literature regarding recommendations for conducting an exploratory factor analysis [19,22], these items were eliminated, and a detailed assessment is required to determine whether their modification is recommended for their inclusion in a new version of the scale [19], or if it is necessary to add new items with similar content to adequately sample the content of the factor [18].

Of the factors resulting from the EFA and CFA, four of these report parental feeding practices associated with the formation of unhealthy eating habits; these are the disposal of non-recommended foods (DNR), the pressure to eat (P), consumption conditioning (Co), and overt restriction (RO), which are considered coercive control practices. On the other hand, the factors associated with the promotion of healthy eating habits are those practices that support autonomy, in this case, nutritional education (EN), praise for healthy eating (El), guided choices (EG), and those relating to structure, namely the structured offer of fruits and vegetables (OFV), monitoring of consumption(Mn), and covert restriction (CR). This classification is based on the reviewed literature [5,9,21] and is supported by the correlations found in the CFA.

The correlations shown by the CFA strengthen the categorization of the practices of open or manifest restriction, the conditioning of consumption, and the pressure to eat as coercive control, since they had positive and high correlations between them but negative correlations with other practices, while the practices of monitoring, the structured offer of fruits and vegetables, nutritional education, praising healthy eating, and guided choices had positive correlations between them and negative correlations with the practices of coercive control, thus strengthening their categorization as practices of autonomy support and structure that, unlike the coercive practices, have been associated in the literature with the formation of healthy eating habits. The disposition of non-recommended foods practice had negative correlations with the structure practices; likewise,: monitoring and the offering of fruits and vegetables had correlations with the practices of overt and covert restriction, but did not correlate with behaviors supporting autonomy, inferring the confusing role that caregivers bringing these foods home can play in promoting healthy eating in children. Regarding covert restriction, positive correlations were obtained with structure practices, such as monitoring and offering fruits and vegetables, and with autonomy support practices, such as guided choices, in addition to a negative correlation with the practice of the disposition of non-recommended food. The preceding result could suggest that this practice, when related to the limited availability of foods not recommended for daily consumption, is considered a practice of structure rather than coercive control, an aspect already discussed in the literature [5,9].

The limitations of this study are the same as those linked to the self-report questionnaires, such as the effects of memory bias or social desire [23], which were taken care of with a frequency scale made explicit in the instructions to consider the events of the last week. Regarding social desirability, care was taken to present the items randomly and to use some reversible ones. However, in the factorial analysis, some of these elements were eliminated. Some authors recently indicated that inverse items could contribute more to confusion than to verifying answers, evidencing that these items required adjustments to the method [24].

Some limitations of this study may be related to the process of selecting samples from social networks, because we considered filters such as having an interest in paternity issues, which represents a bias in the representation of Mexican caregivers, since there may be a significant number of them who do not search for parenting issues on social networks; this might explain the high academic level or low economic level of the sample, which are other possible biases.

Another limitation of this study was the loss of items that evaluated modeling, which is a practice of great interest; a review of the wording of these items is necessary to reduce the response bias of never or always, and conducting a future factorial analysis with them is necessary to be able to include the evaluation of this practice.

Finally, the application of this scale occurred online. Although it is undeniable that this has advantages, such as the possibility of reaching a global population, achieving very large sample sizes, the flexibility of the survey design, the speed and timeliness of administration, and ability to force response completion [25], it is also true that it presents drawbacks. Some prominent factors are the inability to provide clear, one-on-one instructions to respondents, inherent sampling biases, a self-selection bias, variability among respondents in their ability to access the survey due to device limitations, and connectivity issues, among others (for reviews, see [25]).

5. Conclusions

Based on the results previously described and discussed, it is concluded that the instrument presented herein, the Scale on Parental Feeding Behavior (ECOPAL), which contains 40 items in its final version, has adequate internal consistency indexes and shows evidence of construct validity. We consider it adequate and useful for evaluating the frequency of parental eating behaviors, both positive and negative, which factor into the formation of healthy eating habits in children. The above is very useful when planning interventions at both the primary and secondary levels to prevent health problems related to poor nutrition, such as childhood obesity, as well as in the prevention of eating disorders, and more specifically by guiding caregivers on how to deal with or prevent problems with feeding behavior, such as food selectivity, neophobia, emotional eating, or over-eating, more effectively.

Author Contributions: Conceptualization: M.L.G.-T., X.G.-O., G.N.-C. and L.A.G.-O.; formal analysis: M.L.G.-T., X.G.-O. and G.N.-C.; Funding acquisition: M.L.G.-T.; Investigation, M.L.G.-T. and L.A.G.-O.; Methodology: M.L.G.-T. and X.G.-O.; Validation: M.L.G.-T., X.G.-O., G.N.-C. and L.A.G.-O.; Writing—review and editing: M.L.G.-T., X.G.-O. and G.N.-C. All authors have read and agreed to the published version of the manuscript.

Funding: The first author thanks the Gonzalo Rio Arronte Foundation (S.719) and the Autonomous University of Aguascalientes (PIPS22-3) for funding this study.

Institutional Review Board Statement: The present work adhered to the ethical guidelines of the Declaration of Helsinki and was approved by the bioethics committee of the Autonomous University of Aguascalientes CIB-UAA-PIPS22-3 since the informed consent complied with the established guidelines and evidence of the protection of information and ethical treatment of the data was shown.

Informed Consent Statement: Informed consent was obtained from all subjects involved in the study.

Data Availability Statement: Data are available upon request due to privacy restrictions. The data presented in this study are available upon request from the corresponding author.

Acknowledgments: The first author thanks the Gonzalo Rio Arronte Foundation (S.719), the Autonomous University of Aguascalientes (PIPS22-3) for funding this study, and the Technologic of Monterrey for allowing the first author to carry out a research stay with the second author.

Conflicts of Interest: The authors declare no conflict of interest.

References

1. Fondo de las Naciones Unidas para la Infancia (UNICEF). *Estado Mundial de la Infancia 2019—Niños, Alimentos y Nutrición*; UNICEF: Geneva, Switzerland, 2019. Available online: https://www.unicef.org/mexico/media/2436/file/Resumen%20ejecutivo%20espa%C3%B1ol.pdf (accessed on 5 May 2022).
2. Fondo de las Naciones Unidas para la Infancia (UNICEF). *Salud y Nutrición*; UNICEF: Geneva, Switzerland, 2018. Available online: https://www.unicef.org/mexico/spanish/17047_17494.html (accessed on 5 May 2022).
3. Padilla-Vinueza, V.E.P.; Tisalema, H.; Gavilanez, R.I.A.; Cunalata, E.I.J.; Carrión, A.A.M.; Aguilar, A.D.S. Obesidad infantil y métodos de intervención. *Dominio Cienc.* **2022**, *8*, 961–971. [CrossRef]
4. Martínez-Munguía, C.; Navarro-Contreras, G. Factores Psicológicos, Sociales y Culturales del Sobrepeso y la Obesidad Infantil y Juvenil en México. *Rev. Médica Inst. Mex. Seguro Soc.* **2014**, *52*, S94–S101. Available online: https://www.redalyc.org/articulo.oa?id=457745485016 (accessed on 5 May 2022).

5. Vaughn, A.E.; Ward, D.S.; Fisher, J.O.; Faith, M.S.; Hughes, S.O.; Kremers, S.P.; Musher-Eizenman, D.R.; O'connor, T.M.; Patrick, H.; Power, T.G. Fundamental constructs in food parenting practices: A content map to guide future research. *Nutr. Rev.* **2016**, *74*, 98–117. [CrossRef]
6. González-Torres, M.L.; Esqueda, C.N.; Vacio, M.A. Prácticas alimentarias parentales y su relación con la conducta alimentaria infantil: Problemas para la explicación. *Rev. Mex. Trastor. Aliment.* **2018**, *9*, 129–142. [CrossRef]
7. Shloim, N.; Edelson, L.R.; Martin, N.; Hetherington, M.M. Parenting Styles, Feeding Styles, Feeding Practices, and Weight Status in 4–12 Year-Old Children: A Systematic Review of the Literature. *Front. Psychol.* **2015**, *6*, 1849. [CrossRef]
8. Castrillón, I.C.; Giraldo, O. Prácticas de alimentación de los padres y conductas alimentarias en niños: ¿existe información suficiente para el abordaje de los problemas de alimentación? *Rev. Psicol. Univ. Antioq.* **2014**, *6*, 57–74. [CrossRef]
9. González-Torres, M.L.; González, L.A.; Altamirano, A.; Pedroza, F. Interacciones cuidador-niño durante la alimentación y el aprendizaje temprano de hábitos alimentarios. In *Aportaciones Actuales a la Psicología Social (IV)*; Díaz, R., Reyes, L.I., López, F., Eds.; Asociación Mexicana de Psicología Social: Ciudad de México, Mexico, 2018; pp. 2133–2149.
10. Vaughn, A.E.; Dearth-Wesley, T.; Tabak, R.G.; Bryant, M.; Ward, D.S. Development of a comprehensive assessment of food parenting practices: The home self-administered tool for environmental assessment of activity and diet family food practices survey. *J. Acad. Nutr. Diet.* **2017**, *117*, 214–227. [CrossRef]
11. Birch, L.L.; Fisher, J.O.; Grimm-Thomas, K.; Markey, C.N.; Sawyer, R. Confirmatory factor analysis of the Child Feeding Questionnaire: A measure of parental attitudes, beliefs, and practices about child feeding and obesity proneness. *Appetite* **2001**, *36*, 20–201. [CrossRef]
12. Navarro-Contreras, G.; Lagunes, I.R. Validación Psicométrica de la Adaptación Mexicana del Child Feeding Questionnaire. *Acta Investig. Psicol.* **2016**, *6*, 2337–2349. [CrossRef]
13. Musher-Eizenman, D.; Holub, S. Comprehensive Feeding Practices Questionnaire: Validation of a New Measure of Parental Feeding Practices. *J. Pediatr. Psychol.* **2007**, *32*, 960–972. [CrossRef]
14. Ángel, J.G.; Flores, Y.P.; Trujillo, P.E.H.; Ávila, H.A.; Gutiérrez, J.M.V. Confirmatory factor analysis of the Comprehensive Feeding Practices Questionnaire in Mexican mothers of preschool children. *Nutr. Hosp.* **2021**, *38*, 827–832. [CrossRef]
15. Afonso, L.; Castro, J.; Parente, N.; Torres, S. A Comprehensive Assessment of Food Parenting Practices: Psychometric Properties of the Portuguese Version of the HomeSTEAD Family Food Practices Survey and Associations with Children's Weight and Food Intake. *Eur. J. Investig. Health Psychol. Educ.* **2020**, *10*, 424–440. [CrossRef]
16. Escobar-Pérez, J.; Cuervo-Martínez, Á. Validez de Contenido y Juicio de Expertos: Una Aproximación a su Utilización. *Av. Medición* **2008**, *6*, 27–36. Available online: https://gc.scalahed.com/recursos/files/r161r/w25645w/Juicio_de_expertos_u4.pdf (accessed on 1 February 2022).
17. Van Widenfelt, B.M.; Treffers, P.D.A.; de Beurs, E.; Siebelink, B.M.; Koudijs, E. Translation and Cross-Cultural Adaptation of Assessment Instruments Used in Psychological Research with Children and Families. *Clin. Child. Fam. Psychol. Rev.* **2005**, *8*, 135–147. [CrossRef]
18. Costello, A.B.; Osborne, J. Best practices in exploratory factor analysis: Four recommendations for getting the most from your analysis. *Pract. Assess. Res. Eval.* **2005**, *10*, 7. [CrossRef]
19. Lloret-Segura, S.; Ferreres-Traver, A.; Hernández-Baeza, A.; Tomás-Marco, I. El análisis factorial exploratorio de los ítems: Una guía práctica, revisada y actualizada. *An. Psicol. Ann. Psychol.* **2014**, *30*, 1151–1169. [CrossRef]
20. Shamah-Levy, T.; Vielma-Orozco, E.; Heredia-Hernández, O.; Romero-Martínez, M.; Mojica-Cuevas, J.; Cuevas-Nasu, L.; Santaella-Castell, J.A.; Rivera-Dommarco, J. *Encuesta Nacional de Salud y Nutrición [ENSANUT] 2018–19: Resultados Nacionales*; Instituto Nacional de Salud Pública: Cuernavaca, Mexico, 2020. Available online: https://ensanut.insp.mx/encuestas/ensanut2018/doctos/informes/ensanut_2018_informe_final.pdf (accessed on 5 May 2022).
21. Jimeno-Martínez, A.; Maneschy, I.; Rupérez, A.I.; Moreno, L.A. Factores Determinantes del Comportamiento Alimentario y su Impacto Sobre la Ingesta y la Obesidad en Niños. *J. Behav. Feed.* **2021**, *1*, 60–71. Available online: http://148.202.248.171/revistaiican/index.php/JBF/article/view/20 (accessed on 8 July 2022).
22. Ferrando, P.J.; Anguiano-Carrasco, C. El Análisis Factorial Como Técnica de Investigación en Psicología. *Papeles Psicól.* **2010**, *31*, 18–33. Available online: https://www.redalyc.org/pdf/778/77812441003.pdf (accessed on 9 September 2022).
23. Del Valle, M.; Zamora, E.V. El uso de las Medidas de Auto-Informe: Ventajas y Limitaciones en la Investigación en Psicología. *Altern. Psicol.* **2021**, *47*, 22–35. Available online: https://ri.conicet.gov.ar/handle/11336/173600 (accessed on 8 July 2022).
24. Tomás, J.M.; Requena, P.S.; Germes, A.O.; Llinares, L.G.; Moral, J.C.M. Efectos de Método Asociados a Ítems Invertidos vs. Ítems en Negativo. *Rev. Mex. Psicol.* **2012**, *29*, 105–115. Available online: https://www.redalyc.org/articulo.oa?id=243030190001 (accessed on 8 July 2022).
25. Jaeger, S.R.; Cardello, A.V. Factors affecting data quality of online questionnaires: Issues and metrics for sensory and consumer research. *Food Qual. Prefer.* **2022**, *102*, 104676. [CrossRef]

nutrients

MDPI

Article

Prevalence of Feeding Problems in Children and Associated Factors—A Cross-Sectional Study among Polish Children Aged 2–7 Years

Agnieszka Białek-Dratwa [1,*] and Oskar Kowalski [1,2]

[1] Department of Human Nutrition, Department of Dietetics, Faculty of Public Health in Bytom, Medical University of Silesia in Katowice, ul. Jordana 19, 41-808 Zabrze, Poland; okowalski@sum.edu.pl

[2] Department of Cardiology, Congenital Heart Diseases and Electrotherapy, Silesian Center for Heart Diseases, 41-800 Zabrze, Poland

* Correspondence: abialek@sum.edu.pl; Tel.: +48-(0-32)-275-51-95

Abstract: Food neophobia is an aversion to eating or a reluctance to try unfamiliar or new foods. From an evolutionary perspective, this behaviour may minimise the risk of consuming foods that are harmful to health. However, such aversion causes food monotony, which may result in nutritional deficiencies. This study aimed to assess the prevalence of feeding problems among Polish children aged 2–7 years using the Montreal Children's Hospital Feeding Scale and to investigate the correlation between age, gender, mode of feeding in infancy, including complementary feeding, and the prevalence of feeding difficulties in the study group of children. Material and method: The study group consisted of 585 children: 299 boys (51.11%) and 286 girls (48.89%). The study was conducted using a questionnaire-based method, with an indirect survey technique using a web-based form (CAWI). The research tool used was the Montreal Children's Hospital-Pediatric Feeding Program. Results: Groups with the lowest risk feeding problems, risk 0, comprised 445 children (76.06%); group 1, middle difficulties, 59 children (10.08%); group 2, moderate difficulties, 40 children (6.84%); and group 3, most difficulties, 40 children (7.01%). The mean MCH-FS score for the entire study group was calculated and was 37.29 points ± 12.02; for 2 year olds, 35.69 points; for 3 year olds, 37.41 points; for 4 year olds, 38.31 points; for 5 year olds, 38.46 points; for 6 year olds, 37.95 points; and for 7 year olds, 36.06 points. The mean value of the MCH-FS scale for girls was 37.44 points, and for boys, 37.32 points. None of the above parameters correlated with the risk of feeding problems, including age, except with a non-significative tendency to be higher in the youngest age. Conclusion: Breast milk feeding and the time of complementary feeding (CF) in the study group did not influence the risk of feeding problems. Using the full BLW method during CF can protect the child against the occurrence of feeding problems such a food selectivity or picky eating in the future. In our study, children with difficulties during CF, mainly the vomiting reflex, were more likely to develop feeding problems such as food neophobia. Based on our study, we did not observe a correlation between age, gender, and the occurrence of feeding problems, and there was only a non-significant tendency to be higher in the youngest age. However, further research needs to be undertaken to assess how such behaviour affects subsequent feeding difficulties.

Keywords: neophobia; feeding difficulties; children; complementary feeding; baby-led weaning; BLW

1. Introduction

Food neophobia is an aversion to eating or a reluctance to try unfamiliar or new foods [1,2]. From an evolutionary perspective, this behaviour may minimise the risk of consuming foods that are harmful to health. However, such aversion causes food monotony, which may result in nutritional deficiencies [1,3].

One theory of the prevalence of food neophobia is that in early human history, it was beneficial because it helped children avoid potential food hazards, including poisonous foods such as berries or spoiled meat. The ability to detect and avoid unfamiliar foods ensured that children only consumed safe, familiar foods they could trust. This innate preference for familiar foods was significant in the evolutionary pathway because it benefited the species' survival [1,4].

However, the exact aetiology of food neophobia still needs to be determined, and its expression varies with age [5]. During the first period, infants consume one food: breast milk or infant formula. After 4 months of age, solid foods are gradually introduced into the infant's diet, which may provide an opportunity for aversion to unfamiliar foods [6,7]. However, infants under 18–20 months of age readily accept new foods and do not show neophobic behaviour until 20–24 months [5,8]. Food neophobia can be observed in all age groups, but it increases rapidly during the complementary feeding period and peaks at 2–6 years of age [9].

In addition to evolutionary factors, environmental factors may also influence food neophobia in children. Parents and caregivers may inadvertently reinforce a child's reluctance to try new foods by offering only familiar foods or expressing negative attitudes towards unfamiliar foods. This can lead to a vicious circle in which children become increasingly reluctant to try new foods, which can further limit the variety of foods they eat [10–13].

In addition, taste and texture preferences may play a role in food neophobia. Children may be more sensitive to bitter tastes or prefer sweet foods [14–16], making it difficult to savour new or unfamiliar foods. Therefore, it is important to introduce different flavours into the child's diet to shape future food preferences [17]. Some studies suggest that breastfed children accept new foods more readily and have lower levels of food neophobia [18,19].

Babies fed with modified milk tend to become accustomed to the constant and specific taste of milk formula, consequently showing less tolerance or even aversion to new foods and tastes [15,16,20–22]. Studies have also shown that the more authoritarian the parents are during mealtimes, the more often the child rejects the foods offered [23–26].

Food neophobia is a complex phenomenon influenced by many factors, including evolutionary and environmental factors, taste preferences, and cultural norms. Understanding these factors can help parents and carers encourage children to try new foods and develop a more varied and balanced diet. Most studies of food neophobia have examined the prevalence of neophobia in different age groups rather than each year. This has led to broad peak estimates, and whether food neophobia differs between children aged 2 to 7 years remains unclear. Therefore, this study aimed to assess the prevalence of feeding problems among Polish children aged 2–7 years using the Montreal Children's Hospital Feeding Scale and to investigate the correlation between age, gender, mode of feeding in infancy, including complementary feeding, and the prevalence of feeding difficulties in the study group of children.

2. Materials and Methods

2.1. Course of the Study

The study was conducted using a questionnaire-based method, with an indirect survey technique using a web-based form (CAWI). The questionnaire was made available to mothers of children in randomly selected nurseries and kindergartens in Poland through closed groups on instant messaging systems designed for communication between parents and educational institutions and on parent association groups in individual cities and regions in Poland. All survey participants were informed about the purpose of the study, the voluntary nature of their participation, and the preservation of their anonymity, and were asked to accept the data-sharing rules. Adults (mothers of preschool and nursery-aged children) took part in the study. The study period covered the months of January to March 2023.

2.2. Selection of the Study Group

In verifying the study group of parents, it was observed that only one father completed the survey questionnaire; mothers completed the other questionnaires. Therefore, only mothers qualified for the study of feeding children during the period of dietary expansion and feeding during the nursery and preschool period, as they are the ones who are most often at home with their children during the complementary feeding period or in contact with an educational institution such as a nursery/preschool and are responsible for feeding children during this period. The survey was conducted using the CAWI method, so the sample selection was utterly random (according to the adopted inclusion and exclusion criteria of the survey).

2.3. Inclusion and Exclusion Criteria

Mothers taking part in the study gave their informed consent to participate, and the questionnaire was only made available when approval to participate in this study was obtained. The criteria for group selection included the fact that respondents were of legal age, had at least one child of nursery or preschool age, and had no formal knowledge of the behavioural determinants of nutrition (education or profession related to the topics of nutrition, treatment, and upbringing of children and adolescents). Inclusion criteria for the study proper were: being the mother/legal guardian of a child aged between 2 and 7 years, consent to participate in the study, and correct and complete completion of the questionnaire. The criteria for exclusion from the study were: lack of consent to participate in the study; incorrectly completed questionnaire, including non-response to questions; child's age below 2 years and above 7 years; and the presence of a disease determining the method of feeding, e.g., food allergies and intolerances, autism spectrum disorders. After consideration of the inclusion and exclusion criteria, 585 pairs of mothers and their children were included in the final analysis.

The study was conducted according to the Declaration of Helsinki and the Act on the Profession of Physicians and Dentists. A positive opinion of the Bioethics Committee operating at the Medical University of Silesia in Katowice was obtained to conduct the research "Dietary neophobia among infants and children" (BNW/NWN/0052/KB/34/23).

2.4. Research Tool

The research tool was an anonymous survey questionnaire consisting of 5 parts. The first part concerned the parent/guardian and their child; it included data such as age and sex of the parent/guardian, place of residence, education of the parent/guardian, sex of the child, information on delivery, current weight and height, and food intolerances and allergies. Based on the child's current age, weight, length/height using centile grids, and 3 SD BMI for girls and boys aged 0–3 years, the WHO standard body weight of children in terms of underweight, average weight, overweight, and obesity was assessed; for children aged 3–7 years, the developmental norms for girls/boys aged 3–18 years according to OLAF and OLAF studies [27,28] were used. The study asked for information entered in the "Child Health Booklet" such as the week of pregnancy in which the child was born, birth weight, birth length, and mode of delivery (natural, planned caesarean, unplanned caesarean) [29].

According to the Polish law issued by the Polish Ministry of Health, the child health booklet contains standardised information on the child, including the prenatal period; birth; health status after birth; patronage visits; preventive examinations, including dental examinations; history of infectious diseases, allergies, and anaphylactic reactions; radiological procedures; provision of medical devices; exemption from sports activities; and other information relevant to the assessment of the child's normal development from birth, including measurements of weight, length/growth up to adult. All entries in the above document are made by medical staff, including a doctor, midwife, nurse, or other medical professional. This information is entered into the health booklet after providing the health service. If this is not possible, it is completed at the next visit based on the individual's internal records [29].

The next part of the questionnaire focused on the mode of feeding during infancy, taking into account breast milk feeding, exclusive breastfeeding, length of breastfeeding, and the timing and method of CF (when the introduction of CF started; consistency of meals during CF—puree, pureed meals, meals ready to be eaten by the child with fingers; products given to the child as CF; and the method of expanding the infant's diet including the use of the BLW method). In our study, we used the application of the baby-led weaning (BLW) method during complementary feeding. According to the definition of the BLW method, we considered that the child ate completely or mostly independently, so they ate using the BLW method; or the child was occasionally spoon-fed by an adult—approximately 10% feeding, 90% on their own, and also ate using the BLW method.

The third part concerned the child's current diet, including the use of cutlery, food preferences, taste senses, feeding behaviour, and occurrence of food selectivity. The questionnaire was developed based on current dietary recommendations for the group of the youngest children and the method of diet expansion developed by PTGHiŻD [6] based on ESPHGAN recommendations [7], as well as information on diet expansion, including the BLW method and food selectivity occurring in this period of a child's life [4,6,7,10,30,31].

The last part of the questionnaire concerned the prevalence of feeding problems. The research tool used was The Montreal Children's Hospital-Pediatric Feeding Program [32,33]. The Polish version of the Montreal Children's Hospital Feeding Scale (MCH-FS), which was appropriately translated and validated [33], was used in our study.

The Montreal Children's Hospital-Pediatric Feeding Program (MCH-FS) is related to feeding a child from 6 months (receiving a pureed diet) to 6 years of age. It includes questions such as: How would you rate your child's meal pattern? How concerned are you about your child's meal pattern? How do you assess your child's appetite (feeling of hunger)? At what point during a meal does your child start refusing to eat? How long do your child's meals last (in minutes)? How do you assess your child's behaviour during mealtimes? Does your child choke, gag, spit, or vomit at certain foods? Does your child hold food in the mouth without swallowing? Do you have to walk behind your child or distract him/her (toys, TV) to get him/her to eat? Do you have to force your child to eat or drink? How do you assess your child's chewing (or sucking) skills? How do you assess your child's growth (weight, height)? How does feeding your child affect your relationship with your child? How does feeding your child affect your family relationships? [32,33].

The MCH-FS consists of 14 items covering the following feeding characteristics: oral motility, sensory, and appetite. Other items address mothers' concerns about feeding, mealtime behaviour, strategies mothers use, and the family's reaction to the child's feeding [32]. A 7-point Likert scale was included for each question. The meaning of the answers to the questions varied depending on the question [32,33]. Seven items from the MCH-FS scale are scored from a negative to a positive direction, and the remaining seven from a positive to negative direction (reversed scores). The final MCH-FS scale score is obtained by adding the scores for each question and reversing the scores of the seven items from negative to positive. The MCH-FS scale required an appropriate recalculation of the selected responses before adding up each respondent's answers. Questions 1, 3, 4, 8, 10, 12, and 13 had to be reversed in order so that answer 1 had 7 points, answer 2 had 6 points, answer 3 had 5 points, etc. The remaining questions had to be kept in their original order; then, all the points obtained added together. The interpretation of the results was based on the study "The Montreal Children's Hospital Feeding Scale: A brief bilingual screening tool for identifying feeding problems" by Maria Ramsay et al. from 2011 and the study "The Polish version of the Montreal Children's Hospital Feeding Scale (MCH-FS): translation, cross-cultural adaptation, and validation)" by Katarzyna Bąbik et al. from 2019. The interpretation (MCH-FS) is that a score in the range of 14–45 points indicates no feeding difficulties; 46–52 points, middle difficulties; 53–58 points, moderate difficulties; above 59 points, most difficulties. We used the RAVE SCORE MCH-FS in the study, where the maximum score was 98 points [27,32,33].

2.5. Statistical Analysis

The programs used to analyse the collected data were Microsoft Office Word and Microsoft Office Excel. Statistical analysis was performed using Statistica v. 13.3 software (StatSoft Inc., Tulsa, OK, USA). The measured data were characterised by mean and standard deviation (X ± SD), and the range of minimum and maximum values obtained in the study group of children was determined. Statistical tests were used to analyse the variables for statistical inference. The study group of children was divided into 4 subgroups based on the calculation of the MCH-FS scale score: group 0, no risk; group 1, moderate difficulties; group 2, moderate difficulties; and group 3, most difficulties. Bivariate tables were used to compare the group of children in the four groups: 0, no risk; 1, middle difficulties; 2, moderate difficulties; 3, most difficulties, for r non-parametric characteristics Pearson's chi-squared test was used.

The level of statistical significance adopted in the study was set at $p \leq 0.05$.

3. Results

Characteristics of the Study Group

The study group consisted of 585 children: 299 boys (51.11%) and 286 girls (48.89%). Most of the children in the study came from cities with more than 100,000 inhabitants, i.e., 212 children (36.24). In terms of body weight, 404 children (69.06%) were of average weight, 139 children (23.76%) were underweight, 31 children (5.30%) were overweight, and 11 (1.88%) were obese. The study included children aged between 2 and 7 years of age, including 130 two year olds (22.22%), 134 three year olds (22.91%), 91 four year olds (15.56%), 80 five year olds (13.68%), 82 six year olds (14.02%), and 68 seven year olds (11.62%) (Table 1). Throughout the study, the grouping variable was allocated to the group at risk of feeding problems. Groups with the lowest risk of feeding problems (risk 0) comprised 445 children (76.06%); group 1, middle difficulties, 59 children (10.08%); group 2, moderate difficulties, 40 children (6.84%); and group 3, most difficulties, 40 children (7.01%). The correlation of feeding problem risk with gender ($p = 0.988$), place of residence ($p = 0.755$), weight ($p = 0.755$), and age ($p = 0.764$) was analysed. None of the above parameters correlated with the risk of feeding problems, including age, except for a non-significative tendency to be higher in the youngest age.

Table 1. Characteristics of the study group of children with a breakdown according to the MCH-FS scale (0—no risk, 1—middle difficulties, 2—moderate difficulties, 3—most difficulties).

	0—Not at Risk		1—Middle Difficulties		2—Moderate Difficulties		3—Most Difficult		Total		
	n	%	n	%	n	%	n	%	N	%	
The entire group of children surveyed	445	76.06	59	10.08	40	6.84	41	7.01	585	100	
Gender:											
Boy	228	76.25	29	9.69	21	7.02	21	7.02	299	100	$p = 0.988$
Girl	217	75.87	30	10.48	19	6.64	20	6.69	286	100	
Body weight:											
underweight	98	70.50	16	11.51	13	9.35	12	9.63	139	23.76	
normal weight	314	77.72	36	8.91	25	6.18	29	7.17	404	69.06	$p = 0.755$
overweight	25	80.64	5	16.12	1	3.23	0	0.00	31	5.30	
obesity	8	72.72	2	18.18	1	9.09	0	0.00	11	1.88	
Age:											
2 years	110	84.61	12	9.23	4	3.07	4	3.07	130	22.22	
3 years	100	74.62	13	9.70	11	8.20	10	7.46	134	22.91	
4 years	66	72.52	9	9.89	8	8.79	8	8.79	91	15.56	$p = 0.764$
5 years	59	73.75	9	11.25	5	6.25	7	8.75	80	13.68	
6 years	62	75.06	7	8.53	6	7.31	7	8.53	82	14.02	
7 years	48	70.58	9	13.23	6	8.82	5	7.35	68	11.62	

However, it can be seen in the results that the prevalence of feeding problems is lowest in 2 year olds (84.61%), and the level then increases in children aged 7 years.

The mean MCH-FS score for the entire study group was calculated and was 37.29 points ± 12.02; for 2 year olds, it was 35.69 points; for 3 year olds, 37.41 points; for 4 year olds, 38.31 points; for 5 year olds, 38.46 points; for 6 year olds, 37.95 points; and for 7 year olds, 36.06 points. The mean value of the MCH-FS scale for girls was 37.44 points, and for boys, 37.32 points. Age and gender differences were not statistically significant.

By definition, "exclusive breastfeeding" means not giving modified milk to the baby; the baby consumes only breast milk. Both the length of breast milk feeding (p = 0.242), the length of exclusive breast milk feeding (p = 0.296), and the time of initiation of complementary feeding (p = 0.899) did not correlate with the risk of feeding problems.

The mode of complementary feeding in the children studied was also assessed. Children given puree during CF were more likely to have a higher risk of feeding problems (p = 0.010). The administration of puree with lumps did not correlate with the risk of feeding problems (p = 0.240). The study also included the baby-led weaning (BLW) method, which involves child-controlled feeding. It is based on the omission of the spoon-feeding stage by the parents/carers and the feeding of pulpy foods (purees). When the baby can sit up unaided (approx. 6–7 months of age), various solid foods are given in such a form that they can be easily grasped with the hand (e.g., cucumber strips, carrots, pieces of apple, pear, various shapes of pasta, and strips of meat) [6,7]. Children in whom the BLW method was used in dietary expansion did not show a risk of feeding problems (p = 0.026), in contrast to children fed traditionally with a spoon. The study also assessed the difficulties in introducing new foods into the child's diet. Children who experienced difficulties during CF were more likely to be at risk of feeding problems ($p < 0.001$) (Table 2).

Table 2. Mode of complementary feeding in study children with respect to the MCH-FS scale and interpretation of the MCH-FS scale.

Method of Complementary Feeding	0—Not at Risk		1—Middle Difficulties		2—Moderate Difficulties		3—Most Difficult		Total		
	n	%	n	%	n	%	n	%	N	%	
puree	369	82.92	57	96.61	38	95.00	39	95.12	503	85.98	p = 0.010
puree with lumps	316	71.01	44	74.58	30	75.00	28	68.29	418	71.45	p = 0.240
Feeding/spoon fed: The child ate completely or mostly independently (BLW)	69	88.46	3	3.85	2	2.56	4	5.13	78	13.33	p = 0.026
Child occasionally spoon-fed by an adult (approximately 10% feeding, 90% on their own) (BLW)	11	100.00		0.00		0,00		0.00	11	1.88	
Baby fully or mostly spoon-fed by an adult	106	68.83	17	11.04	13	8.44	18	11.69	154	26.32	
The child was half fed by an adult with a spoon. half ate independently	259	75.73	39	11.40	25	7.31	19	5.56	342	58.46	
Difficulties in introducing new foods in the child: I don't remember	19	57.58	6	18.18	3	9.09	5	15.15	33	5.64	$p < 0.001$
No, there were no problems in expanding the baby's diet	349	84.50	36	8.72	16	3.87	12	2.91	413	70.60	
Yes, there were problems in expanding the child's diet	77	55.40	17	12.23	21	15.11	24	17.27	139	23.76	

Table 3 shows the results for the occurrence of problems during CF. Children who had a vomiting reflex during CF were more likely to have feeding problems (p = 0.001). In contrast, spitting food out of the mouth (p = 0.085), gagging (p = 0.244), choking (p = 0.590), and choking and needing medical attention (p = 0.121) did not correlate with the risk of feeding problems.

Table 3. Incidence of problems during complementary feeding in the study group of children with respect to the MCH-FS scale and interpretation.

Problems during CF		0—Not at Risk	1—Middle Difficulties	2—Moderate Difficulties	3—Most Difficult	Total						
		n	%	n	%	n	%	n	%	N	%	
Vomiting reflex	yes	113	25.39	14	23.73	16	40.00	21	51.22	164	28.03	$p = 0.001$
spat food out of its mouth	yes	270	60.67	38	64.41	29	72.50	32	78.05	369	63.08	$p = 0.085$
Gagging	yes	142	31.91	12	20.34	14	35.00	15	36.59	183	31.28	$p = 0.244$
Choking	yes	33	7.42	4	6.78	4	10.00	1	2.44	42	7.18	$p = 0.590$
Choked and needed medical attention	yes	1	0.22	0	0.00	0	0.00	1	2.44	2	0.34	$p = 0.121$

Tables 4 and 5 show the mothers' subjective assessment of their child's food intake and appetite and of the fact that their child was a picky eater. In both cases, the majority of mothers correctly assessed their child's appetite and the fact of being a picky eater ($p < 0.001$) and ($p < 0.001$).

Table 4. Mothers' subjective assessment towards her child's food intake and appetite score ($p < 0.001$).

	0—Not at Risk		1—Middle Difficulties		2—Moderate Difficulties		3—Most Difficult		Total	
	n	%	n	%	n	%	n	%	N	%
The child often does not want to eat and I have to encourage/force him to do so	36	28.80	33	26.40	28	22.40	28	22.40	125	21.37
The child has an appetite and eats almost everything he is given.	297	98.67	3	1.00	0	0.00	1	0.33	301	51.45
The child has an appetite but eats a severely limited amount of food (up to 20 dishes)	8	61.54	1	7.69	3	23.08	1	7.69	13	2.22
The child has an appetite, but eats a limited amount of food	23	85.19	2	7.41	2	7.41	0	0.00	27	4.62
The child doesn't want to eat, but I don't force him to.	63	64.95	19	19.59	6	6.19	9	9.28	97	16.58
Child has no appetite, but eats because he is very hungry (eats only a limited amount of food)	1	50.00	0	0.00	0	0.00	1	50.00	2	0.34
Baby has no appetite, but eats because he is very hungry (eats everything)	0	0.00	0	0.00	1	100.00	0	0.00	1	0.17
I didn't pay attention to it.	17	89.47	1	5.26		0.00	1	5.26	19	3.25

Table 5. Mother's subjective assessment of their child being a picky eater ($p < 0.001$).

The Fact of Being a Picky Eater	0—Not at Risk		1—Middle Difficulties		2—Moderate Difficulties		3—Most Difficult		Total	
	n	%	n	%	n	%	n	%	N	%
no	372	92.08	23	5.69	9	2.23		0.00	404	69.06
I don't know	31	62.00	10	20.00	4	8.00	5	10.00	50	8.55
yes	42	32.06	26	19.85	27	20.61	36	27.48	131	22.39

Among the children surveyed, the consumption of foods with specific tastes was assessed. In the surveyed group, most children consume products with different flavours (90.43%). A total of 4.44% of the children surveyed consume products with selected flavours (Table 6).

Table 6. Consumption of flavoured meals in the study group of children ($p < 0.001$).

	0—Not at Risk		1—Middle Difficulties		2—Moderate Difficulties		3—Most Difficulties		Final Total	
	n	%	n	%	n	%	n	%	n	%
I don't know/ difficult to say	13	46.43	5	17.86	6	21.43	4	14.29	28	4.79
No, he consumes products from different taste groups.	419	79.21	51	9.64	30	5.67	29	5.48	529	90.43
Yes, he eats only bitter-tasting products	0	0.00	0	0.00	1	100.00	0	0.00	1	0.17
Yes, he eats only sweet-tasting products	0	0.00	0	0.00	0	0.00	1	100.00	1	0.17
Yes, he only consumes products with the flavour of his choice.	13	50.00	3	11.54	3	11.54	7	26.92	26	4.44

The study assessed current problems related to children's eating patterns. Both the vomiting reflex ($p < 0.001$, V Cramer = 0.274), spitting food out of the mouth ($p < 0.001$, V Cramer = 0.289), playing with food ($p = 0.004$, V Cramer = 0.149), and burying cutlery in food ($p = 0.001$, V Cramer = 0.186) correlated positively with the occurrence of feeding problem risk. Choking did not correlate with feeding problems ($p = 0.278$, V Cramer = 0.0810) (Table 7).

Table 7. Current problems related to the child's eating patterns.

Problems Related to Eating		0—Not at Risk		1—Middle Difficulties		2—Moderate Difficulties		3—Most Difficult		Total		
		n	%	n	%	n	%	n	%	n	%	
vomiting reflex	yes	6	1.35	3	5.08	5	12.50	8	19.51	22	3.76	$p < 0.001$
spitting food out of mouth	yes	31	6.97	13	22.03	11	27.50	15	36.59	70	11.97	$p < 0.001$
playing with food	yes	131	29.44	23	38.98	17	42.50	22	53.66	193	32.99	$p = 0.004$
burying cutlery in food	yes	129	28.99	27	45.76	23	57.50	18	43.90	197	33.68	$p = 0.001$
whooping	yes	2	0.45	1	1.69	1	2.50	1	2.44	5	0.85	$p = 0.278$

Table 8 analyses the principal components of the Montreal Children's Hospital Feeding Scale (MCH-FS) for the entire sample of children. The mean, along with the standard deviation obtained for each question, and the median, were assessed. The higher the mean and median, the more frequent the behaviour. In the study group, the most frequent behaviour occurred in the aspect of walking behind the child or distracting the child (toys, TV) in order for the child to eat a meal (mean 5.67 ± 1.80, median = 7). Frequent behaviours were as follows: the child refusing to eat a meal (mean 3.19 ± 1.91, median = 3), extending the meal time (mean 3.13 ± 1.41, median = 3), and forcing the child to eat and drink (mean 3.16 ± 2.48, median = 3).

Table 8. Principal component analysis of the Montreal Children's Hospital Feeding Scale (MCH-FS) for the whole children sample.

Factors and Items	Construct	Mean	Median
1. how do you find mealtimes with your child?	Parental concern	2.93 ± 1.52	3
2. how worried are you about your child's eating?	Parental concern	2.67 ± 1.83	2
12. how do you find your child's growth?	Parental concern	1.86 ± 1.43	1
3. how much appetite (hunger) does your child have?	Appetite	2.70 ± 1.61	2
4. when does your child start refusing to eat during mealtimes?	Appetite	3.19 ± 1.91	3
9. Do you have to follow your child around or use distractions (toys, TV) so that your child will eat?	Compensatory strategies	5.67 ± 1.80	7
10. Do you have to force your child to eat or drink?	Compensatory strategies	3.16 ± 2.48	1
6. how does your child behave during mealtimes?	Mealtime behaviour	2.79 ± 1.07	1
13. How does your child's feeding influence your relationship with him/her?	Family relations	2.07 ± 1.47	1
14. How does your child's feeding influence your family relationships?	Family relations	2.26 ± 1.72	1
5. how long do mealtimes take for your child (in minutes)?	Compensatory strategies	3.13 ± 1.41	3
7. does your child gag or spit or vomit with certain types of food?	Oral sensors	1.55 ± 1.07	1
11. how are your child's chewing (or sucking) abilities?	Oral motor	1.46 ± 1.15	1
8. Does your child hold food in his/her mouth without swallowing it?	Oral sensory, oral motor, mealtime behaviour	1.83 ± 1.38	1

4. Discussion

There is no precise formal definition of picky eating, although it is generally accepted that it includes the rejection or restriction of familiar and unfamiliar foods, and thus includes an element of neophobia; these factors are associated with feeding problems in children [9,31]. The most common definition offered by Dovey et al. is that picky/fussy eaters are children "who consume an inappropriate variety of foods, rejecting a significant amount of foods that are familiar (as well as unfamiliar) to them". They see food neophobia (food aversion or avoidance of new foods) as a somewhat distinct construct, while observing that the two factors of food aversion and avoidance of new foods are interrelated and both contribute to food rejection or acceptance, especially of fruit and vegetables [9]. Hence, the terms feeding neophobia (used according to Dovey's definition), feeding problems, and picky eating will appear frequently in our study and in this discussion. One would consider food neophobia to be a fear of new, unfamiliar foods, but many of the authors of the studies cited below consider children with food neophobia to be children who have an aversion to eating or who avoid new foods (according to Dovey's definition). Food aversion and avoidance of new foods, in turn, lead to a variety of feeding problems such as refusal to eat particular foods because of their texture, taste, colour, or shape, reflexes such as the vomiting reflex, or spitting out food or closing the mouth.

A high prevalence of food neophobia and pickiness has been reported previously among children aged 3 to 7 years in a study by Hafsrad G. et al. [34]. An exceptionally high prevalence of picky eating and food neophobia has been reported previously in China (59%) and the United States (60%) [35]. In contrast, a study in the Netherlands showed a very low prevalence of picky eating (5.6%) among 4 year old children [36]. A Polish study by Kozieł-Kozakowska et al. conducted among children aged 2.5–7 years showed low neophobia in 12.3% and high neophobia in 10.8% of the children studied [14]. In the meta-analysis by Torres et al. [2], the prevalence of food neophobia was present in 10 (53%) of the studies analysed and ranged from 12.8% to 100%.

In diagnosing feeding difficulties, including pickiness and feeding neophobia, the Montreal Children's Hospital Feeding Scale (MCH-FS) may be applicable [33,37]. The Children's Feeding Related Scale (MCH-FS Scale) is used to screen children with feeding difficulties adding challenges for preventive and diagnostic purposes. It can be used as a perfect tool to identify possible feeding difficulties in children aged 6 months to 6 years.

The MCH consists of 14 questions addressing issues related to the course of the meal, assessment of appetite evaluation, meal duration, problems within the orofacial sphere, or the parent's perception of the child's average weight and height. Each question is answered on a 7-point Likert-type scale [33]. The MCH-FS can be used in the nutritional interview and can be extended to include questions about the child's diet.

Feeding problem, selective eating, and food neophobia can lead to deficiencies in some essential nutrients, especially vitamins and minerals [1]. Children with high levels of food neophobia and other different feeding problems showed reduced adherence to standard eating patterns, which can negatively affect dietary diversity and lead to imbalanced nutrient intake [38]. This is supported by studies by Yong [39], Schmidt [40], Bell [41], and Kaar [13] Falciglia [3].

The results of the Di Nucci study showed a low intake of foods typical of the Mediterranean model, such as fruit, vegetables, and legumes, and conversely, a high intake of foods typical of the Western dietary model, such as sweets, sugary drinks, and red meat [42].

Food neophobia tends to occur with highly recommended and health-promoting foods such as fruit, vegetables, and legumes, which taste bitter or sour. Lower intake also occurs in the group of animal products, such as fish [43]. Children with high food neophobia were more likely to consume ultra-processed, sugar-rich foods (snacks, filled and unfilled cakes and sweets), as well as protein-rich foods (white meat, cheese and yoghurt) [38].

Some studies indicate that neophobic children are less likely to meet the recommended intake standards, especially the need for vitamin E [3]. In addition, children who only eat selected foods may not acquire specific eating skills, especially if they only eat soft-textured or pureed foods [1]. The negative health consequences of food neophobia should be seen in the context of the lost potential health benefits of a poor or poorly varied diet and, above all, the consumption of too few vegetables and fruits compared to recommendations [3,44]. A review of publications shows that neophobic children have a deficient intake of fruit and vegetables, which are health-promoting. This is supported by most epidemiological studies that demonstrate the health-promoting effects of fruit and vegetable consumption [45].

Nutritional neophobia is highly relevant to the concept of metabolic programming, especially in the nutritional aspect, which is understood as the long-term or lifelong effect of a stimulus or signal affecting the structures or functions of the organism during a critical period of development. It has been shown that the occurrence of factors such as malnutrition, or nutrient deficiency or excess, during so-called critical periods can reprogram the metabolism, leading to irreversible consequences. The first 1000 days of a child's life is when the metabolism is programmed, and many of the physiological processes responsible for appetite control and energy regulation are fixed. During the first three years of a child's life, there is less activity of enzymes produced in the liver, which is responsible for the metabolism of harmful compounds. The immature kidneys do not yet excrete toxins efficiently. The child's diet should include, above all, products rich in vitamins A, D, C, and B. Micronutrients such as zinc, selenium, iron, and copper should also be present. Polyunsaturated fatty acids, including DHA, cod liver oil, probiotics, and prebiotics, are also essential to the diet [46–49]. Therefore, it seems essential to minimise the occurrence of nutritional neophobia in the youngest children. The above study aimed to answer questions on how feeding neophobia can be minimised through early modification of feeding behaviour from birth through CF.

The origin of food neophobia can be traced back to evolution when a neophobic attitude protected children from eating potentially contaminated food [14]. Humans, as an omnivorous species, had to distinguish between safe and poisonous food to survive [50]. Although this skill has now lost its value, it can still be observed in children around and after the age of 2 years, when unfamiliar foods or foods given in a different way than before cause anxiety in the child and a relative preference for familiar foods is apparent [51].

Although food neophobia is genetically determined, environmental factors that underlie individual differences in taste preferences can also influence its occurrence [50]. Genetic factors influencing food choice are related to taste receptors, which can differentiate the perception of sweet, umami, or bitter tastes depending on individual gene differences [51]. Thus, some children tolerate bitter-tasting green vegetables such as broccoli or cabbage better, others will not care for them, and some will reject these foods at the mere sight of them [51]. In our study, regardless of the level of risk of feeding problems, the majority of the children (90.43%) consumed products from different taste groups, 4.44% of the children only consumed products with selected tastes, and only one child out of the entire group consumed products with a sweet or bitter taste.

Food preferences are highly variable, resulting in a reluctance to eat new foods, and those less accepted may be reduced in the child. This is influenced by several factors, including the diet during pregnancy and lactation [52] or the mode of exposure and its repetition [51]. These are essential factors that may indirectly influence feeding difficulties and the course of food neophobia, which, depending on individual characteristics, may go unnoticed.

In our study, the length of breast milk feeding ($p = 0.242$), the length of exclusive breast milk feeding ($p = 0.296$), and the time of initiation of complementary feeding ($p = 0.899$) did not correlate with the risk of feeding problems. The Øverby study found no significant association between feeding problems and any breastfeeding nor a significant correlation between exclusive breastfeeding [53]. Maier's study compared the acceptance of new foods by milk-formula-fed and breastfed infants when they received different foods at different frequencies. They found that breastfeeding and milk formula feeding and giving a variety of foods during the early weaning period, rather than giving a specific food, often resulted in better acceptance of new foods, as measured several weeks after the intervention [18].

There are not many studies linking the method of dietary expansion and the occurrence of feeding problems. In our study, we verified the use of the BLW method by assessing the estimated percentage of spoon-feeding during CF. The children we included in the group of children who were fully fed using the BLW method were labelled as entirely or mostly independent eaters, and children who were occasionally spoon-fed by an adult (approximately 10% adult feeding 90% independent) (full-BLW). Children using the complete BLW method in CF did not show a risk of feeding problems ($p = 0.026$), unlike children fed traditionally with a spoon. It should be emphasised that we assessed the full use of the BLW method in the present analysis. The mixed BLW method (50% adult feeding and 50% self-feeding) already indicated a higher risk of feeding problems. Since our study was not aimed at verifying the BLW method as a superior method, we believe that the study should be extended in this respect to fully assess in which aspect the BLW method helps avoid the occurrence of feeding problems.

Other factors also influenced the course of feeding problems. In a study by An M. et al., the main factors were urging the child to eat with a firm refusal on the child's part, unpleasant emotions during mealtimes (e.g., parent's nervousness, stress, child's crying), and high levels of neophobia in the mother [54]. Similar conclusions were reached by de Oliveira Torres et al. [2] in a systematic review of the literature, stating that the level of neophobia in children is influenced by, among other things, the eating habits of the parents, children's innate preference for sweet and salty tastes, the mismatch between texture and the child's psychomotor skills, pressure during meals, failure to read hunger and satiety signals, and monotony in child feeding. In our study, children who experienced a vomiting reflex during complementary feeding were at higher risk of developing food neophobia ($p = 0.001$), whereas spitting food out of the mouth ($p = 0.085$), gagging ($p = 0.244$), choking ($p = 0.590$), and choking and needing medical intervention ($p = 0.121$) did not directly affect the risk of developing feeding problems at a later stage of development.

The high prevalence of feeding problems between the ages of 2 and 6 years may also be because children tend to behave assertively and try to become independent from their parents. Therefore, refusing certain foods is a way of asserting their authority and presence. Another reason for this higher figure may be that older children are influenced by their peers and family, making them more likely to accept new foods [55,56].

The factors influencing food neophobia and feeding problems vary widely. On the one hand, it is a natural developmental stage; on the other hand, some factors may influence the perpetuation of inappropriate behaviour [54]. Therefore, appropriate intervention should be undertaken if neophobic behaviours do not subside but intensify. As in the case of eating disorders, the patient should be managed by a team of specialists, including a paediatrician/gastroenterologist, a clinical dietician, a neurologist, a psychologist, a sensory integration therapist, and a feeding therapist [2,37].

5. Conclusions

The following conclusions can be drawn from this study:

1. Breast milk feeding and the time of CF in the study group did not influence the risk of feeding problems.
2. Using the full BLW method during CF can protect the child against the occurrence of feeding problems, such a food selectivity or picky eating, in the future.
3. In our study, children with difficulties during CF, mainly the vomiting reflex, were more likely to develop feeding problem such as food neophobia.
4. In our study, we did not observe a correlation between age, gender, and the occurrence of feeding problems; there was only a non-significant tendency to be higher in the youngest age.
5. However, further research needs to be undertaken to assess how such behaviour affects subsequent feeding difficulties.

6. Strengths and Limitations of the Study

The results of our study should be interpreted with its limitations in mind. The study should expect some risk of error due to the greater interest of study participants in their children's diets.

Our study was a retrospective study, which may influence the occurrence of the false memory effect, especially in the group of mothers of older children, particularly 4–7 year olds, regarding the details of CF and infancy.

Additionally, the survey was conducted using the CAWI method, which is repeatedly criticised for lacking insight into the data collection process. However, it is worth noting that this type of data collection is widely accepted and convenient for collecting large amounts of information in groups that are often difficult to reach.

The MCH-FS tool was not developed primarily for screening and diagnosing neophobia; however, using the questions in this questionnaire, we believe that many of the questions and answers provided can be a tool for initial screening of food neophobia.

The advantage of the study is the size of the group; to date, most studies on food neophobia among children have been conducted on smaller groups of subjects. It is also worth mentioning that very few studies have been conducted on this topic, especially in Poland, and the above study is also currently being continued. In addition, to date, no cross-sectional study has examined the relationship between the use of the BLW method and difficulties during CF and the CF method, and the occurrence of food neophobia in the preschool age group.

Author Contributions: Conceptualization, A.B.-D. methodology, A.B.-D.; formal analysis, A.B.-D.; investigation, A.B.-D.; resources, A.B.-D.; data curation, A.B.-D.; writing—original draft preparation, A.B.-D.; writing—review and editing, A.B.-D.; visualization, A.B.-D.; supervision, O.K.; project administration, A.B-D. All authors have read and agreed to the published version of the manuscript.

Funding: This research received no external funding.

Institutional Review Board Statement: The Declaration of Helsinki and the Act on the Profession of Physicians and Dentists conducted the study. A positive opinion of the Bioethics Committee operating at the Medical University of Silesia in Katowice was obtained for conducting the research "Dietary neophobia among infants and children" (BNW/NWN/0052/KB/34/23).

Informed Consent Statement: Informed consent was obtained from all subjects involved in the study.

Data Availability Statement: The data presented in this study are available on request from the corresponding author. The data are not publicly available due to restrictions that apply to the availability of these data.

Conflicts of Interest: The authors declare no conflict of interest.

References

1. Pliner, P. Development of measures of food neophobia in children. *Appetite* **1994**, *23*, 147–163. [CrossRef]
2. Torres, T.D.O.; Gomes, D.R.; Mattos, M.P. Factors Associated with Food Neophobia in Children: Systematic review. *Rev. Paul. Pediatr.* **2020**, *39*, e2020089. [CrossRef] [PubMed]
3. Falciglia, G.A.; Couch, S.C.; Gribble, L.S.; Pabst, S.M.; Frank, R. Food neophobia in childhood affects dietary variety. *J. Am. Diet Assoc.* **2000**, *100*, 1474–1481. [CrossRef] [PubMed]
4. Karaağaç, Y.; Bellikci-Koyu, E. A narrative review on food neophobia throughout the lifespan: Relationships with dietary behaviours and interventions to reduce it. *Br. J. Nutr.* **2022**. *ahead of print*. [CrossRef]
5. Hazley, D.; Stack, M.; Walton, J.; McNulty, B.A.; Kearney, J.M. Food neophobia across the life course: Pooling data from five national cross-sectional surveys in Ireland. *Appetite* **2022**, *171*, 105941. [CrossRef] [PubMed]
6. Szajewska, H.; Socha, P.; Horvath, A. Zasady żywienia zdrowych niemowląt. Stanowisko Polskiego Towarzystwa Gastroenterologii, Hepatologii i Żywienia Dzieci. *Stand. Med.* **2021**, *18*, 7–24.
7. Fewtrell, M.; Bronsky, J.; Campoy, C.; Domellöf, M.; Embleton, N.; Mis, N.F.; Hojsak, I.; Hulst, J.M.; Indrio, F.; Lapillonne, A.; et al. Complementary Feeding: A Position Paper by the European Society for Paediatric Gastroenterology, Hepatology, and Nutrition (ESPGHAN) Committee on Nutrition. *J. Pediatr. Gastroenterol. Nutr.* **2017**, *64*, 119–132. [CrossRef]
8. Harris, G. *Food Neophobia: Behavioral and Biological Influences: Neophobia at 20 Months: A Visual Categorization Problem?* Woodhead Publishing: New Delhi, India, 2018; pp. 193–217. [CrossRef]
9. Dovey, T.M.; Staples, P.A.; Gibson, E.L.; Halford, J.C. Food neophobia and 'picky/fussy' eating in children: A review. *Appetite* **2008**, *50*, 181–193. [CrossRef]
10. Szakály, Z.; Kovács, B.; Soós, M.; Kiss, M.; Balsa-Budai, N. Adaptation and Validation of the Food Neophobia Scale: The Case of Hungary. *Foods* **2021**, *10*, 1766. [CrossRef]
11. Capiola, A.; Raudenbush, B. The effects of food neophobia and food neophilia on diet and metabolic processing. *Food Nutr. Sci.* **2012**, *3*, 1397–1403. [CrossRef]
12. Galloway, A.T.; Lee, Y.; Birch, L.L. Predictors and consequences of Food neophobia and pickiness in young girls. *J. Am. Diet Assoc.* **2003**, *103*, 692–698. [CrossRef] [PubMed]
13. Kaar, J.L.; Shapiro, A.L.B.; Fell, D.M.; Johnson, S.L. Parental feeding practices, food neophobia, and child food preferences: What combination of factors results in children eating a variety of foods? *Food Qual. Prefer.* **2016**, *50*, 57–64. [CrossRef]
14. Kozioł-Kozakowska, A.; Piórecka, B.; Pediatrii, K.; Gastroenterologii, I.; Żywienia, P.; Pediatrii, I. Neofobia żywieniowa, jej uwarunkowania i konsekwencje zdrowotne. *Stand Med. Pediatr.* **2013**, *1*, 1–6.
15. Blissett, J.; Fogel, A. Intrinsic and extrinsic influences on children's acceptance of new foods. *Physiol. Behav.* **2013**, *121*, 89–95. [CrossRef]
16. Scaglioni, S.; De Cosmi, V.; Ciappolino, V.; Parazzini, F.; Brambilla, P.; Agostini, C. Factors influencing children's eating behaviours. *Nutrients* **2018**, *10*, 706. [CrossRef]
17. Perry, R.A.; Mallan, K.M.; Koo, J.; Mauch, C.E.; Daniels, L.A.; Magarey, A.M. Food neophobia and its association with diet quality and weight in children aged 24 months: A cross sectional study. *Int. J. Behav. Nutr. Phys. Act.* **2015**, *12*, 13. [CrossRef]
18. Maier, A.S.; Chabanet, C.; Schaal, B.; Leathwood, P.D.; Issanchou, S.N. Breastfeeding and experience with variety early in weaning increase infants' acceptance of new foods for up to two months. *Clin. Nutr.* **2008**, *27*, 849–857. [CrossRef]
19. Hausner, H.; Nicklaus, S.; Issanchou, S.; Mølgaard, C.; Møller, P. Breastfeeding facilitates acceptance of a novel dietary flavour compound. *Clin. Nutr.* **2010**, *29*, 141–148. [CrossRef]
20. Lafraire, J.; Rioux, C.; Giboreau, A.; Picard, D. Food rejections in children: Cognitive and social/environmental factors involved in food neophobia and picky/fussy eating behavior. *Appetite* **2016**, *96*, 347–357. [CrossRef]
21. Mennella, J.A.; Beauchamp, G.K. Beauchamp. Understanding the origin of flavor preferences. *Chem. Senses* **2005**, *30*, i242–i243. [CrossRef]
22. Cooke, L. Genetic and environmental influences on food neophobia. In *Woodhead Publishing Series in Foodscience, Technology and Nutrition. Food Neophobia: Behavioral and Biological Influences*; Reilly, S., Ed.; Woodhead Publishing: Cambridge, MA, USA, 2018; pp. 237–254.
23. Howard, A.J.; Mallan, K.M.; Byrne, R.; Margarey, A.; Daniels, L.A. Toddlers food preferences. The impact of novel food exposure, maternal preferences and food neophobia. *Appetite* **2012**, *59*, 818–825. [CrossRef] [PubMed]
24. Kral, T.V.; Rauh, E.M. Eating behaviors of children in the context of the ir family environment. *Physiol. Behav.* **2010**, *100*, 567–573. [CrossRef] [PubMed]
25. Mitchell, G.L.; Farrow, C.; Haycraft, E.; Meyer, C. Parental influences on children's eating behaviour and characteristics of successful parent-focussed interventions. *Appetite* **2013**, *60*, 85–94. [CrossRef] [PubMed]

26. Rigal, N.; Chabanet, C.; Issanchou, S.; Monnery-Patris, S. Links between maternal feeding practices and children's eating difficulties. Validation of French tools. *Appetite* **2012**, *58*, 629–637. [CrossRef]
27. Kułaga, Z.; Litwin, M. Media-Press sp. z o.o. Warszawa 2018. Normy rozwojowe dziewcząt/chłopców urodzonych przedwcześnie według T.R. Fenton. Normy rozwojowe dziewcząt/chłopców w wieku 0–3 lat według WHO. Normy rozwojowe dziewcząt/chłopców w wieku 3–18 lat oraz normy ciśnienia tętniczego dziewcząt/chłopców według badań OLAF i OLA. Red.
28. WHO. *Multicentre Growth Reference Study WHO Child Growth Standards: Length/Height-for-Age, Weight-for-Age, Weight-for-Length, Weight-for-Height and Body Mass Index-for-Age: Methods and Development*; WHO: Geneva, Switzerland, 2006.
29. Rozporządzenie Ministra Zdrowia z Dnia 6 Kwietnia 2020 r. w Sprawie Rodzajów, Zakresu i Wzorów Dokumentacji Medycznej Oraz Sposobu jej Przetwarzania. Dz.U. 2020 poz. 666. 2022. Available online: https://isap.sejm.gov.pl/isap.nsf/DocDetails.xsp?id=WDU20200000666 (accessed on 16 July 2023).
30. Bocquet, A.; Brancato, S.; Turck, D.; Chalumeau, M.; Darmaun, D.; De Luca, A.; Feillet, F.; Frelut, M.L.; Guimber, D.; Lapillonne, A.; et al. "Baby-led weaning"–Progress in infant feeding or risky trend? *Arch. Pediatr.* **2022**, *29*, 516–525. [CrossRef]
31. Białek-Dratwa, A.; Szczepańska, E.; Trzop, P.; Grot, M.; Grajek, M.; Kowalski, O. Practical Implementation of the BLW Method During the Expansion of the Infant Diet-A Study Among Polish Children. *Front. Nutr.* **2022**, *9*, 890843. [CrossRef]
32. Ramsay, M.; Martel, C.; Porporino, M.; Zygmuntowicz, C. The Montreal Children's Hospital Feeding Scale: A brief bilingual screening tool for identifying feeding problems. *Paediatr. Child Health* **2011**, *16*, 147–151. [CrossRef]
33. Bąbik, K.; Dziechciarz, P.; Horvath, A.; Ostaszewski, P. The Polish version of the Montreal Children's Hospital Feeding Scale (MCH-FS): Translation, cross-cultural adaptation, and validation. *Pediatr. Pol.* **2019**, *94*, 299–305. [CrossRef]
34. Hafstad, G.S.; Abebe, D.S.; Torgersen, L.; von Soest, T. Picky eating in preschool children: The predictive role of the child's temperament and mother'snegative affectivity. *Eat. Behav.* **2013**, *14*, 274–277. [CrossRef]
35. Xue, Y.; Lee, E.; Ning, K.; Zheng, Y.; Ma, D.; Gao, H.; Yang, B.; Bai, Y.; Wang, P.; Zhang, Y. Prevalence of picky eating behavior in Chinese school-age children and associations with anthropometric parameters and intelligence quotient. A cross-sectional study. *Appetite* **2015**, *91*, 248–255. [CrossRef]
36. Tharner, A.; Jansen, P.; Jong, J.K.-d.; Moll, H.; van der Ende, J.; Jaddoe, V.; Hofman, A.; Tiemeier, H.; Franco, O. Toward an operative diagnosis of fussy/picky eating: A latent profile approach in a population-based cohort. *Int. J. Behav. Nutr. Phys. Act.* **2014**, *11*, 14. [CrossRef] [PubMed]
37. Białek-Dratwa, A.; Szczepańska, E.; Szymańska, D.; Grajek, M.; Krupa-Kotara, K.; Kowalski, O. Neophobia—A Natural Developmental Stage or Feeding Difficulties for Children? *Nutrients* **2022**, *14*, 1521. [CrossRef] [PubMed]
38. Anjos, L.A.D.; Vieira, D.A.D.S.; Siqueira, B.N.F.; Voci, S.M.; Botelho, A.J.; Silva, D.G.D. Low adherence to traditional dietary pattern and food preferences of low-income preschool children with food neophobia. *Public Health Nutr.* **2021**, *24*, 2859–2866. [CrossRef] [PubMed]
39. Yong, C.; Kuang, X.; Liu, Y.; Xiang, C.; Xi, Y.; Huo, J.; Liang, J.; Zou, H.; Lin, Q. Parental food neophobia, feeding practices, and preschooler's food neophobia: A cross-sectional study in China. *Appetite* **2023**, *185*, 106547. [CrossRef] [PubMed]
40. Schmidt, R.; Hiemisch, A.; Kiess, W.; von Klitzing, K.; Schlensog-Schuster, F.; Hilbert, A. Macro- and Micronutrient Intake in Children with Avoidant/Restrictive Food Intake Disorder. *Nutrients* **2021**, *13*, 400. [CrossRef]
41. Bell, L.K.; Jansen, E.; Mallan, K.; Magarey, A.M.; Daniels, L. Poor dietary patterns at 1–5 years of age are related to food neophobia and breastfeeding duration but not age of introduction to solids in a relatively advantaged sample. *Eat. Behav.* **2018**, *31*, 28–34. [CrossRef]
42. Di Nucci, A.; Scognamiglio, U.; Grant, F.; Rossi, L. The impact of COVID-19 pandemic on food habits and neophobia in children in the framework of the family context and parents' behaviors: A study in an Italian central region. *Front. Nutr.* **2022**, *9*, 1070388. [CrossRef]
43. Cooke, L.; Wardle, J.; Gibson, E. Relationship between parental report of food neophobia and everyday food consumption in 2–6-year-old children. *Appetite* **2003**, *41*, 205–206. [CrossRef]
44. Flight, I.; Leppard, P.; Cox, D.N. Food neophobia and associations with cultural diversity and socio-economic status amongst rural and urban Australian adolescents. *Appetite* **2003**, *41*, 51–59. [CrossRef]
45. Patel, M.D.; Donovan, S.M.; Lee, S.-Y. Considering Nature and Nurture in the Etiology and Prevention of Picky Eating: A Narrative Review. *Nutrients* **2020**, *12*, 3409. [CrossRef]
46. Kimber-Trojnar, Ż.; Marciniak, A.; Patro-Małysza, J.; Marciniak, B.; Mielnik-Niedzielska, G.; Leszczyńska-Gorzelak, B. Programowanie płodowe. *Ginekologia Perinatologia Praktyczna* **2018**, *3*, 2.
47. Fall CH, D.; Kumaran, K. Metabolic programming in early life in humans. Philosophical transactions of the Royal Society of London. *Ser. B Biol. Sci.* **2019**, *374*, 20180123. [CrossRef] [PubMed]
48. Fernandez-Twinn, D.S.; Ozanne, S.E. Early life nutrition and metabolic programming. *Ann. N. Y. Acad. Sci.* **2010**, *1212*, 78–96. [CrossRef] [PubMed]
49. Godfrey, K.M.; Costello, P.M.; Lillycrop, K.A. Development, Epigenetics and Metabolic Programming. *Nestle Nutr. Inst. Workshop Ser.* **2016**, *85*, 71–80. [CrossRef]
50. Wardle, J.; Cooke, L. Genetic and environmental determinants of children's food preferences. *Br. J. Nutr.* **2008**, *99* (Suppl. S1), S15–S21. [CrossRef]
51. Feeney, E.; O'Brien, S.; Scannell, A.; Markey, A.; Gibney, E.R. Genetic variation in taste perception: Does it have a role in healthy eating? *Proc. Nutr. Soc.* **2011**, *70*, 135–143. [CrossRef]

52. Spahn, J.; Callahan, E.; Spill, M.; Wong, Y.P.; Benjamin-Neelon, S.; Birch, L.; Black, M.; Cook, J.; Faith, M.; Mennella, J.; et al. Influence of maternal diet on flavor transfer to amniotic fluid and breast milk and children's responses: A systematic review. *Am. J. Clin. Nutr.* **2019**, *109* (Suppl. S7), 1003S–1026S. [CrossRef]
53. Øverby, N.C.; Blomkvist EA, M.; Hillesund, E.R. Associations between breastfeeding mode and duration and food neophobia in toddlerhood: A cross-sectional study among Norwegian toddlers. *Food Nutr. Res.* **2020**, *64*, 10–29219. [CrossRef]
54. An, M.; Zhou, O.; Younger, K.M.; Liu, X.; Kearney, J.M. Are Maternal Feeding Practices and Mealtime Emotions Associated with Toddlers' Food Neophobia? A Follow-Up to the DITCoombe Hospital Birth Cohort in Ireland. *Int. J. Environ. Res. Public Health* **2020**, *17*, 8401. [CrossRef]
55. El Mouallem, R.; Malaeb, D.; Akel, M.; Hallit, S.; Fadous Khalife, M.C. Food neophobia in Lebanese children: Scale validation and correlates. *Public Health Nutr.* **2021**, *24*, 5015–5023. [CrossRef]
56. Taylor, C.M.; Emmett, P.M. Picky eating in children: Causes and consequences. *Proc. Nutr. Soc.* **2019**, *78*, 161–169. [CrossRef] [PubMed]

nutrients

Article

Infants Fed Breastmilk or 2′-FL Supplemented Formula Have Similar Systemic Levels of Microbiota-Derived Secondary Bile Acids

David R. Hill and Rachael H. Buck *

Abbott, Nutrition Division, Columbus, OH 43219, USA; david.hill1@abbott.com
* Correspondence: rachael.buck@abbott.com; Tel.: +1-614-624-3148

Abstract: Human milk represents an optimal source of nutrition during infancy. Milk also serves as a vehicle for the transfer of growth factors, commensal microbes, and prebiotic compounds to the immature gastrointestinal tract. These immunomodulatory and prebiotic functions of milk are increasingly appreciated as critical factors in the development of the infant gut and its associated microbial community. Advances in infant formula composition have sought to recapitulate some of the prebiotic and immunomodulatory functions of milk through human milk oligosaccharide (HMO) fortification, with the aim of promoting healthy development both within the gastrointestinal tract and systemically. Our objective was to investigate the effects of feeding formulas supplemented with the HMO 2′-fucosyllactose (2′-FL) on serum metabolite levels relative to breastfed infants. A prospective, randomized, double-blinded, controlled study of infant formulas (64.3 kcal/dL) fortified with varying levels of 2′-FL and galactooligosaccharides (GOS) was conducted [0.2 g/L 2′-FL + 2.2 g/L GOS; 1.0 g/L 2′-FL + 1.4 g/L GOS]. Healthy singleton infants age 0–5 days and with birth weight > 2490 g were enrolled (n = 201). Mothers chose to either exclusively formula-feed or breastfeed their infant from birth to 4 months of age. Blood samples were drawn from a subset of infants at 6 weeks of age (n = 35–40 per group). Plasma was evaluated by global metabolic profiling and compared to a breastfed reference group (HM) and a control formula (2.4 g/L GOS). Fortification of control infant formula with the HMO 2′-FL resulted in significant increases in serum metabolites derived from microbial activity in the gastrointestinal tract. Most notably, secondary bile acid production was broadly increased in a dose-dependent manner among infants receiving 2′-FL supplemented formula relative to the control formula. 2′-FL supplementation increased secondary bile acid production to levels associated with breastfeeding. Our data indicate that supplementation of infant formula with 2′-FL supports the production of secondary microbial metabolites at levels comparable to breastfed infants. Thus, dietary supplementation of HMO may have broad implications for the function of the gut microbiome in systemic metabolism. This trial was registered at with the U.S. National library of Medicine as NCT01808105.

Keywords: breastfeeding; human milk oligosaccharide; pediatric nutrition; metabolomics

1. Introduction

Medical consensus has long held that exclusive breastfeeding is the best source of nutrition and immune protection during early life. Exclusive breastfeeding through 12 months of age is strongly encouraged by prominent medical advisory groups including the American Academy of Pediatrics [1] and the World Health Organization [2]. However, access to healthcare, cultural expectations, and employment outside the home can present significant challenges to exclusive and prolonged breastfeeding [3]. In addition, there are uncommon but compelling instances in which breastfeeding may be contraindicated, such as in infants with significant metabolic disorders, in mothers undergoing radiotherapy, or taking certain pharmacologic agents that may be transferred through milk, the presence of some transmissible infectious disease, or in following mastectomy [1]. Therefore, the provision of nutritionally complete infant formula to support the developing immune system remains an essential goal for pediatric nutrition research.

Significant progress has been made in recent years regarding the fortification of some infant formulas with Human Milk Oligosaccharides (HMOs). HMOs are the 3rd largest solid component of human milk with a broad range of potential benefits, including prebiotic effects and enhanced gut maturation, gut motility, immunity, and cognition [4]. More than 150 unique HMO structures have been identified [5]. Although the individual composition is highly variable, 2′-FL is among the most abundant naturally occurring HMOs with levels ranging from 0.06–4.65 g/L in human milk [6]. Pioneering in vitro experiments indicated that 2′-FL inhibits the binding of gastrointestinal and respiratory pathogens [7–9] and further work in animal models has demonstrated that 2′-FL feeding also attenuates pro-inflammatory signaling within the gastrointestinal tract [10,11]. Epidemiologic studies have demonstrated that the presence of certain HMOs, including 2′-FL, in breastmilk is associated with protection from infectious disease [12] and that premature infants who carry the non-secretor trait have a greater risk of morbidity and mortality due to necrotizing enterocolitis [13].

Recent improvements in the efficiency of HMO synthesis have allowed for the production of HMOs on an industrial scale, making supplementation of infant formula with oligosaccharides that are chemically and structurally identical to those found in human milk more feasible [14,15]. Clinical studies have demonstrated that supplementation of infant formula with 2′-FL is well tolerated [16] and promotes systemic reduction in inflammatory cytokine levels relative to control formula and comparable to breastfed infants [17]. Additional data from the same patient cohort indicated that infants fed formula fortified with 2′-FL experienced fewer respiratory infections relative to infants fed control formula [18]. A similar study suggests that fortification of infant formula with 2′-FL and LNnT may be associated with lower rates of antibiotic use in young children [19].

HMOs, including 2′-FL, readily cross the epithelium of the gastrointestinal tract [20] and have been measured in both plasma and urine from breastfed infants [21–23]. HMOs and their secondary metabolites circulate systemically, affecting multiple organ systems and processes [24]. Given the known role of 2′-FL as a prebiotic capable of influencing the composition and metabolic function of the gut microbiome [25–28], we hypothesized that supplementation of 2′-FL may have substantial effects on the metabolic output of the intestinal microbiome, which contributes significantly to the systemic benefits associated with breastfeeding [29]. We conducted a prospective, randomized, and double-blinded study in a previously studied cohort [16,17] to examine circulating metabolite composition in infants fed one of several formula matrices differing only in their oligosaccharide content and relative to age-matched infants who were exclusively breastfed. We found differences in circulating metabolite composition between breastfed infants and those who were fed a control infant formula. Fortification of infant formula with 2′-FL was associated with an increase in the abundance of microbial fermentation products. We also observed that 2′-FL fortification resulted in a dose-dependent increase in the circulation of microbe-derived secondary bile acids. Secondary bile acids in circulation were associated with changes in circulating cytokine concentrations, suggesting changes to the systemic immune environment. Taken together, these results suggest that 2′-FL fortification of infant formula may support aspects of microbial metabolism typically associated with breastfeeding.

2. Materials and Methods

2.1. Study Design and Population

The present report is a new component of a previously described clinical study [16,17]. Blood samples were collected from a subset of healthy, full-term infants who participated in a prospective growth study, conducted at 28 sites throughout the United States from April 2013 through January 2014. Prior to enrollment, a parent or legally authorized representative of each enrolled infant gave written informed consent. The protocol, informed consent, and all study procedures were reviewed and approved by Schulman Institutional

Review Board, Cincinnati, OH under the ethical approval code 201300836. This trial was registered at clinicaltrials.gov as NCT01808105.

- The inclusion criteria were as follows:
- singleton birth;
- gestational age 37 to 42 weeks;
- birth weight 2490 g;
- 0 and 5 days of age at enrollment;
- exclusive formula or breastfeeding since birth;
- overall good health in the infant's medical history and parental report;
- A resident of a smoke-free home.

Exclusion criteria were the medical history of either the mother or child that might be considered to have potential developmental or growth effects including potential maternal substance abuse. Gestational diabetes was not considered exclusion criteria in cases where infant weight was within the 95th percentile [30]. The use of antibiotics was also considered a cause for exclusion, with the exception of routine antibiotic eye drops used at birth.

Infants whose parents intended to exclusively feed their infants formula were randomized to receive one of three formulas, all containing a total amount of 2.4 g/L of oligosaccharides, according to randomization schedules stratified by site and sex. A non-randomized breastfed (BF) group was also enrolled. A flow diagram illustrating the study group assignments is given in Figure 1. The control formula (CF) contained galactooligosaccharides (GOS; Vivinal® GOS, FrieslandCampina, Amersfoort, The Netherlands) only [CF: 0 g/L 2′-FL + 2.4 g/L GOS]; the experimental formulas (EFs) were fortified with varying levels of 2′-FL and GOS [EF1: 0.2 g/L 2′-FL + 2.2 g/L GOS; EF2: 1 g/L 2′-FL + 1.4 g/L GOS]. The three formulas contained 64.3 kcal/dL (19 kcal/fl oz) (Table 1).

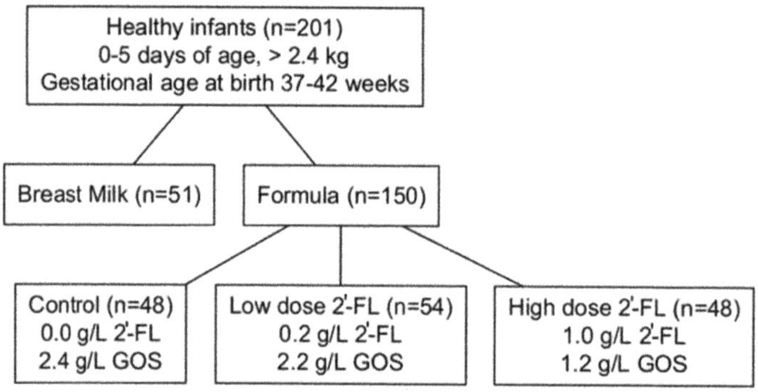

Figure 1. Flow diagram of participants recruited in this substudy. 2′-FL, 2′-fucosyllactose. GOS, galactooligosaccharides.

Table 1. Composition of study formulas. GOS, galactooligosaccharides.

Ingredient	Control Formula	Low Dose 2′-FL	High Dose 2′-FL
Energy, kcal/dL	64.3	64.3	64.3
Protein, g/L	13.3	13.3	13.3
Fat, g/L	34.7	34.7	34.7
Total carbohydrate, g/L	69.0	69.0	69.0
GOS, g/L	2.4	2.2	1.4
2′-FL, g/L	0.0	0.2	1.0

"Exclusively fed" was defined as the sole use of breast milk or assigned formula, and no other liquids or solids. An exception was made for the use of non-antibiotic prescriptions, mineral supplements, and vitamins. Occasional use of alternative feedings, defined as less than 5 times during the study period, was considered consistent with exclusive feeding.

Participant selection for the substudy. Selection for the substudy was determined on the sole basis of parental or legal guardian authorization for the collection of blood samples. Participation in blood sample collection was entirely optional for all study participants

2.2. *Anthropometric, Demographic Data, and Blood Sample Collection*

At the enrollment visit, pre-study feeding regimens, birth anthropometric measurements, gestational age, and demographic data were collected, including race, number, and ages of siblings in the home, and mode of delivery. At 6 weeks (±3 days) of age parents were questioned to determine eligibility for optional blood sampling. The following exclusion criteria were applied:

- >240 mL per week of an alternate feeding other than the assigned study formula or >2 breastfeedings;
- Use of any alternate feeding in the preceding 48 h;
- Maternal or infant use of any oral anti-inflammatory medication.

2.3. *Assays*

2.3.1. Metabolic Profiling

Sample Storage and Preparation. 2–3 mL of non-fasting venous blood was drawn into sodium heparin vacutainer tubes, shipped at ambient temperature to the laboratory, and received within 24 h of collection. Plasma was obtained by standard centrifugation procedure, dispensed into small plastic vials, and stored at −80 °C until analysis. Plasma samples were shipped frozen for analysis to Metabolon, Inc. (Durham, NC, USA). A total of 201 plasma samples were analyzed belonging to the treatment groups listed in Figure 1. Sample collection and analysis were both completed at the conclusion of the clinical study in 2014.

Metabolomic profiling was performed as described previously [31–33]. Metabolites were extracted from 100 μL plasma by the addition of cold methanol. The precipitated extract was split into five aliquots and dried under n_2. The samples were re-suspended in platform-specific solutions before they were applied to the instruments. The untargeted metabolomic profiling platform employed for this analysis was based on a combination of four independent platforms: ultrahigh performance liquid chromatography/tandem mass spectrometry (UHPLC/MS/MS) optimized for basic species, UHPLC/MS/MS optimized for acidic species, UHPLC/MS/MS optimized for polar species and gas chromatography/mass spectrometry (GC/MS) [31–33]. LC-MS was performed on a Waters ACQUITY ultra-performance liquid chromatography (UPLC) and a Thermo Scientific Q-Exactive high resolution/accurate mass spectrometer interfaced with a heated electrospray ionization (HESI-II) source and Orbitrap mass analyzer operated at 35,000 mass resolution [31,32]. Samples destined for GC/MS analysis were derivatized under dried nitrogen using bistrimethyl-silyl-trifluoroacetamide (BSTFA). Samples were analyzed on a Thermo-Finnigan Trace DSQ fast-scanning single-quadrupole mass spectrometer using electron impact ionization at a unit mass resolution [33]. Metabolites were identified by matching the ions' chromatographic retention index and mass spectral fragmentation signatures with reference library entries created from authentic standard metabolites. For ions that were not covered by the standards, additional library entries were added based on their unique retention time and ion signatures. Peak ion counts for each compound in each sample were used for statistical analysis, resulting in the comparisons of relative concentrations. A given compound was reported from only one of the four platforms.

2.3.2. Targeted Assay of 2′-Fucosyllactose

2′-Fucosyllactose (2′-FL) was quantitated by LC-MS/MS. Human heparinized plasma was spiked with the internal standard, melezitose, and subjected to protein precipitation with methanol. After centrifugation, the organic supernatant was removed, evaporated, and reconstituted in Methanol/Water (75:25). An aliquot of the reconstituted extract was injected into Agilent 1290/AB Sciex QTrap 5500 LC-MS/MS system equipped with a BEH Amide normal phase UHPLC column. The peak area of the m/z 487→205 product ion of 2′-Fucosyllactose was measured against the peak area of the Internal Standard (Melezitose) production of m/z 503→323. Quantitation was performed using a weighted linear least squares regression analysis generated from freshly prepared calibration standards.

2.3.3. Plasma Cytokine Measurements

Plasma cytokine levels were measured according to the methods previously published [17]. Among qualifying research subjects, 2–3 mL of non-fasting venous blood was drawn into sodium heparin tubes. Blood samples were shipped overnight to Lovelace Biomedical. Samples were transferred to frozen storage within 24 h of collection. Cytokine concentrations were measured in thawed plasma samples using a multiplex kit according to the manufacturer's protocol (HCYTOMAG-60K-10, custom 10 analyte kit; EMD Millipore).

2.4. Statistical Analysis

Demographic characteristics were analyzed using GraphPad Prism 6.02. Continuous values were compared by 1-factor ANOVA or Kruskal-Wallis test. Categorical variables were compared by χ^2 and adjusted for multiple comparisons). All metabolomics analysis was conducted in R [34] using GNU Emacs v26.2 [35] on Windows 10. Plots were constructed using the R package ggplot2 [36]. Data analysis scripts documenting the complete statistical analysis are available by request from the authors.

3. Results

There were no significant differences among feeding groups for age at enrollment, gender, weight, length, incidence of Cesarian section, or head circumference at birth. There was a significant difference between the high dose 2′-FL and exclusive breastfeeding groups with respect to race, with the breastfed group having more infants that were white and the high dose 2′-FL formula fed having more infants that were black (Table 2). In the original study, 9 of the total 424 participants violated the criteria of "exclusively fed" (1 control formula, 3 low dose 2′-FL, 1 high dose 2′-FL, 4 breastfed) [16]. These numbers did not impact the mean birth weight of any of the groups.

3.1. Breastfeeding Is Associated with Significant Differences in Circulating Metabolites Relative to Control Formula

Although previous studies have examined the metabolic profiles of breastfed infants compared to formula-fed infants [37], improvements in HPLC/MS methodologies have expanded the range of measured metabolites. Thus we set out to broadly characterize the systemic metabolite profile of breastfed infants relative to formula-fed infants. Blood plasma was collected from all study participants at 6 weeks postpartum and blood metabolites were extracted for parallel analysis via GC/MS, LC/MS/MS, and Polar LC to ensure a broad range of metabolite identification. These measurements were matched to a library of metabolite standards for identification, and 743 out of 1113 metabolites were assigned chemical identities with a high degree of precision.

To better understand the differences in systemic metabolites between breastfed and infants fed control formula, we computed the $\log_2$-transformed fold change in the relative abundance of 1113 metabolites among all breastfed infants relative to all infants fed control formula at 6 weeks postpartum and utilized a two-tailed Wald test [38] to evaluate the statistical significance of the observed differences ($p < 0.05$). This analysis resulted in 178 metabolites that were significantly higher among breastfed infants and 238 metabolites that were significantly lower relative to infants fed the control formula (Figure 2, Supplemental Table S1). These analyses revealed differences in systemic metabolites between breastfed infants and infants who were exclusively fed control infant formula.

Table 2. Baseline characteristics of infants enrolled in this sub-study. Values are means ± SEM or mean with percentages of the total in parentheses. 2′-FL, 2′-fucosyllactose. Weight, length, and head circumference were measured at birth. Data on Weight, Length, and head circumference are stratified by gender. Continuous variables were compared between study groups by ANOVA. Categorical variables were compared by Chi-squared test according to the methods described above.

	Control Formula (n = 48)	Breastfed (n = 51)	Low Dose 2′-FL (n = 54)	High Dose 2′-FL (n = 48)	p
Age at enrollment, days	38.1 ± 0.1	3.5 ± 0.2	3.4 ± 0.2	3.8 ± 0.2	0.30
Males, n (%)	27 (56)	31 (61)	24 (44)	23 (48)	0.32
Gestational age, weeks	39.3 ± 0.2	39.4 ±0.1	39.2 ± 0.1	39.4 ± 0.2	0.51
Weight, g					
Male	3338 ± 70	3498 ± 92	3248 ±75	3322 ± 86	0.17
Female	3269 ± 94	3354 ±78	3188 ± 83	3191 ± 69	0.27
Length, cm					
Male	50.5 ± 0.3	51.2 ±0.4	50.5 ± 0.4	51.2 ± 0.5	0.32
Female	50.6 ± 0.3	50.9 ± 0.6	49.7 ± 0.4	50.1 ± 0.4	0.26
Head circumference, cm					
Male	34.8 ± 0.5	35.2 ± 0.4	34.5 ± 0.4	34.4 ± 0.5	0.49
Female	34.1 ± 0.4	33.9 ± 0.5	33.2 ± 0.4	33.5 ± 0.4	0.44
Race, n (%)					0.02
White	30 (63)	35 (69)	29 (54)	20 (42)	
Black	12 (25)	7 (14)	12 (22)	21 (44)	
Other	6 (13)	9 (18)	13 (24)	7 (15)	
Mode of delivery, n (%)					0.58
Vaginal	30 (63)	38 (75)	38 (70)	35 (73)	
C-Section	18 (38)	13 (25)	16 (30)	12 (27)	
Siblings in home	1.3 ± 0.2	1.2 ± 0.2	1.5 ± 0.2	1.2 ± 0.2	0.55

3.2. *Fortification of Formula with 2′-FL Increases Levels of Circulating Microbiota-Derived Metabolites*

Given that our data demonstrated significant differences in systemic metabolites in breastfed infants relative to infants who were exclusively formula fed, we asked whether targeted fortification of infant formula could be utilized to support a metabolic profile that more closely resembled that seen among breastfed infants. HMOs, and 2′-FL in particular, have been established as potent prebiotic compounds both in vitro [24–26] and in vivo [19]. We hypothesized that fortification of infant formula with prebiotic 2′-FL might result in emergent effects on systemic metabolites due to its influence on the composition of the developing microbiota, and the subsequent influence of those microorganisms on the metabolic activity of the gut.

We examined plasma metabolite composition among infants fed formula fortified with 2′-FL at 0.2 g/L (n = 36) or 1.0 g/L (n = 35) relative to matched infants who were fed control formula without 2′-FL (n = 37) or who were exclusively breastfed (n = 40) at 6 weeks postpartum. Analysis of plasma 2′-FL levels revealed a linear correlation with the level of 2′-FL fortification among formula-fed infants (Figure 2A, $r^2 = 0.4$, $p = 2.7 \times 10^{-13}$), indicating that 2′-FL was absorbed into the circulation in proportion with the dietary intake. Similarly, plasma fucose levels were correlated with 2′-FL supplementation in a dose-dependent manner among formula-fed infants (Figure 2A, $r^2 = 0.15$, $p = 2.743 \times 10^{-5}$). 2′-FL fortification was not associated with any change in plasma lactose concentrations in formula-fed infants.

However, the potential impact of 2′-FL fortification on plasma metabolites extends well beyond the increase in 2′-FL and its immediate catabolic products, fucose, and lactose. We examined the fold change in plasma metabolites in infants fed formula containing 0.2–1.0 g/L 2′-FL relative to infants fed control formula (Figure 2B). In comparison to the metabolic changes associated with breastfeeding relative to the control formula, the impact of 2′-FL fortification alone is substantial and accounts for 48 differentially abundant plasma metabolites. Gene Set Enrichment Analysis (GSEA) [39] revealed that these differences in plasma metabolites were consistent with a general increase in markers of benzoate metabolism, a process associated with many dairy products [40], and bile acid metabolism (Figure 2C). Markers of dipeptide metabolism, purine metabolism, and lysophospholipid metabolism were somewhat lower among infants fed 2′-FL-containing formula relative to breastfed infants fed control formula.

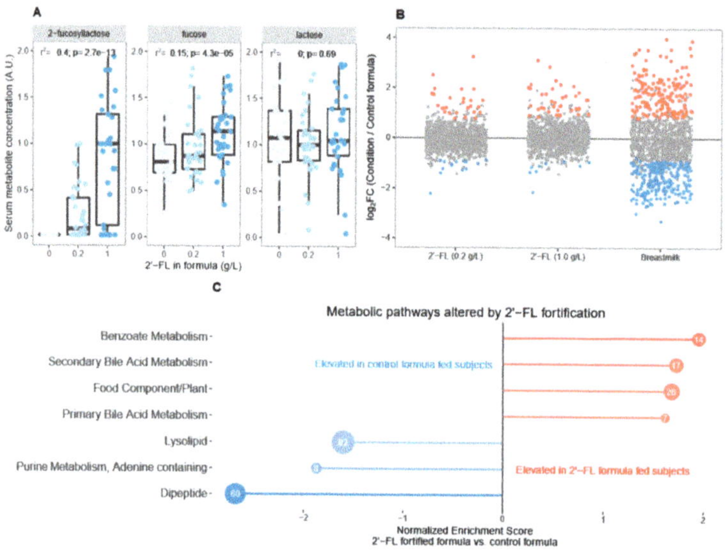

Figure 2. (**A**) Plasma 2′-FL levels are elevated in a dose-dependent manner among infants fed formula containing 0.2–1.0 g/L 2′-FL relative to infants fed formula without 2′-FL. Linear regression analysis demonstrated a strong correlation between formula 2′-FL concentration and relative abundance of 2′-FL (r^2 = 0.4, $p = 2.7 \times 10^{-13}$) and fucose (r^2 = 0.15, $p = 4.3 \times 10^{-5}$) in the plasma but was not correlated with plasma lactose concentration. (**B**) Differentially expressed plasma metabolites in infants fed formula containing 0.2–1 g/L 2′-FL or breastfed infants relative to infants fed control formula that did not contain 2′-FL. Red indicates metabolites that are significantly increased relative to infants fed control infant formula. Blue indicates metabolites that are significantly lower relative to infants fed control infant formula. (**C**) GSEA analysis was conducted using a list of all significantly different metabolites ranked according to the average log2-transformed fold change in 2′-FL fed infants relative to infants fed control formula. This ranked list was evaluated for the enrichment of metabolites in known KEGG metabolic pathways and a NES was computed to evaluate the relative enrichment of metabolites in 2′-FL fed infants relative to infants fed control formula. NES > 0 indicates relative enrichment in infants fed formula containing any amount of 2′-FL and NES < 0 indicates relative enrichment among infants fed control formula relative to 2′-FL enriched formula. The number of metabolites in each pathway is indicated in the bubble. Only pathways with statistically significant ($p < 0.05$) NES are shown.

Given prior data establishing 2′-FL as a potent and selective prebiotic oligosaccharide [24–26], we examined broad changes in bacterial fermentation products in infants fed formula containing 2′-FL, infants fed control formula, and infants who were exclusively breastfed (Figure 3). This analysis revealed increases in microbial fermentation products such as dicarboxylic acids, and both medium- and short-chain fatty acids (SCFA) that were associated with the level of 2′-FL fortification (Figure 3). Remarkably, some SCFAs were present in 2′-FL fed infants at levels comparable to the levels in breastfed infants. We also noted an apparent trend towards dose-dependent increases in microbial fermentation products, with 1 g/L 2′-FL fortification supporting higher levels of some microbial metabolites relative to infants fed formula containing 0.2 g/L of 2′-FL.

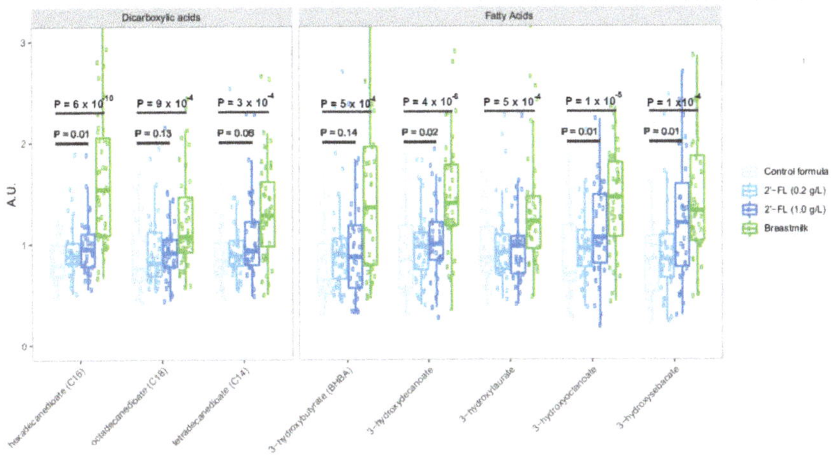

Figure 3. Relative levels of key microbial metabolites dicarboxylic acids, medium- and short-chain fatty acids in each study group. Statistical results represent a one-tailed Wilcoxon ranked-sum test for the comparisons indicated by black bars.

3.3. Levels of Circulating Secondary Bile Acids Differ Significantly in Breastfed Infants Compared to Infants Fed Control Formula

Significant metabolic differences associated with the 2′-FL fortification of infant formula occur in processes associated with or dependent upon the intestinal microbiota (Figures 2 and 3). The most notable among these differences are the changes we observed in secondary bile acid metabolism. Secondary bile acids are exclusively generated by the intestinal microbiota through the action of bile salt hydrolases that convert a limited pool of primary bile acids produced in the liver into a highly heterogeneous mix of derivative structures [41,42]. In the gut, secondary bile acids emulsify dietary lipids [42], suppress the growth of pathogenic microbes [43,44], and promote epithelial cell renewal [45]. The majority of bile acids are reabsorbed by the small intestine and circulate systemically, where they regulate immune homeostasis [46]. Given the importance of secondary bile acids to human health, we first wanted to understand how the bile acid profile of breastfed infants might differ from the bile acids circulating within infants fed control infant formula. We found that many secondary bile acids differed between breastfed infants and infants fed control formula, including 12-dehydrocholate, hyocholate, tau- rolithocholate 3-sulfate, taurocholenate sulfate, and glycolithocholate sulfate which were higher in the plasma of breastfed infants relative to infants fed control formula (Figure 4A). Other secondary bile acids, such as glycoursodeoxycholate, hyodeoxycholate, and ursodeoxycholate were more abundant in control formula-fed infants in comparison to breastfed infants.

3.4. 2′-FL Fortification Is Associated with Dose-Dependent Increase in Circulating Secondary Bile Acids

We next examined the dose-dependent influence of 2′-FL fortification on plasma secondary bile acid levels relative to control formula feeding or breastfeeding (Figure 4B,C). Here it became apparent that 2′-FL fortification of infant formula changes the levels of many secondary bile acids in plasma to levels similar to those seen among breastfed infants, as shown in Figure 4B. The concentration of secondary bile acids in plasma was clearly dependent upon the level of 2′-FL fortification in infant formula (Figure 4C). Thus, 2′-FL fortification impacts aspects of microbial metabolism in the gut compared to control infant formula and increases the production of key bile acid metabolites that may be involved in systemic immune homeostasis.

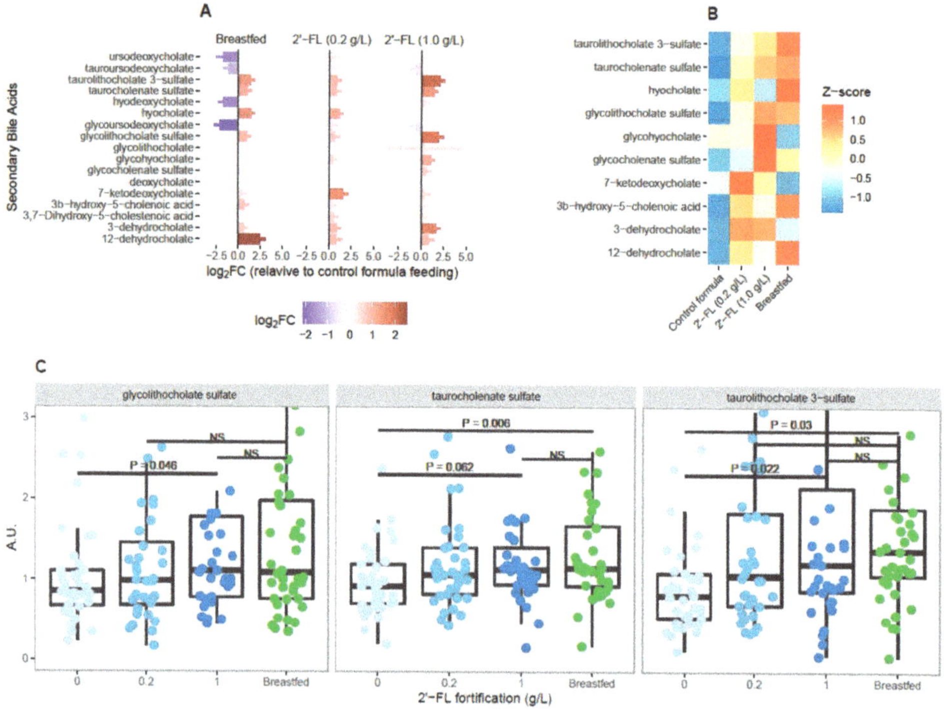

Figure 4. (**A**) Mean log2-transformed fold change in secondary bile acids detected in breastfed infants relative to infants fed control formula that did not contain 2′-FL. Red indicates bile acids that are higher relative to infants fed control formula. Blue indicates metabolites that are lower relative to infants fed control infant formula. (**B**) Heat map showing normalized Z-scores for plasma secondary bile acids among infants fed control formula, formula containing 0.2–1.0 g/L 2′-FL, or infants who were exclusively breastfed. (**C**) Box-plot showing relative abundance of key secondary bile acids in plasma among formula fed infants at two levels of 2′-FL fortification and in the plasma of breastfed infants. Statistical results represent a one-tailed Student's *t*-test for the comparisons indicated by black bars.

3.5. Elevated Secondary Bile Acids Are Correlated with Immunoregulatory Cytokine Levels in Plasma

Given the potential significance of changes in secondary bile acid metabolism for systemic immunity, we hypothesized that secondary bile acid metabolism might be associated with changes in immune mediators in our study participants. The study design included the measurement of plasma cytokine levels in a portion of the blood drawn at 6 weeks post-partum. Notably, these were the same blood samples used to measure plasma metabolites for our other analyses. The following cytokines were measured in plasma via ELISA in all study participants: interferon-α2, interferon-γ, Interleukin 10 (IL-10), Interleukin-1 receptor antagonist (IL-1ra), Interleukin-1α (IL-1α), Interleukin-1β (IL-1β), Interleukin-6 (IL-6), C-X-C motif chemokine ligand 10 (CXCL10, i.e., IP-10), RANTES i.e., CCL5, and tumor necrosis factor α (TNF-α). We then applied a linear regression analysis to examine the potential correlation between secondary bile acid levels in plasma and plasma cytokine levels across all study participants (Figure 5). We found that plasma levels of the secondary bile acid glychocholenate sulfate were significantly and positively correlated with concentrations of the cytokines interferon-α2, IL-10, RANTES, and the chemokine CXCL10. Other secondary bile acid structures, including glycohyocholate, taurocholenate sulfate, and taurolithocholenate 3-sulfate exhibited significant and positive statistical correlations with plasma concentrations of CXCL10 and interferon-α2. These observations suggest that increased circulation of secondary bile acids may promote certain aspects of systemic immune signaling involved in antigen recognition and immune cell trafficking.

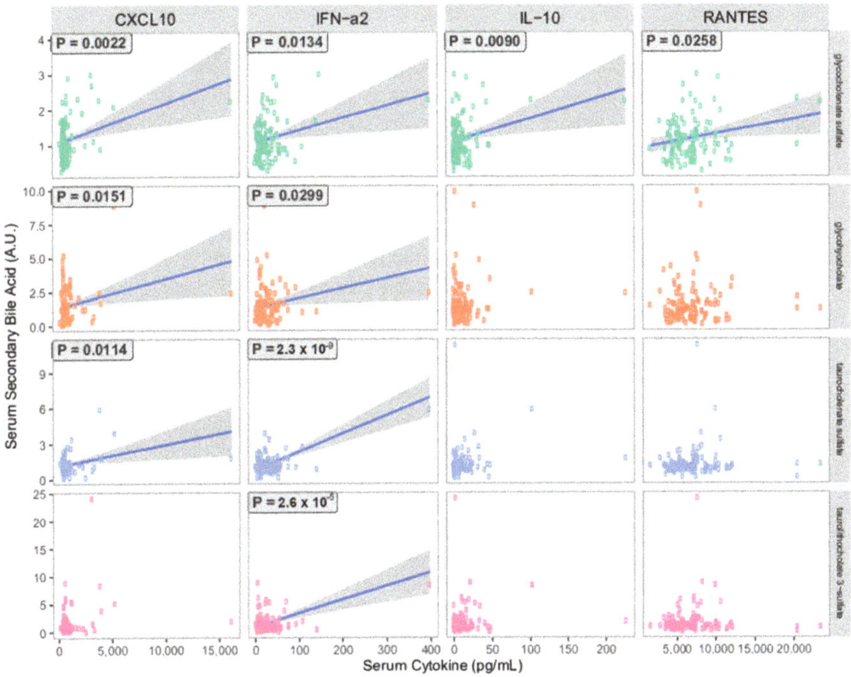

Figure 5. Linear regression analysis comparing plasma secondary bile acid levels and plasma cytokine concentrations among all study participants at 6 weeks postpartum. A p-value is given for combinations that meet the level of statistical significance ($p < 0.05$). Additional cytokines evaluated but not found to have any statistically significant correlation to plasma secondary bile acids include: interferon-γ, IL-1ra, IL-1α, IL-1β, and TNF-α.

4. Discussion

In the present study, we characterized circulating plasma metabolites in breastfed infants relative to infants who were fed one of multiple formula preparations that differed only in their oligosaccharide content. Our data demonstrate that there are multiple differences in circulating metabolites between breastfed infants and infants who were exclusively fed control infant formula (Figure 2). Fortification of infant formula with 2′-FL was associated with an increase in the production of circulating metabolites derived from gut microbial metabolism (Figures 2–5). In particular, 2′-FL fortification resulted in a dose-dependent increase in circulating levels of secondary bile acids relative to the control formula and reaching concentrations comparable to our observations in breastfed infants (Figure 4). Previous reports have demonstrated that secondary bile acid metabolism regulates systemic immunity [46,47] and in the present study, secondary bile acid metabolites in plasma were correlated with plasma cytokine and chemokine concentrations (Figure 5). To the best of our knowledge, these findings represent the first report linking human milk oligosaccharide consumption to the production of secondary bile acids by the gut microbiota in infants.

Metabolomics is a growing field of research utilizing high throughput liquid and gas chromatography, mass spectrometry, and nuclear magnetic resonance techniques to independently quantify and analyze vast numbers of unique metabolites in biological samples [48]. Previous studies have compiled broad surveys of the metabolites present in breastmilk itself [49,50] as well as the differences in circulating metabolites between breastfed and formula-fed infants [37]. Studies examining the differences between formula-fed and breastfed infants have utilized a variety of techniques to measure 356 metabolite composition in stool [51,52], urine [21,52–54], and plasma [21,55,56] samples collected from infants aged 0–24 months. However, wide variations in methodology, sample collection, and study populations have limited the generalizability and reproducibility of these studies [37]. To the best of our knowledge, the present study represents one of the largest surveys of the infant metabolome with 200 enrolled participants. This dataset also includes a wider survey of metabolites (743 known metabolites) than any of the previous reports (<200) [37]. The results are broadly consistent with previous reports associating variation in amino acid metabolism [37] and lipid metabolism [51] with the mode of feeding (Figure 2).

Importantly, the large study cohort and range of metabolites measured have facilitated insights into the metabolic differences between the metabolism of breastfed and formula-fed infants. Given the large number of differentially expressed metabolites that we observed, we applied Gene Set Enrichment Analysis (GSEA) [39] to evaluate the potential for coordinated shifts in metabolites that might be influenced by the mode of feeding. This analysis confirmed previous reports [37,51,55,57] suggesting that steroid metabolism, lipid metabolism and biosynthesis, and amino acid metabolism vary somewhat according to the mode of feeding (Figure 2C). These data characterizing changes in metabolites according to the mode of feeding provide a basis against which to evaluate the benefits of changes to infant formula feeding regimens.

The addition of human milk oligosaccharides (HMOs) is perhaps the most significant recent innovation in infant formula. New methods of production have enabled the cost-effective fortification of some infant formulas with oligosaccharides that are biochemically identical to those that occur in nature [14,15]. Fortification of infant formula with 2′-FL is safe [16,18] and has been shown to confer important benefits to immunity [17] and gut health [19]. Pre-clinical data suggest additional benefits of 2′-FL, which serves as a potent prebiotic [24–26,28] and anti-inflammatory immune modulator [10,11,58–61]. We hypothesized that 2′-FL fortification of control infant formula might alter some systemic metabolic markers and recapitulate metabolic features associated with the consumption of HMOs during breastfeeding. Previous reports have demonstrated that 2′-FL is present in the plasma of breastfed infants at levels that correlate with the concentrations found in the corresponding breast milk; 2′-FL was not detected in plasma samples from infants fed control formula [21]. Our results are entirely consistent with those of Goerhing et al. [21] in that infants fed control formula do not have detectable levels of 2′-FL in the circulation. However, our results also demonstrate that the fortification of infant formula with 2′-FL resulted in a highly significant dose-dependent increase in circulating 2′-FL and free fucose (Figure 2A). This offers additional evidence that dietary 2′-FL is readily absorbed in the GI tract and circulates systemically where it may exert immunoregulatory benefits [24].

The differences in metabolite profiles between infants fed control formula and those fed 2′-FL fortified formula extended beyond 2′-FL and its immediate catabolic products fucose and lactose (Figure 2B). This suggested that the addition of 2′-FL might support additional metabolic activity. Given the known role of 2′-FL as a potent prebiotic and substrate for fermentation by the gut microbiota [24–26,28], we examined the levels of multiple bacterial fermentation products in formula-fed and breastfed infants (Figure 3). 2′-FL fortification was associated with elevated levels of dicarboxylic acids, and medium and short-chain fatty acids typically associated with bacterial fermentation. In some cases, 2′-FL fortification resulted in the production of these metabolites at levels comparable to our observations in breastfed infants. This suggested that dietary 2′-FL acts as either a direct substrate for bacterial fermentation or that it supports the growth of strains that are participating in the fermentation of other dietary compounds.

Other metabolites associated with microbial activity were elevated in infants fed 2′-FL fortified formula. We applied GSEA to analyze the coordinated regulation of metabolites within known metabolic pathways and found that 2′-FL fortification was associated with a significant increase in bile acid metabolism (Figure 2C). Primary bile acids are synthesized from cholesterol in the liver and released into the duodenum via the gallbladder. They play an essential role in the emulsification of dietary lipids, allowing for the efficient absorption of fats in the proximal bowel [62]. At least 95% of bile acids released into the intestinal lumen are reabsorbed by the intestinal epithelium and enter the circulation where they can be reduced to cholesterol and recycled by hepatocytes [63]. This includes a diverse pool of structures known as secondary bile acids. These are generated through a two-step process that involves first the deconjugation of glycine or taurine by intestinal microbes expressing bile salt hydrolases followed by a wide variety of dihydroxylation reactions that result in structural heterogeneity [41,42]. Mode of feeding in infancy has been associated with changes in lipid metabolism [37] and there is some preclinical evidence to suggest that at least one bile acid, cholic acid, is altered in formula-fed primates [64].

We conducted an extensive characterization of differentially expressed secondary bile acids in breastfed infants relative to infants fed the control formula (Figure 4A). Several secondary bile acids, notably 12-dehydrocholate, hyocholate, taurolithocholate 3-sulfate, taurocholenate sulfate, and glycolithocholate sulfate were significantly higher in the circulation of breastfed infants relative to control formula-fed infants. A smaller subset of deoxycholate structures were elevated in control formula-fed infants relative to breastfed infants (Figure 4A). These results indicate that the composition of the circulating pool of secondary bile acids is dependent upon the mode of feeding in infants, a finding that has recently been independently observed in stool samples by Sillner et al. [65]. Upon further examination, it became clear that fortification of infant formula with 2′-FL resulted in the increased abundance in plasma of many of the secondary bile acids associated with breastfeeding (Figure 5B). In many cases, this relationship was dose-dependent with higher levels of 2′-FL fortification being correlated with higher levels of circulating secondary bile acids (Figure 5C). Thus, 2′-FL fortification of infant formula supports the generation of secondary bile acid metabolites at levels typically associated with breastfed infants.

The absence of data on the composition of the fecal microbiota and fecal secondary bile acids in these study participants is a significant limitation of this study. Given the known prebiotic activity of HMOs and 2′-FL in particular [24–26,28], it is possible that the changes in secondary bile acid levels associated with 2′-FL feeding are caused by changes in the composition of the microbiota. Alternatively, 2′-FL may activate alternate metabolic activity by the existing microbiota. Finally, differences in intestinal absorption of secondary bile acids under different feeding conditions cannot be ruled out as a contributing factor in the observed differences in plasma secondary bile acids.

The physiologic significance of secondary bile acids has undergone significant reevaluation in recent years. Emerging pre-clinical studies have demonstrated that these microbe-derived metabolites play a key role in regulating systemic immunity [41,42,47,62]. Secondary bile acids are innate ligands of G protein-coupled bile acid receptor 1 (GPBAR1) and Farnesoid X-Receptor (FXR), expressed by intestinal epithelial cells, and macrophages, dendritic cells, and natural killer T-cells found throughout the gastrointestinal-associated lymphoid tissue (GALT) [66]. Activation of these pathways by secondary bile acids is broadly anti-inflammatory, inhibiting NF-κB mediated cytokine secretion and NLPR3 Inflammasome activity [66–69]. Dysbiosis, or the dysfunctional composition of the intestinal microbiota, alters the pool of available secondary bile acids [41,42,70] and may result in increased susceptibility to inflammatory disease and infection [43,71–73]. Recently, secondary bile acids have been shown to play an essential role in the development of immune homeostasis through the proliferation of a robust population of anti-inflammatory RORγ^+ T regulatory cells within the GI tract [46]. We hypothesized that the changes in circulating secondary bile acids that we observed across our infant feeding cohort might be associated with systemic changes in immune function. We identified multiple secondary bile acids that were positively correlated with concentrations of immune modulators in plasma (Figure 5). In particular, increased plasma levels of glycocholenate sulfate were associated with elevated levels of CXCL10, interferon-α, interleukin-10, and RANTES. This profile may be consistent with a state of gut immune homeostasis associated with robust secondary bile acid signaling [46,62,66,72]. For example, CXCL10 and IFN-α play an important role in the formation of long-lived memory T-cell populations which are critical to immune homeostasis [74,75]. IL-10 is a well-characterized mediator of anti-inflammatory regulatory T cell function [76,77]. RANTES (CCL5) is a multifunctional chemotactic cytokine that serves as one of the key signals for regulatory T cell homing [78]. Future studies may investigate whether the restoration of secondary bile acid metabolites through the fortification of infant formula with 2′-FL could mitigate the risk of allergy, autoimmunity, or inflammatory disease among formula-fed infants.

In summary, the present study demonstrates that fortification of infant formula with the HMO 2′-FL results in the dose-dependent restoration of certain metabolites derived from microbial activity in the gastrointestinal tract, particularly secondary bile acids. These secondary bile acids play a putative role in the development and maintenance of immune homeostasis [41,42,46,47,62] and our data supports a correlation between increased levels of circulating secondary bile acids and the activation of systemic immune mediators.

Supplementary Materials: The following supporting information can be downloaded at: https://www.mdpi.com/article/10.3390/nu15102339/s1, Supplementary Table S1: Differentially expressed metabolites.

Author Contributions: Conceptualization, D.R.H. and R.H.B.; methodology, D.R.H. and R.H.B.; validation, D.R.H. and R.H.B.; formal analysis, D.R.H. and R.H.B.; investigation, D.R.H. and R.H.B.; resources, R.H.B.; data curation, D.R.H.; writing—original draft preparation, D.R.H. and R.H.B.; writing—review and editing, D.R.H. and R.H.B.; visualization, D.R.H.; supervision, R.H.B.; project administration, R.H.B.; funding acquisition, R.H.B. All authors have read and agreed to the published version of the manuscript.

Funding: This research was funded by Abbott, Division of Nutrition.

Institutional Review Board Statement: The protocol, informed consent, and all study procedures were reviewed and approved by Schulman Institutional Review Board, Cincinnati, OH under the ethical approval code 201300836.

Informed Consent Statement: Prior to enrollment, a parent or a legally authorized representative of each enrolled infant gave written informed consent. This trial was registered at clinicaltrials.gov as NCT01808105.

Data Availability Statement: The data presented in this study are available on request from the corresponding author.

Acknowledgments: The authors would like to thank all study participants and their families for their contributions to this research. We also acknowledge the many clinic staff members who helped facilitate study participation and who ensured accurate data collection at each step. Finally, we thank our colleagues Grace Niemiro, and Anice Sabag-Daigle, for their critical revision of the manuscript.

Conflicts of Interest: The authors are employees of Abbott Nutrition, which manufactures Similac® infant formulas containing HMOs.

References

1. Section on Breastfeeding; Eidelman, A.I.; Schanler, R.J.; Johnston, M.; Landers, S.; Noble, L.; Szucs, K.; Viehmann, L. Breastfeeding and the use of human milk. *Pediatrics* **2012**, *129*, e827–e841. [CrossRef]
2. Haroon, S.; Das, J.K.; Salam, R.A.; Imdad, A.; Bhutta, Z.A. Breastfeeding promotion interventions and breastfeeding practices: A systematic review. *BMC Public Health* **2013**, *13* (Suppl. 3), S20. [CrossRef] [PubMed]
3. Office of the Surgeon General; Center for Disease Control. Barriers to Breastfeeding in the United States; Office of the Surgeon General (US), Publication Title: The Surgeon General's Call to Action to Support Breastfeeding. 2011. Available online: https://www.ncbi.nlm.nih.gov/books/NBK52682/ (accessed on 9 March 2023).
4. Bode, L. Human milk oligosaccharides: Every baby needs a sugar mama. *Glycobiology* **2012**, *22*, 1147–1162. [CrossRef] [PubMed]
5. Thurl, S.; Munzert, M.; Boehm, G.; Matthews, C.; Stahl, B. Systematic review of the concentrations of oligosaccharides in human milk. *Nutr. Rev.* **2017**, *75*, 920–933. [CrossRef] [PubMed]

6. Castanys-Munoz, E.; Martin, M.J.; Prieto, P.A. 2′-fucosyllactose: An abundant, genetically determined soluble glycan present in human milk. *Nutr. Rev.* **2013**, *71*, 773–789. [CrossRef]
7. Ruiz-Palacios, G.M.; Cervantes, L.E.; Ramos, P.; Chavez-Munguia, B.; Newburg, D.S. Campylobacter jejuni binds intestinal H(O) antigen (Fuc alpha 1, 2Gal beta 1, 4GlcNAc), and fucosyloligosaccharides of human milk inhibit its binding and infection. *J. Biol. Chem.* **2003**, *278*, 14112–14120. [CrossRef] [PubMed]
8. Weichert, S.; Jennewein, S.; Hüfner, E.; Weiss, C.; Borkowski, J.; Putze, J.; Schroten, H. Bioengineered 2′-fucosyllactose and 3-fucosyllactose inhibit the adhesion of Pseudomonas aeruginosa and enteric pathogens to human intestinal and respiratory cell lines. *Nutr. Res.* **2013**, *33*, 831–838. [CrossRef]
9. Duska-McEwen, G.; Senft, A.P.; Ruetschilling, T.L.; Barrett, E.G.; Buck, R.H. Human Milk Oligosaccharides Enhance Innate Immunity to Respiratory Syncytial Virus and Influenza in Vitro. *Food Nutr. Sci.* **2014**, *5*, 48796. [CrossRef]
10. He, Y.; Lawlor, N.T.; Newburg, D.S. Human Milk Components Modulate Toll-Like Receptor-Mediated Inflammation. *Adv. Nutr.* **2016**, *7*, 102–111. [CrossRef]
11. He, Y.; Liu, S.; Kling, D.E.; Leone, S.; Lawlor, N.T.; Huang, Y.; Feinberg, S.B.; Hill, D.R.; Newburg, D.S. The human milk oligosaccharide 2′-fucosyllactose modulates CD14 expression in human enterocytes, thereby attenuating LPS-induced inflammation. *Gut* **2016**, *65*, 33–46. [CrossRef]
12. Newburg, D.S.; Ruiz-Palacios, G.M.; Altaye, M.; Chaturvedi, P.; Meinzen-Derr, J.; Guerrero, M.L.; Morrow, A.L. Innate protection conferred by fucosylated oligosaccharides of human milk against diarrhea in breastfed infants. *Glycobiology* **2004**, *14*, 253–263. [CrossRef] [PubMed]
13. Morrow, A.L.; Meinzen-Derr, J.; Huang, P.; Schibler, K.R.; Cahill, T.; Keddache, M.; Kallapur, S.G.; Newburg, D.S.; Tabangin, M.; Warner, B.B.; et al. Fucosyltransferase 2 non-secretor and low secretor status predicts severe outcomes in premature infants. *J. Pediatr.* **2011**, *158*, 745–751. [CrossRef] [PubMed]
14. Zeuner, B.; Jers, C.; Mikkelsen, J.D.; Meyer, A.S. Methods for improving enzymatic trans-glycosylation for synthesis of human milk oligosaccharide biomimetics. *J. Agric. Food Chem.* **2014**, *62*, 9615–9631. [CrossRef] [PubMed]
15. Walsh, C.; Lane, J.A.; van Sinderen, D.; Hickey, R.M. From lab bench to formulated ingredient: Characterization, production, and commercialization of human milk oligosaccharides. *J. Funct. Foods* **2020**, *72*, 104052. [CrossRef]
16. Marriage, B.J.; Buck, R.H.; Goehring, K.C.; Oliver, J.S.; Williams, J.A. Infants Fed a Lower Calorie FormulaWith 2′FL Show Growth and 2′FL Uptake Like Breast-Fed Infants. *J. Pediatr. Gastroenterol. Nutr.* **2015**, *61*, 649–658. [CrossRef]
17. Goehring, K.C.; Marriage, B.J.; Oliver, J.S.; Wilder, J.A.; Barrett, E.G.; Buck, R.H. Similar to Those Who Are Breastfed, Infants Fed a Formula Containing 2′-Fucosyllactose Have Lower Inflammatory Cytokines in a Randomized Controlled Trial. *J. Nutr.* **2016**, *146*, 2559–2566. [CrossRef]
18. Reverri, E.J.; Devitt, A.A.; Kajzer, J.A.; Baggs, G.E.; Borschel, M.W. Review of the Clinical Experiences of Feeding Infants Formula Containing the Human Milk Oligosaccharide 2′-Fucosyllactose. *Nutrients* **2018**, *10*, 1346. [CrossRef]
19. Berger, B.; Porta, N.; Foata, F.; Grathwohl, D.; Delley, M.; Moine, D.; Charpagne, A.; Siegwald, L.; Descombes, P.; Alliet, P.; et al. Linking Human Milk Oligosaccharides, Infant Fecal Community Types, and Later Risk To Require Antibiotics. *mBio* **2020**, *11*, e03196-19. [CrossRef]
20. Gnoth, M.J.; Rudloff, S.; Kunz, C.; Kinne, R.K. Investigations of the in vitro transport of human milk oligosaccharides by a Caco-2 monolayer using a novel high performance liquid chromatography-mass spectrometry technique. *J. Biol. Chem.* **2001**, *276*, 34363–34370. [CrossRef]
21. Goehring, K.C.; Kennedy, A.D.; Prieto, P.A.; Buck, R.H. Direct evidence for the presence of human milk oligosaccharides in the circulation of breastfed infants. *PLoS ONE* **2014**, *9*, e101692. [CrossRef]
22. Rudloff, S.; Pohlentz, G.; Diekmann, L.; Egge, H.; Kunz, C. Urinary excretion of lactose and oligosaccharides in preterm infants fed human milk or infant formula. *Acta Paediatr.* **1996**, *85*, 598–603. [CrossRef] [PubMed]
23. Ruhaak, L.R.; Stroble, C.; Underwood, M.A.; Lebrilla, C.B. Detection of milk oligosaccharides in plasma of infants. *Anal. Bioanal. Chem.* **2014**, *406*, 5775–5784. [CrossRef] [PubMed]
24. Eiwegger, T.; Stahl, B.; Haidl, P.; Schmitt, J.; Boehm, G.; Dehlink, E.; Urbanek, R.; Szépfalusi, Z. Prebiotic oligosaccharides: In vitro evidence for gastrointestinal epithelial transfer and immunomodulatory properties. *Pediatr. Allergy Immunol.* **2010**, *21*, 1179–1188. [CrossRef] [PubMed]
25. Yu, Z.T.; Chen, C.; Newburg, D.S. Utilization of major fucosylated and sialylated human milk oligosaccharides by isolated human gut microbes. *Glycobiology* **2013**, *23*, 1281–1292. [CrossRef] [PubMed]
26. Yu, Z.T.; Chen, C.; Kling, D.E.; Liu, B.; McCoy, J.M.; Merighi, M.; Heidtman, M.; Newburg, D.S. The principal fucosylated oligosaccharides of human milk exhibit prebiotic properties on cultured infant microbiota. *Glycobiology* **2013**, *23*, 169–177. [CrossRef] [PubMed]
27. Thongaram, T.; Hoeflinger, J.L.; Chow, J.; Miller, M.J. Human milk oligosaccharide consumption by probiotic and humanassociated bifidobacteria and lactobacilli. *J. Dairy Sci.* **2017**, *100*, 7825–7833. [CrossRef] [PubMed]
28. Garrido, D.; Ruiz-Moyano, S.; Lemay, D.G.; Sela, D.A.; German, J.B.; Mills, D.A. Comparative transcriptomics reveals key differences in the response to milk oligosaccharides of infant gut-associated bifidobacteria. *Sci. Rep.* **2015**, *5*, 13517. [CrossRef] [PubMed]
29. Mueller, N.T.; Bakacs, E.; Combellick, J.; Grigoryan, Z.; Dominguez-Bello, M.G. The infant microbiome development: Mom matters. *Trends Mol. Med.* **2015**, *21*, 109–117. [CrossRef] [PubMed]

30. Grummer-Strawn, L.M.; Reinold, C.; Krebs, N.F.; Centers for Disease Control and Prevention (CDC). Use of World Health Organization and CDC growth charts for children aged 0–59 months in the United States. *MMWR Recomm. Rep.* **2010**, *59*, 1–15.
31. Evans, A.M.; Bridgewater, B.R.; Liu, Q.; Mitchell, M.W.; Robinson, R.J.; Dai, H.; Stewart, S.J.; DeHaven, C.D.; Miller, L.A.D. High Resolution Mass Spectrometry Improves Data Quantity and Quality as Compared to Unit Mass Resolution Mass Spectrometry in High- Throughput Profiling Metabolomics. *Metabolomics* **2014**, *4*, 1–7. [CrossRef]
32. Evans, A.M.; DeHaven, C.D.; Barrett, T.; Mitchell, M.; Milgram, E. Integrated, nontargeted ultrahigh performance liquid chromatography/electrospray ionization tandem mass spectrometry platform for the identification and relative quantification of the small-molecule complement of biological systems. *Anal. Chem.* **2009**, *81*, 6656–6667. [CrossRef] [PubMed]
33. Sha, W.; da Costa, K.A.; Fischer, L.M.; Milburn, M.V.; Lawton, K.A.; Berger, A.; Jia, W.; Zeisel, S.H. Metabolomic profiling can predict which humans will develop liver dysfunction when deprived of dietary choline. *FASEB J.* **2010**, *24*, 2962–2975. [CrossRef]
34. R Core Team. *R: A Language and Environment for Statistical Computing*; R Foundation for Statistical Computing: Vienna, Austria, 2017.
35. Stallman, R.M. EMACS the Extensible, Customizable Self-documenting Display Editor. *ACM SIGOA Newsl.* **1981**, *2*, 147–156. [CrossRef]
36. Wickham, H. *ggplot2: Elegant Graphics for Data Analysis*; Springer: New York, NY, USA, 2009.
37. Phan, M.; Momin, S.R.; Senn, M.K.; Wood, A.C. Metabolomic Insights into the Effects of Breast Milk Versus Formula Milk Feeding in Infants. *Curr. Nutr. Rep.* **2019**, *8*, 295–306. [CrossRef] [PubMed]
38. Love, M.I.; Huber, W.; Anders, S. Moderated estimation of fold change and dispersion for RNA-seq data with DESeq. *Genome Biol.* **2014**, *15*, 550. [CrossRef] [PubMed]
39. Subramanian, A.; Tamayo, P.; Mootha, V.K.; Mukherjee, S.; Ebert, B.L.; Gillette, M.A.; Paulovich, A.; Pomeroy, S.L.; Golub, T.R.; Lander, E.S.; et al. Gene set enrichment analysis: A knowledge-based approach for interpreting genome-wide expression profiles. *Proc. Natl. Acad. Sci. USA* **2005**, *102*, 15545–15550. [CrossRef]
40. Park, S.Y.; Yoo, M.Y.; Paik, H.D.; Lim, S.D. Production of benzoic acid as a natural compound in fermented skim milk using commercial cheese starter. *J. Dairy Sci.* **2017**, *100*, 4269–4275. [CrossRef]
41. Winston, J.A.; Theriot, C.M. Diversification of host bile acids by members of the gut microbiota. *Gut Microbes* **2020**, *11*, 158–171. [CrossRef]
42. Foley, M.H.; O'Flaherty, S.; Barrangou, R.; Theriot, C.M. Bile salt hydrolases: Gatekeepers of bile acid metabolism and hostmicrobiome crosstalk in the gastrointestinal tract. *PLoS Pathog.* **2019**, *15*, e1007581. [CrossRef]
43. Theriot, C.M.; Bowman, A.A.; Young, V.B. Antibiotic-Induced Alterations of the Gut Microbiota Alter Secondary Bile Acid Production and Allow for Clostridium difficile Spore Germination and Outgrowth in the Large Intestine. *mSphere* **2016**, *1*, e00045-15. [CrossRef]
44. Tam, J.; Icho, S.; Utama, E.; Orrell, K.E.; Gomez-Biagi, R.F.; Theriot, C.M.; Kroh, H.K.; Rutherford, S.A.; Lacy, D.B.; Melnyk, R.A. Intestinal bile acids directly modulate the structure and function of of C. difficile TcdB toxin. *Proc. Natl. Acad. Sci. USA* **2020**, *117*, 6792–6800. [CrossRef] [PubMed]
45. Zeng, H.; Umar, S.; Rust, B.; Lazarova, D.; Bordonaro, M. Secondary Bile Acids and Short Chain Fatty Acids in the Colon: A Focus on Colonic Microbiome, Cell Proliferation, Inflammation, and Cancer. *Int. J. Mol. Sci.* **2019**, *20*, 1214. [CrossRef]
46. Song, X.; Sun, X.; Oh, S.F.; Wu, M.; Zhang, Y.; Zheng, W.; Geva-Zatorsky, N.; Jupp, R.; Mathis, D.; Benoist, C.; et al. Microbial bile acid metabolites modulate gut RORγ+ regulatory T cell homeostasis. *Nature* **2020**, *577*, 410–415. [CrossRef] [PubMed]
47. Fiorucci, S.; Cipriani, S.; Mencarelli, A.; Renga, B.; Distrutti, E.; Baldelli, F. Counter-regulatory role of bile acid activated receptors in immunity and inflammation. *Curr. Mol. Med.* **2010**, *10*, 579–595. [CrossRef] [PubMed]
48. Nicholson, J.K.; Lindon, J.C. Systems biology: Metabonomics. *Nature* **2008**, *455*, 1054–1056. [CrossRef] [PubMed]
49. Cesare Marincola, F.; Dessì, A.; Corbu, S.; Reali, A.; Fanos, V. Clinical impact of human breast milk metabolomics. *Clin. Chim. Acta* **2015**, *451*, 103–106. [CrossRef]
50. Gay, M.; Koleva, P.T.; Slupsky, C.M.; Toit, E.D.; Eggesbo, M.; Johnson, C.C.; Wegienka, G.; Shimojo, N.; Campbell, D.E.; Prescott, S.L.; et al. Worldwide Variation in Human Milk Metabolome: Indicators of Breast Physiology and Maternal Lifestyle? *Nutrients* **2018**, *10*, 1151. [CrossRef]
51. Bazanella, M.; Maier, T.V.; Clavel, T.; Lagkouvardos, I.; Lucio, M.; Maldonado-Gomez, M.X.; Autran, C.; Walter, J.; Bode, L.; Schmitt-Kopplin, P.; et al. Randomized controlled trial on the impact of early-life intervention with bifidobacteria on the healthy infant fecal microbiota and metabolome. *Am. J. Clin. Nutr.* **2017**, *106*, 1274–1286. [CrossRef]
52. Martin, F.P.; Moco, S.; Montoliu, I.; Collino, S.; Da Silva, L.; Rezzi, S.; Prieto, R.; Kussmann, M.; Inostroza, J.; Steenhout, P. Impact of breast-feeding and high- and low-protein formula on the metabolism and growth of infants from overweight and obese mothers. *Pediatr. Res.* **2014**, *75*, 535–543. [CrossRef]
53. Chiu, C.Y.; Yeh, K.W.; Lin, G.; Chiang, M.H.; Yang, S.C.; Chao, W.J.; Yao, T.C.; Tsai, M.H.; Hua, M.C.; Liao, S.L.; et al. Metabolomics Reveals Dynamic Metabolic Changes Associated with Age in Early Childhood. *PLoS ONE* **2016**, *11*, e0149823. [CrossRef]
54. Dessi, A.; Murgia, A.; Agostino, R.; Pattumelli, M.G.; Schirru, A.; Scano, P.; Fanos, V.; Caboni, P. Exploring the Role of Different Neonatal Nutrition Regimens during the First Week of Life by Urinary GC-MS Metabolomics. *Int. J. Mol. Sci.* **2016**, *17*, 265. [CrossRef] [PubMed]
55. He, X.; Parenti, M.; Grip, T.; Domellöf, M.; Lönnerdal, B.; Hernell, O.; Timby, N.; Slupsky, C.M. Metabolic phenotype of breast-fed infants, and infants fed standard formula or bovine MFGM supplemented formula: A randomized controlled trial. *Sci. Rep.* **2019**, *9*, 339. [CrossRef]

56. Slupsky, C.M.; He, X.; Hernell, O.; Andersson, Y.; Rudolph, C.; Lönnerdal, B.; West, C.E. Postprandial metabolic response of breast-fed infants and infants fed lactose-free vs regular infant formula: A randomized controlled trial. *Sci. Rep.* **2017**, *7*, 3640. [CrossRef] [PubMed]
57. Hellmuth, C.; Uhl, O.; Demmelmair, H.; Grunewald, M.; Auricchio, R.; Castillejo, G.; Korponay-Szabo, I.R.; Polanco, I.; Roca, M.; Vriezinga, S.L.; et al. The impact of human breast milk components on the infant metabolism. *PLoS ONE* **2018**, *13*, e0197713. [CrossRef] [PubMed]
58. Noll, A.J.; Yu, Y.; Lasanajak, Y.; Duska-McEwen, G.; Buck, R.H.; Smith, D.F.; Cummings, R.D. Human DC-SIGN binds specific human milk glycans. *Biochem. J.* **2016**, *473*, 1343–1353. [CrossRef] [PubMed]
59. Sodhi, C.P.; Wipf, P.; Yamaguchi, Y.; Fulton, W.B.; Kovler, M.; Niño, D.F.; Zhou, Q.; Banfield, E.; Werts, A.D.; Ladd, M.R.; et al. The human milk oligosaccharides 2′-fucosyllactose and 6′-sialyllactose protect against the development of necrotizing enterocolitis by inhibiting toll-like receptor 4 signaling. *Pediatr. Res.* **2020**, *89*, 91–101. [CrossRef]
60. Werts, A.D.; Fulton, W.B.; Ladd, M.R.; Saad-Eldin, A.; Chen, Y.X.; Kovler, M.L.; Jia, H.; Banfield, E.C.; Buck, R.H.; Goehring, K.; et al. A Novel Role for Necroptosis in the Pathogenesis of Necrotizing Enterocolitis. *Cell. Mol. Gastroenterol. Hepatol.* **2020**, *9*, 403–423. [CrossRef]
61. Good, M.; Sodhi, C.P.; Yamaguchi, Y.; Jia, H.; Lu, P.; Fulton, W.B.; Martin, L.Y.; Prindle, T.; Nino, D.F.; Zhou, Q.; et al. The human milk oligosaccharide 2′-fucosyllactose attenuates the severity of experimental necrotising enterocolitis by enhancing mesenteric perfusion in the neonatal intestine. *Br. J. Nutr.* **2016**, *116*, 1175–1187. [CrossRef]
62. Chiang, J.Y. Recent advances in understanding bile acid homeostasis. *F1000Research* **2017**, *6*, 2029. [CrossRef]
63. Staels, B.; Fonseca, V.A. Bile acids and metabolic regulation: Mechanisms and clinical responses to bile acid sequestration. *Diabetes Care* **2009**, *32* (Suppl. 2), S237–S245. [CrossRef]
64. Jackson, E.M.; Lewis, D.S.; McMahan, C.A.; Mott, G.E. Preweaning diet affects bile lipid composition and bile acid kinetics in infant baboons. *J. Nutr.* **1993**, *123*, 1471–1479. [CrossRef] [PubMed]
65. Sillner, N.; Walker, A.; Lucio, M.; Maier, T.V.; Bazanella, M.; Rychlik, M.; Haller, D.; Schmitt-Kopplin, P. Longitudinal Profiles of Dietary and Microbial Metabolites in Formula- and Breastfed Infants. *Front. Mol. Biosci.* **2021**, *8*, 660456. [CrossRef] [PubMed]
66. Fiorucci, S.; Biagioli, M.; Zampella, A.; Distrutti, E. Bile Acids Activated Receptors Regulate Innate Immunity. *Front Immunol* **2018**, *9*, 1853. [CrossRef] [PubMed]
67. Gadaleta, R.M.; van Erpecum, K.J.; Oldenburg, B.; Willemsen, E.C.; Renooij, W.; Murzilli, S.; Klomp, L.W.; Siersema, P.D.; Schipper, M.E.; Danese, S.; et al. Farnesoid X receptor activation inhibits inflammation and preserves the intestinal barrier in inflammatory bowel disease. *Gut* **2011**, *60*, 463–472. [CrossRef] [PubMed]
68. Guo, C.; Xie, S.; Chi, Z.; Zhang, J.; Liu, Y.; Zhang, L.; Zheng, M.; Zhang, X.; Xia, D.; Ke, Y.; et al. Bile Acids Control Inflammation and Metabolic Disorder through Inhibition of NLRP3 Inflammasome. *Immunity* **2016**, *45*, 802–816. [CrossRef] [PubMed]
69. Hao, H.; Cao, L.; Jiang, C.; Che, Y.; Zhang, S.; Takahashi, S.; Wang, G.; Gonzalez, F.J. Farnesoid X Receptor Regulation of the NLRP3 Inflammasome Underlies Cholestasis-Associated Sepsis. *Cell Metab* **2017**, *25*, 856–867.e5. [CrossRef]
70. Khan, T.J.; Hasan, M.N.; Azhar, E.I.; Yasir, M. Association of gut dysbiosis with intestinal metabolites in response to antibiotic treatment. *Hum. Microbiome J.* **2019**, *11*, 100054. [CrossRef]
71. Duboc, H.; Rajca, S.; Rainteau, D.; Benarous, D.; Maubert, M.A.; Quervain, E.; Thomas, G.; Barbu, V.; Humbert, L.; Despras, G.; et al. Connecting dysbiosis, bile-acid dysmetabolism and gut inflammation in inflammatory bowel diseases. *Gut* **2013**, *62*, 531–539. [CrossRef]
72. Sinha, S.R.; Haileselassie, Y.; Nguyen, L.P.; Tropini, C.; Wang, M.; Becker, L.S.; Sim, D.; Jarr, K.; Spear, E.T.; Singh, G.; et al. Dysbiosis-Induced Secondary Bile Acid Deficiency Promotes Intestinal Inflammation. *Cell Host Microbe* **2020**, *27*, 659–670.e5. [CrossRef]
73. Staley, C.; Weingarden, A.R.; Khoruts, A.; Sadowsky, M.J. Interaction of gut microbiota with bile acid metabolism and its influence on disease states. *Appl. Microbiol. Biotechnol.* **2017**, *101*, 47–64. [CrossRef]
74. Huber, J.P.; Farrar, J.D. Regulation of effector and memory T-cell functions by type I interferon. *Immunology* **2011**, *132*, 466–474. [CrossRef] [PubMed]
75. Alanio, C.; Barreira da Silva, R.; Michonneau, D.; Bousso, P.; Ingersoll, M.A.; Albert, M.L. CXCR3/CXCL10 axis shapes tissue distribution of memory phenotype CD8+ T cells in nonimmunized mice. *J. Immunol.* **2018**, *200*, 139–146. [CrossRef] [PubMed]
76. Chaudhry, A.; Samstein, R.M.; Treuting, P.; Liang, Y.; Pils, M.C.; Heinrich, J.M.; Jack, R.S.; Wunderlich, F.T.; Brüning, J.C.; Müller, W.; et al. Interleukin-10 signaling in regulatory T cells is required for suppression of Th17 cell-mediated inflammation. *Immunity* **2011**, *34*, 566–578. [CrossRef] [PubMed]
77. Murai, M.; Turovskaya, O.; Kim, G.; Madan, R.; Karp, C.L.; Cheroutre, H.; Kronenberg, M. Interleukin 10 acts on regulatory T cells to maintain expression of the transcription factor Foxp3 and suppressive function in mice with colitis. *Nat. Immunol.* **2009**, *10*, 1178–1184. [CrossRef] [PubMed]
78. Tan, M.C.; Goedegebuure, P.S.; Belt, B.A.; Flaherty, B.; Sankpal, N.; Gillanders, W.E.; Eberlein, T.J.; Hsieh, C.S.; Linehan, D.C. Disruption of CCR5-dependent homing of regulatory T cells inhibits tumor growth in a murine model of pancreatic cancer. *J. Immunol.* **2009**, *182*, 1746–1755. [CrossRef]

nutrients

Review

Bovine Colostrum in Pediatric Nutrition and Health

Ahmet Alperen Canbolat [1], Mauro Lombardo [2], Alicia del Carmen Mondragon [3], Jose Manuel Miranda López [3], Mikhael Bechelany [4,5] and Sercan Karav [1,*]

1 Department of Molecular Biology and Genetics, Çanakkale Onsekiz Mart University, Çanakkale 17000, Türkiye; ahmetalperencanbolat@stu.comu.edu.tr
2 Department for the Promotion of Human Science and Quality of Life, San Raffaele Open University, Via di 11 Val Cannuta 247, 00166 Rome, Italy; mauro.lombardo@uniroma5.it
3 Laboratorio de Higiene Inspección y Control de Alimentos, Departamento de Química Analítica, Nutrición Bromatología, Universidade de Santiago de Compostela, Campus Terra, 27002 Lugo, Spain; alicia.mondragon@usc.es (A.d.C.M.); josemanuel.miranda@usc.es (J.M.M.L.)
4 Institut Européen des Membranes (IEM), UMR 5635, University Montpellier, ENSCM, CNRS, F-34095 Montpellier, France; mikhael.bechelany@umontpellier.fr
5 Functional Materials Group, Gulf University for Science and Technology (GUST), Masjid Al Aqsa Street, Mubarak Al-Abdullah 32093, Kuwait
* Correspondence: sercankarav@comu.edu.tr

Abstract: Bovine colostrum (BC), the first milk secreted by mammals after birth, is a trending alternative source for supplementing infants and children, offering benefits for gut and immune health. Its rich components, such as proteins, immunoglobulins, lactoferrin, and glycans, are used to fortify diets and support development. Preterm development is crucial, especially in the maturation of essential systems, and from 2010 to 2020, approximately 15% of all premature births occurred at less than 32 weeks of gestation worldwide. This review explores the composition, benefits, and effects of BC on general infants and children, along with preterm infants who require special care, and highlights its role in growth and development. BC is also associated with specific pediatric diseases, including necrotizing enterocolitis (NEC), infectious diarrhea, inflammatory bowel disease (IBD), short-bowel syndrome (SBS), neonatal sepsis, gastrointestinal and respiratory infections, and some minor conditions. This review also discusses the clinical trials regarding these specific conditions which are occasionally encountered in preterm infants. The anti-inflammatory, antimicrobial, immunomodulatory, and antiviral properties of BC are discussed, emphasizing its mechanisms of action. Clinical trials, particularly in humans, provide evidence supporting the inclusion of BC in formulas and diets, although precise standards for age, feeding time, and amounts are needed to ensure safety and efficacy. However, potential adverse effects, such as allergic reactions to caseins and immunoglobulin E, must be considered. More comprehensive clinical trials are necessary to expand the evidence on BC in infant feeding, and glycans, important components of BC, should be further studied for their synergistic effects on pediatric diseases. Ultimately, BC shows promise for pediatric health and should be incorporated into nutritional supplements with caution.

Keywords: colostrum; dairy foods; pediatric nutrition; disease; glycan; preterm infants; milk; necrotizing enterocolitis

1. Introduction

Bovine colostrum (BC) is the first milk secreted by the mammary glands of mammalian species after parturition and has a thicker texture than milk [1]. BC possesses diverse components, including macro and micronutrients, biological peptides, immunoglobulins, and growth factors, along with other ingredients that function primarily in antimicrobial activity [2]. The high nutritional value of BC provides a broad range of food and functional applications [3]. BC is crucial to neonates because of the presence of key nutrients essential for energy, development, and growth. If human milk is limited or unavailable, BC is often preferred as an alternative source of nutrients, such as glucose, amino acids, lactose, and proteins, for infants [4]. In addition to providing developmental support, BC offers constitutional immune protection to newborns, building their innate immunity until the adaptive immunity of neonates matures to match their specific environment.

The colostrum is essential for neonates and provides the nutrients required for essential vital activities. One of the vital functions of milk and colostrum for newborns is to prepare the innate immune system for external environmental conditions, resulting in the onset of adaptive immunity [5]. As an antimicrobial, immunological, and nutritional conditioner, colostrum transitions the newborn from the mostly sterile conditions of fetal life to diverse microbial exposures and nutrients from postnatal breast milk intake. In this context, humans and other mammals share common external environmental conditions and are exposed to similar microorganisms, such as microbes, fungi, and viruses, through the external surfaces of the body (such as the gut, skin, or lungs) [6]. The functional development of the gastrointestinal tract is driven by colostrum consumption in mammalian infants. A range of complex glycans are abundantly found in bovine milk and its products. Glycans are key components of milk glycoproteins and shape microbiota by selectively promoting the growth of beneficial bacterial strains, based on the results of previous research [7]. BC influences metabolism and the hormonal system in neonatal calves and infants [8–10]. The muscular and skeletal repair system is also supported by BC because of its rich composition of bioactive contents [11]. BC consumption prevents injuries and strengthens muscles, which are results of the positive impact of BC on muscle and bone development because of its growth factors [12]. In general, BC has been evaluated as a nutraceutical and has been used in clinical trials to analyze its antiviral and antibacterial potential, with the finding that the antimicrobial properties of colostrum from one species may be effective in another species [13–15]. Undoubtedly, colostrum is essential for the survival of newborns in distinct mammals, such as cows and goats, whereas for human infants, it is considered important but not vital for survival.

Both BC and human colostrum (HC) and their milk products have highly similar compositions, but there are considerable nutritional differences in terms of carbohydrate, lipid, mineral, protein, and vitamin concentrations along with bioactive components (i.e., immunoglobulins) [16]. Nonetheless, the precise and functional immunological support of dairy products in infants and children has not been fully elucidated. In BC applications, safety and tolerability for age groups, including neonates and infants as well as children with allergies, is the first emerging concern. Although prominent studies exist, the mechanisms of bioactive components are still not fully clarified. Current evidence and standard dosage and administration guidelines remain also insufficient in this regard. After optimizing milk products in terms of nutrition for infants and children, evidence from preterm infants in the following years has revealed several serious concerns about these milk products. According to affiliated studies, processed cow milk formulas cause more necrotizing enterocolitis (NEC), inflammatory bowel syndrome (IBD), sepsis (late-onset sepsis, LOS), food intolerance (FI), and allergies compared to either infant-fed formula or a combination with human milk [6,17–21]. The reason for the observable adverse effects of formula products in comparison with milk remains unclear, whether due to their bovine origin, the inclusion of vegetable products, or industrial processing (serial heat treatment or filtration). Additionally, it is not clear whether the risk conditions for infants vary between term and preterm infants, between bovine dairy products and those from different mammalian species (i.e., camels, donkeys, and goats), or between colostrum and milk [6]. New approaches for the production of hypoallergenic infant formulas are important factors in infant nutrition and are currently being investigated. Commercially available formulas frequently promote classical symptoms of cow milk allergy (CMA), and one of the most commonly applied methods to overcome related allergic reactions is the elimination of these allergens from the infant diet; however, the most crucial allergens of milk products are milk proteins, and alternative compensation methods must be investigated since the isolation of milk proteins severely decreases the benefits of milk products [22]. BC is also present in these milk products and should be investigated in this regard.

This review covers the significance, applications, and participation of bovine colostrum (BC) in pediatric conditions and diseases, focusing on its nutritional, preventive, or therapeutic properties for supplementation in severe pediatric or immunologic diseases, particularly in premature infants. The review also comprises clinical animal models and specific human studies. The extent of colostrum in the context of utilization, risk factors, and specific diseases are discussed in detail. Additionally, glycan, one of the most important and common components of colostrum and dairy products, is discussed in detail, as have its applications under several conditions.

2. Components of Colostrum

The composition of BC is close to that of mature bovine milk products; the only difference is the variable rates of bioactive components, making BC a key component for biological processes (Figure 1). BC offers a rich compositional similarity which makes BC a suitable alternative source compared to HC [23]. BC includes higher amounts of IgG content, growth factors, and protein content, promoting muscle growth, tissue repair, and adaptive immunity (see later sections). Although BC is less species-specific than HC, its more abundant contents result in the particularly effective general wellness and recovery of essential systems. Also, the abundance of BC over HC should be noted in the context of availability. Since essential developmental progress in preterm infants is often insufficient, the benefits of BC may aid in their improvements and adjust the insufficient systems when properly used.

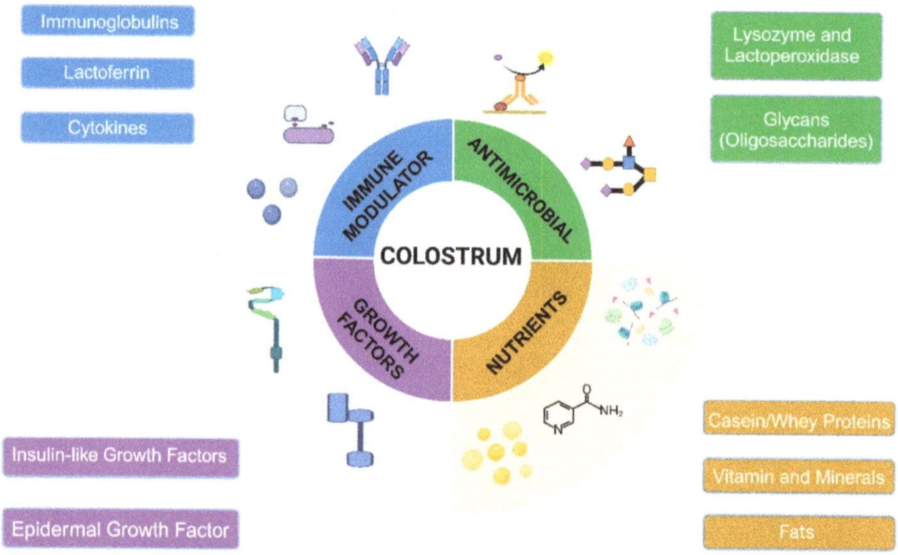

Figure 1. The key components of bovine colostrum. The antimicrobial and immune-modulating properties, growth factors, and nutrients of BC are essential for infants. The relative concentrations of BC differ daily and transform into milk 7 days after parturition (created with BioRender.com, accessed on 27 August 2024).

2.1. Macronutrients

Both human and bovine colostrum consist of analogous structures and components in terms of their nutritional ingredients; the only difference between them is the relative concentration of major macronutrients, in which the protein and fat contents of BC are highly concentrated [23]. At the onset of lactation, the protein and fat concentrations of colostrum are relatively higher than those of lactose, but over time, the protein and fat concentrations decrease as lactose increases [24]. As the lactose content of milk increases over time and as offspring mature, the immunological and trophic role of colostrum transforms into a more nutritional role, ultimately becoming milk [25]. As time passes, the contents of colostrum decrease in favor of nutritional properties other than protective properties. The total carbohydrate composition of colostrum and milk also includes oligosaccharides, which have larger molecular structures than mono- and disaccharides do [6]. As mentioned above, the protein concentrations of BC and milk are much greater than those of HC and milk. This difference also leads to key differences in amino acid concentrations and availability (Figure 2) [6,25].

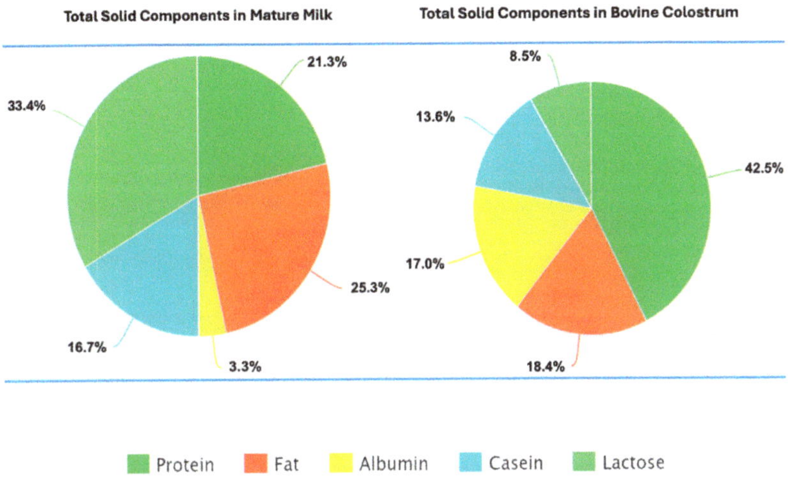

Figure 2. This chart shows the mean (±) levels of total solid components present in BC and mature milk [2]. The difference between BC and mature milk indicates that while BC supports immunity and growth in newborn infants, mature milk is prevalent in terms of its nutritional ingredients. (Created with meta-chart.com, accessed on 24 August 2024).

Milk proteins are generally classified as whey or casein proteins, and throughout mammalian species, their total protein fractions vary [26]. In bovine milk, casein proteins make up 80% of the total protein, and whey proteins make up 20% [27]. In contrast, overall, human milk is dominated by whey proteins (60%) rather than caseins (40%) [28]. Further inspection of milk protein fractions revealed that the milk composition of this species is highly homologous. Specifically, the most common and studied bioactive components of colostrum are immunoglobulins (Igs), lactoferrin (LF), lysozyme, α-lactalbumin, and growth factors [6]. Colostrum contains growth factors such as epidermal growth factor (EGF), transforming growth factor β (TGF-β), platelet-derived growth factor (PDGF), and insulin-like growth factor (IGF), which contribute to wound healing and cell proliferation [29]. The nutritional value of colostrum stems from both its amino acid content and how its proteins are digested in the stomach and upper intestine [30]. Casein proteins create a gel-like structure (or clots) in the upper intestinal compartments, slowing the release of amino acids for absorption, whereas whey proteins dissolve more rapidly and are transferred to the small intestine for faster digestion and absorption [6]. Whey proteins are resistant to protease enzymes, which degrade proteins, and this ability keeps whey proteins functional throughout the GI tract. The variations in resistance levels depend on the age of the infant, as preterm infants are not able to produce enough gastric acid and digestive enzymes. As a result of this lack, preterm infants on breast milk absorb fewer beneficial proteins in the GI tract. It can be assumed that colostrum proteins are not intended merely for growth. The unique feature of colostrum also provides essential immune protection [31].

The diverse components of colostrum affect almost every compartment of the system. According to the current literature, several studies have investigated the potential benefits of whole BC and its distinct components in susceptible newborn infants, as well as their therapeutic effects on pediatric diseases.

2.2. Lactoferrin

Lactoferrin is a glycoprotein that is specifically capable of iron binding and is present in various biological fluids. The highest concentration of LF is found in milk, which means that HC is a valuable source of LF at even higher concentrations. Compared with milk, which has a concentration of 1 mg/mL, HC has an LF concentration ranging from 5 to 6 mg/mL [32]. BC, on the other hand, also includes LF at concentrations ranging from 1.5 to 5 mg/mL, which decreases from 0.02 to 0.35 mg/mL in bovine milk [33]. Some of the remarkable capabilities of LF are its antimicrobial, antioxidant, antitumor, and antiviral properties [34,35]. According to previous studies, LF performs its cellular functions via LF receptor (LFR) interactions. These receptors are located mainly in the microvilli of the intestinal cell membrane, maintaining their presence significantly in the jejunum during the early months of life, as observed in piglet models for the first time [36]. As soon as LF binds to the LFR, it is able to translocate into the cell nucleus, where it triggers gene transcription, resulting in increased cellular proliferation within the intestine [37]. Additionally, LF is capable of binding and sequestering iron (a crucial nutrient for both commensal and pathogenic bacteria), thereby enhancing its antimicrobial properties [6]. This selective antimicrobial ability allows for the elimination of pathogens and stimulates the growth of beneficial microorganisms such as *Lactobacillus* and *Bifidobacterium* in the GI tract [38]. Additionally, in another study, the selective deglycosylation pathway of LF affected the extent of the antimicrobial activity of LF. Sialylated glycans are responsible for the antimicrobial activity of LF, whereas neutral glycans do not have any significant effect [39]. It was also shown that bovine LF (BLF) stimulated the growth of *B. infantis* and *B. brevis*, whereas human LF (HLF) stimulated the growth of *B. infantis* much more effectively [40]. Both the promoting and hindering mechanisms of LF contribute to beneficial health effects, especially in the GI tract, and affect the whole organism.

Similarly, BHL and HLF share approximately 69% of their amino acid identity [41]. Owing to this high homology and the costs of BLF being much lower than those of HLF, BLF has been the most investigated LF species in clinical in vivo trials. Several studies have explored the potential of BLF in preventing inflammatory diseases in premature infants, including necrotizing enterocolitis (NEC) and late-onset sepsis (LOS) [42]. Randomized controlled trials have shown that daily supplementation with BLF in 472 infants or recombinant human LF in 120 infants can protect against NEC and LOS. However, the trial with the largest scale to date included 2203 infants, and LF failed to exert any protective effect [42,43]. A Cochrane meta-analysis with 12 randomized clinical trials and 5425 participants revealed low-certainty evidence that LF supplementation in enteral feeds decreases the LOS but not the NEC in preterm infants [44]. LF also has consistent treatment effects on viruses such as SARS-CoV-1. In addition, it has a special role in recovery because of its benefits to the overall immune system [45]. The vulnerability of preterm infants to respiratory system diseases is also a systemic and severe condition requiring special care, and LF has elimination and recovery effects, indicating its importance in viral infections. LF may support protective mechanisms and trigger the onset of immune response repair. LF also plays a role in dopaminergic cell mechanisms by hindering the Fenton reaction, causing damage with the help of its relative oxygen species (ROS)-modulating properties [46].

2.3. Lysozyme and α-Lactalbumin

Lysozyme is an enzyme belonging to the glycoside hydrolase family and is abundant in animal species. Owing to its antimicrobial properties (Figure 3), it plays a role in innate immune system functions and is found in various body secretions, including tears, saliva, human milk, and mucus [47,48]. This enzyme is broadly distributed in body fluids, as mentioned above, but is found at high concentrations in human breast milk, ranging from 200 to 400 μg/mL, whereas it is present at much lower concentrations in bovine milk, ranging from 0.05 to 1.5 μg/mL [6]. Some studies have reported that lysozyme promotes the protection of the intestinal wall by inhibiting the growth of harmful microorganisms (primarily bacteria) in the GI tract [49]. It also contributes to maintaining a healthy balance in the gut microbiota, which is essential for proper digestive functions and overall gut behaviors.

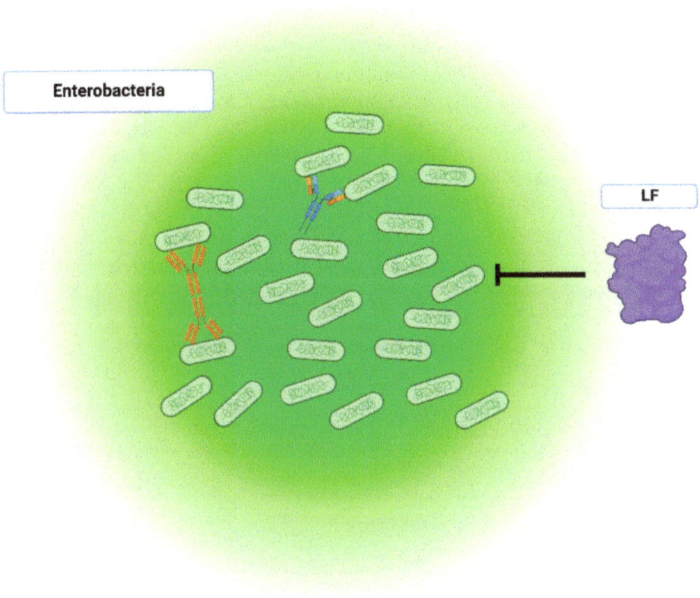

Figure 3. The hindering mechanism between *Enterobacteriaceae* and specific colostrum components. The figure illustrates the regulation of *Enterobacteriaceae* species in the infant gut, including pathogenic bacteria such as *E. coli* and *Salmonella*. Its bioactive components, particularly immunoglobulin A (IgA) and lactoferrin (LF), have strong antimicrobial properties. IgA binds to pathogenic bacteria, neutralizing them and preventing their attachment to the gut lining, whereas LF inhibits bacterial growth by sequestering iron, a nutrient essential for these bacteria. (Created with BioRender.com, access date: 7 September 2024).

α-Lactalbumin is a whey milk protein that plays an important role in lactose synthesis in the mammary glands and serves as a source of bioactive components and amino acids that aid in infant development. Many biochemical and nutritional studies have revealed that α-lactalbumin is an important factor in early infant development [50]. Its concentrations vary from 1.2 to 1.5 mg/mL in bovine milk. Owing to its unique amino acid composition, especially tryptophan, lysine, sulfur-containing amino acids, and branched-chain amino acids, this protein is also believed to contribute to the infant intestinal system and brain development [51]. An improvement in the amino acid composition of bovine milk and its products can be achieved by adjusting the levels of α-lactalbumin and β-lactoglobulin in bovine milk to more closely match those in human milk [6]. Studies investigating the effects of α-lactalbumin also show that this protein has antibacterial potential [52]. In a study attributed to this property, α-lactalbumin, isolated from camels in its apo form, exhibited antibacterial effects on a bacterial strain named *P. aeruginosa* [53]. The isolated form of this protein may not be efficient against most harmful microorganisms, but a combination with enhancers may increase its effectiveness, and further studies should be designed to reveal its potential effects [52,54].

2.4. Immunoglobulins

The immunoglobulin distribution in BC consists of three distinct immunoglobulins, namely IgG (also divided into two subisotypes, IgG1 and IgG2), IgA, and IgM, and bovine milk also contains minor amounts of these immunoglobulins [31] (Table 1). Compositionally, approximately 90% of BC immunoglobulins are IgG, whereas the remaining immunoglobulins are IgM, IgA, and IgG2 [13,55,56]. The primary function of immunoglobulins is to provide essential immune system compartments for the survival of calves by hindering harmful microorganisms, including bacteria, microbes, and viruses [31]. These immunoglobulins are crucial for the survival of calves since without intake, calves are susceptible to pathogenic infections, leading to a high level of morbidity and mortality. Interactions among BC components are not unique to calves but may also have effects on various mammalian species [6]. Immunoglobulin studies indicate that the function and transport of immunoglobulins are not species-specific when BC effects are considered [57,58]. Calves and other mammalian species are born without immunoglobulins, and proper feeding of colostrum is thought to be necessary for the establishment of an immunoglobulin supply; the absorption of immunoglobulins is nonspecific in the first 12–36 h after parturition [59,60]. For preterm infants, the importance of immunoglobulins is much greater since they are developed insufficiently and need special care. Immunoglobulins are a major source of immune system functions. Colostrum feeding and absorption are more important for activating immunity and eliminating disease agents in the first weeks after birth [61]. The administration of colostrum just after birth helps calves eliminate infections such as *E. coli* [62].

Table 1. The mean (±) concentrations of immunoglobulins in BC and bovine milk are shown. After parturition, the concentration of Igs is at its highest. Consequently, the primary role of milk shifts from protection to nutrition, with mature milk containing significantly lower concentrations of Igs.

Immunoglobulin (g/L)	Bovine Colostrum	Bovine Milk
IgG1	60.5	0.355
IgM	4.9	0.045
IgA	4.7	0.05
IgG2	3.8	0.055

2.5. Milk Fat Globule Membranes

Lipid droplets containing triacylglycerols are secreted by integration with the plasma membrane of alveolar epithelial cells, where they acquire a bilayer membrane composed of lipids and proteins, which is referred to as the milk fat globule membrane (MFGM) [6,63]. The bioactive ingredients of these droplets have antimicrobial, anti-inflammatory, and anticarcinogenic properties [64,65]. MFGM proteins are suggested to have nutritional and systemic benefits by assisting in the formation of healthy microbiota and exhibiting anti-infectious and anti-inflammatory properties [66,67]. Environmental factors, maternal genetics, gestation and lactation periods, body composition, and diet have radical influences on the composition of the MFGM [63]. The total MFGM content of BC, which is an abundant source of bioactive proteins, is attributed to the health of neonatal calves, indicating that it may be beneficial for preterm infants [68]. Bovine and human MFGMs are structurally and functionally similar; both have polar lipids in comparable amounts in both species. The lipid groups present in the MFGM are mainly phospholipids and sphingolipids. The MFGM proteome is also highly homologous, with some proteins being more abundant in the bovine MFGM [6].

MFGM proteins show very diverse and beneficial effects on human systems. Research has shown that adding MFGM-enriched protein fractions to milk and formula can aid in protection against infections [69]. For the prevention of diarrhea, certain MFGM proteins in whey protein concentrate inhibit pathogens caused by bacterial or viral strains [70]. In the context of neurobiology, studies involving premature infants indicate that sphingomyelin-fortified milk induces neurobehavioral development [71]. Additionally, sphingolipids such as gangliosides play crucial roles in neurodevelopmental pathways [72,73]. The MFGM proteome has diverse bioactivities, ranging from the antimicrobial functions of mucins and xanthine oxidase to the anticancer properties of fatty acid-binding proteins (FABPs) [74,75]. Mucins and xanthine oxidase act as decoys in the GI tract, preventing pathogens from interacting with epithelial cells. In addition, xanthine oxidase generates ROS and reactive nitrogen species (RNS) that have bactericidal effects. In the context of antiviral activity, one of the components of bovine whey protein with a high molecular weight exhibits antiviral effects on rotavirus in vitro [68]. MFGM glycoproteins are also considered potentially effective against other viruses, such as HIV [76]. When the composition of MFGM proteins is considered, butyrophilin is the most abundant protein and plays several roles in immune-modulation activities, namely, anti-infectious and anti-inflammatory activities [77,78]. Another point to consider is that MFGM supplementation in formula-fed infants has been shown to reduce the presence of *Moraxella catarrhalis*, a common pathogen causing ear infections in young children [79]. Considering the biodiversity of MFGM proteins and their affiliated properties, infant formulas supplemented with these proteins have great potential, leading to more complex and complementary feeding. For preterm infants, more precise and certain studies and trials are essential, yet the potential effects of MGFM proteins provide a trustworthy potential pool for the supplementation of formulas.

2.6. Glycans (Oligosaccharides)

The carbohydrates present in colostrum are predominantly lactose, and several oligosaccharides have more than three monosaccharides structurally [80]. The core structure of oligosaccharides is either lactose or *N*-acetyl lactosamine [81]. Their classification is determined by the presence of a sialic acid, and they can be neutral or acidic [82,83]. A variety of oligosaccharides are present in bovine milk and colostrum, and different types of monosaccharides are bound to the core lactose of *N*-acetyl lactosamine [84]. Carbohydrates exist as free saccharides (such as glucose [Glc], milk oligosaccharides, and glycosaminoglycans [GAGs]) or as glycoconjugates (such as glycoproteins, proteoglycans, and glycolipids) [85,86]. Proteoglycans contain conjugated GAGs in their structure. Heparin, heparan sulfate (HS), and chondroitin sulfate are crucial for the immune system. The most important difference between proteoglycans and glycoproteins is the nature of the glycan [87]. Additionally, oligosaccharides are not digested in the upper GI tract; instead, they are fermented by gut microorganisms in the small intestine and colon [83,88]. The selective prebiotic activity of glycans makes them unique in shaping the composition of the gut microbiome (Figure 4) [89]. Colostrum has the highest levels of oligosaccharides, and after delivery, the levels diminish gradually [88]. Oligosaccharides are mostly abundant in human milk, ranging from 7 to 10 g/L, accounting for 10% of the total calories of milk. In HC, the amount of oligosaccharides increases to 22–24 g/L (1 g/L in BC) but decreases gradually at 48 h postpartum [80]. In a dedicated study by Karav et al. (2016), BC whey proteins were also reported to cleave a significant amount of complex milk glycans that are active biologically, indicating that the variability of glycans is very diverse and unpredictable [7].

GAGs consist of repeating disaccharide units with hexosamine and with diverse acetylation and sulfation activities, along with either uronic acid or galactose (Gal). However, glycoproteins are proteins with glycans that sequentially consist of one residue at a time, not repeating units. The glycosylation of proteins involves several kinds of modifications, including asparagine (*N*-linked glycans), *O*-GalNAc (*O*-linked *N*-acetylgalactosamine), or mucin-type glycans, and, finally, smaller glycan modifications, such as *O*-GlcNAc and *O*-fucose. *N*-glycans play roles particularly in protein folding quality control in the ER, whereas *O*-GlcNAc modifications play roles in signaling modulation, which is complementary, competes with, and acts independently from phosphorylation itself. Most importantly, *O*-fucose, or fucose (Fuc), which is located on serine or threonine residues, is crucial for lymphocyte development through the Notch pathway [87]. These fucosylated oligosaccharides provide developmental support for the nervous system and its healthy functions [90].

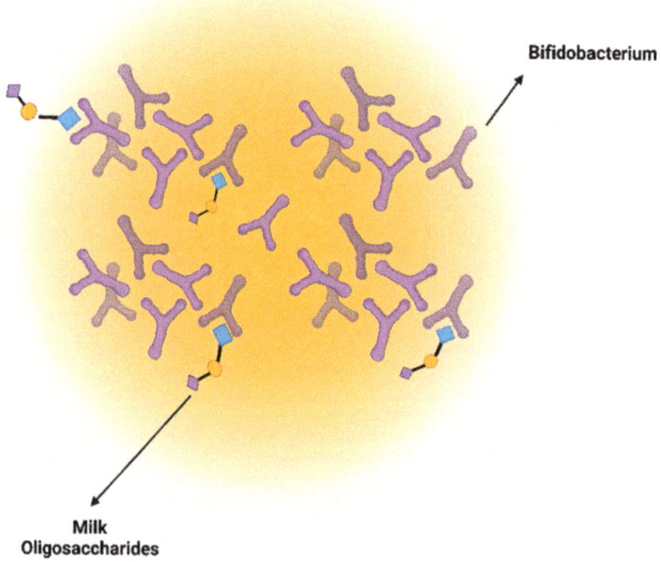

Figure 4. The interaction between milk oligosaccharides and Bifidobacteria species. Human milk oligosaccharides (HMOs), such as those found in human or bovine milk and colostrum, play a critical role in promoting the growth of *Bifidobacterium* in the infant gut, acting as selective prebiotics. *Bifidobacterium* ferments these oligosaccharides, producing short-chain fatty acids (SCFAs) such as acetate and butyrate, which help maintain gut health by lowering the pH and inhibiting pathogenic bacteria. This interaction also enhances the gut barrier, preventing harmful microbes from entering the bloodstream and supporting immune system development.

The microbiota can also synthesize glycans and glycoconjugates (e.g., peptidoglycan, lipopolysaccharides, and glycoproteins) [85,86]. As a key example, *Campylobacter jejuni* is capable of functioning via a basic *N*-linked glycosylation pathway, even though its glycan structure does not share a mammalian structure and composition. Another microorganism, *Mycobacterium tuberculosis*, can synthesize various glycan molecules, such as lipoarabinomannan, in its outer wall, neutralizing oxidizing agents. Fungi, on the other hand, synthesize β-glucans that target pattern recognition receptors (Dectin-1 and Dectin-2, which are part of the C-type lectin family (CTLF)). Additionally, viruses are also related to the production of glycans and are essential for mammals because of their viral life cycle. Viral proteins and their conjugated molecules are synthesized by the host cell replication machinery; thus, viral glycan structures generally mimic the glycome of infected cells [87].

Glycans are essential components of anti-inflammatory pathways in which tumor cells evade immune surveillance to protect themselves. The complexities of these mechanisms have been discovered through glycomic studies of autoimmunity disorders such as rheumatoid arthritis (RA). In a case study conducted in 1985, almost 1400 IgG-derived oligosaccharides from RA patients indicated that IgG glycans changed with the progression of autoimmune disease [91]. RA is related to a relative loss of galactose (Gal) and the exposure of terminal GlcNAc branching points in IgG *N*-glycans. Interestingly, female RA patients who were pregnant achieved remission of RA and had normal IgG glycosylation and sialylation during pregnancy [92]. However, after giving birth, these female subjects lost IgG Gal and sialic acid once again [93]. In addition to RA, certain autoimmune diseases also show significant changes in antibody glycosylation pathways. For example, increased IgG4 fucosylation has been detected in Hashimoto's thyroiditis patients [94,95]. Crohn's disease displays a correlation between the loss of IgG galactosylation and the severity of the disease [96]. In IgA nephropathy, on the other hand, the decrease in *O*-GalNAc glycan galactosylation within the hinge region of IgA1 heavy chains is closely associated [97]. In a different context, Sjögren syndrome triggers the loss of IgG sialylation, as in RA. Studies have shown that patients with allergies exhibit increased levels of sialic acid in total IgE [98]. Research by Shade et al. (2020) revealed that desialylation, the removal of sialic acid, reduced both effector cell degranulation and anaphylaxis in model organisms. Notably, the specific effect of sialic acid on IgE is poorly understood [99]. The colostrum, which is rich in bioactive molecules such as antibodies, immunoglobulins, and immune factors that can help support the development of the immune system in children, has potential therapeutic effects on related autoimmune diseases. These mechanisms include the modulation of immune responses, the improvement of antibody glycosylation, the promotion of gut health, and a reduction in inflammation. This situation may indicate that colostrum may be beneficial for managing the immune dysregulation associated with these diseases. The immunomodulatory and anti-inflammatory properties of colostrum may restore normal glycosylation patterns and mitigate disease symptoms; however, further investigation is needed to reveal the clinical benefits and optimal use of colostrum.

It remains uncertain in many situations whether changes in antibody glycosylation are merely indicators of disease, play a role in disease causation, or influence disease modulation. In the context of RA, the loss of sialic acid and Gal on IgG is not only indicative of disease but also that the proinflammatory nature of a galactosylated IgG actively contributes to the progression of the disease [100]. Notably, high-dose intravenous immunoglobulin (IVIg) therapy, which delivers sialylated IgG, effectively suppresses autoimmunity, demonstrating that the mechanism of action for IVIg therapy involves, at least partially, changes in IgG glycosylation [101,102].

The altered glycan theory is prompted by profound modifications in glycosylation pathways associated with inflammation, infection, and autoimmunity [103]. According to this theory, any form of autoimmunity creates a specific and unique glycan fingerprint on the basis of the relative presence of various glycoforms on tissues, cells, and glycoproteins. In summary, the altered glycan theory provides a framework for the exploration of glycosylation changes in autoimmune diseases, including those affecting children [104]. By applying this theory, researchers may identify unique glycan biomarkers for the early detection, monitoring, and treatment of pediatric autoimmune conditions such as T1D, JIA, pSLE, and autoimmune hepatitis. These advances might hold promise for improving pediatric autoimmunity management through targeted therapeutic and diagnostic innovations.

As mentioned, colostrum can colonize beneficial bacterial species in the colon. In a study by Karav and Mills, *B. infantis* exhibited significant growth by consuming released *N*-glycans as the sole carbon source from milk, although *B. lactis* did not exhibit any growth due to the lack of homologous enzymes. Infant-associated *Bifidobacterium* species, such as *B. infantis*, *B. breve*, and *B. bifidum*, are able to consume these released *N*-glycans and vastly colonize the colon [105,106]. In addition to their symbiotic effects, HC and BC may also be able to function as competitive inhibitors for pathogenic and harmful bacteria by hindering their binding to mucosal surfaces of the GI tract, resulting in the protection of neonates from bacterial infections [6,83]. Human milk oligosaccharides (HMOs) have also been proven to have anti-infectious effects against a wide range of pathogenic microorganisms, such as *Helicobacter pylori*, *Neisseria meningitidis*, and influenza virus, in a variety of models [107]. Recent studies have investigated the potential roles of HMOs in the protection of preterm infants from necrotizing enterocolitis (NEC). In a study using rodent models, the results indicated that the protective effects of HMOs are highly specific to their molecular structure [108]. The structural and prosperous specificity of oligosaccharides highlights the necessity for versatile and further research on milk oligosaccharide supplementation in infant formulas, specifically for vulnerable preterm populations.

3. Bovine Colostrum in the Context of Growth, Development, and Immune Function

The nutritional requirements of infants (6 months and above) are fulfilled by designed and developed follow-up or growing-up formulas. The necessity of the growth, development, and establishment of a long-term diet can be provided by the complementary feeding period, especially when solid foods are introduced into enteral pathways alongside a milk-based diet. Milk from various species (mostly bovine, buffalo, camel, and goat) is utilized to produce dairy products such as fermented milk, kefir, cheese, and yogurt. These products are rich in bioactive components and nutritional benefits and are utilized in infant diets for different durations [109]. Infants have high vitamin and mineral requirements, particularly for iron and zinc. In recent decades, numerous modifications have been made to conventional infant formulas to better match the nutrient content of human milk [6]. These changes reduce overall protein and casein contents, increase α-lactalbumin, and lead to the use of essential oils instead of bovine milk lipids. The purpose is to mimic human milk, which is uniquely tailored to the requirements of infants and, in fact, is even individualized between a mother and her infant. To achieve this goal, novel ingredients such as lactoferrin, osteopontin, lutein, oligosaccharides, MFGMs, and essential fatty acids have been added to manufacture humanized formulas [110]. Despite these efforts, the replication of the exact nutritional and bioactive properties of human milk has proven to be harsh, primarily because of the instability and heat sensitivity of the bioactive components of colostrum. However, since breast milk or alternative milk-based formulas provides most of infants' vital requirements, complementary foods should be nutrient-dense and diverse, including animal-source foods [6]. At this point, colostrum may be a powerful formula component, because as colostrum ingredients meet the essential requirements for infants, there may be a growing trend in the exploitation of colostrum in novel formulations (Figure 5).

Current studies suggest that BC should be used as a supplement for infants under certain conditions, such as the optimal age, time, and standardization for efficient and safe use [111–113]. BC can protect against gastrointestinal diseases, i.e., rotaviral diarrhea, necrotizing enterocolitis, sepsis, and chemotherapy-induced mucositis (all of these diseases will be discussed in detail in the next sections), specifically after pasteurization, and can be used as a supplement to infant formulas [114,115]. Considering the significant promise of BC, infant formulas can be fortified with BC or its components. The promotion of the gastrointestinal tract, the enhancement of the absorption of nutrients, and the strengthening of the defense mechanism of infants may be possible with the fortification of formulas with BC. It is also crucial to standardize the composition of BC fortifiers and design sufficient clinical trials to establish their safety and effectiveness before their introduction into preterm infant nutrition diets. Even if BC is beneficial because of its immunoglobulins and bioactive factors along with other components, it is not recommended for use as a sole nutritional source for infants because of nutritional imbalances compared with human or bovine milk. Adverse effects are minimal in the case of appropriate nutritional guidelines for infants; in fact, these guidelines may support therapies such as probiotics for immunocompromised children [6]. However, BC supplementation is recommended only when a mother's own milk or donor milk is unavailable or insufficient to feed infants.

Bovine colostrum is extensively utilized as a nutritional and immunological supplement for piglets, specifically in modern pig farming, where sows often produce more offspring than they have functional teats for feeding [116]. According to clinical trials with piglets, supplementation with intact BC has been proven to improve piglet survival rates compared with feeding them only with standard formulas, even though it is not as efficient as providing a sow's colostrum from the mother or a foster mother [117]. Like in human infants, BC enhances immunity in piglets through interactions with gut pathogens and the mucosa. Moreover, combining BC with porcine plasma can increase GI health and even promote development in piglets, demonstrating that BC can act as a partly species-specific substitute for porcine colostrum and can sometimes exceed the benefits of porcine colostrum in terms of gut trophic effects and enzyme maturation [6,112]. Humans have discovered the health benefits of BC in the past and have used BC as an alternative dietary option. Recent studies have explored its use in infant nutrition. A clinical trial performed on preterm pigs indicated that the addition of BC to human milk reduced the risk of gut dysfunction and NEC compared with formula-based fortifiers [118]. In a randomized controlled pilot trial, BC powder in combination with human milk and donor milk was proven to be tolerated by preterm infants, increasing protein intake and plasma tyrosine levels without any significant effects. BC has been suggested as a promising alternative to infant formula because of its potential for promoting intestinal health, enhancing nutrient absorption, and supporting immune defense [119]. It is also advised that standardization of the fortifier composition and the performance of more clinical trials are essential before general use. In addition, compared with traditional bovine milk fortifiers, BC fortifiers have been shown to increase antimicrobial activity in vitro and are considered a viable option for preterm infants [119,120].

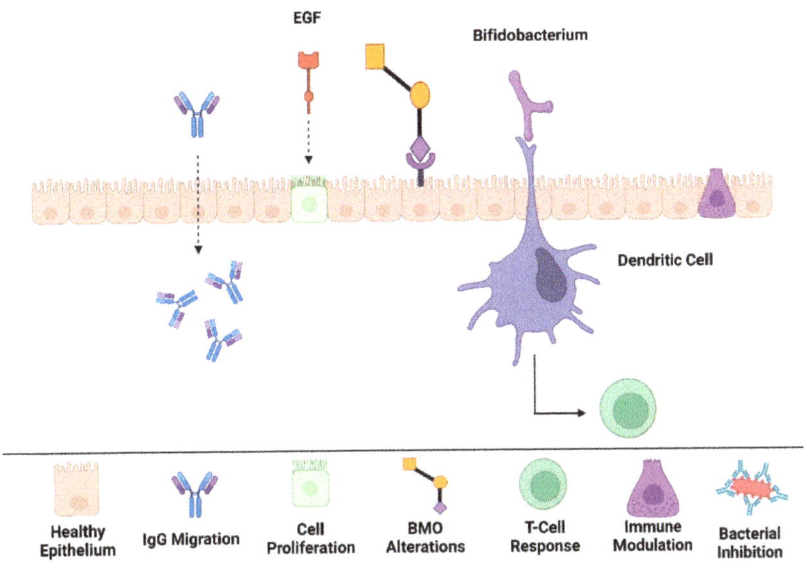

Figure 5. The biological effects of BC and its mechanisms of action. BC supports a healthy epithelium and administers immunoglobulins and growth factors to support immunity and induce cell proliferation. Milk oligosaccharides strengthen the gut barrier by promoting the development of the gut lining. The colostrum also contains immunoglobulins that help prime dendritic cells (DCs). Antibodies can bind to pathogens, making them easier for DCs to recognize, process, and present as antigens to T cells. This mechanism enhances the ability of the immune system to establish an effective response to infections in newborn infants. (Created with BioRender.com, accessed on 7 September 2024).

4. The Potential Roles of Bovine Colostrum in the Context of Pediatric Diseases

4.1. Necrotizing Enterocolitis

Necrotizing enterocolitis is a prevalent and severe condition and is the primary cause of GI-related infant deaths, affecting approximately 3–10% of hospitalized preterm infants globally, with a 50% mortality rate [121–123]. The disease is the most common GI disease, and the primary victims are premature infants who have managed to survive in the early neonatal periods [124]. NEC was first defined more than a hundred years ago following a set of case studies concerning this disease published between the 1940s and 1950s [125,126]. To date, a sufficient number of clinical and scientific studies have been conducted to elucidate the pathogenetic pathways of NEC, develop therapeutic applications and interventions to prevent NEC disease, and advance the management of this disease [127]. Among the aims of these studies, intervention is the most important factor, and surgical application is required in 20–40% of NEC patients to achieve lower morbidity rates. With respect to the triggering factors of NEC, situations such as the prematurity of infants, the presence of a gut microbiome, and enteral feeding, especially with formulations, are notable. The occurrence of multiple combinations leads to the increased severity of NEC. The essential factor that sufficiently reduces the incidence of NEC in preterm infants is feeding with breast milk, according to current studies. This situation can be explained by the ingredients of HC and milk, which are rich in immune factors [6]. Bovine colostrum, as a substitute for HC, may be a promising source for the intervention of NEC incidence. Some remarkable trials have been conducted to investigate the potential effects of BC in preterm infants.

The results of an open-label randomized controlled trial conducted on 120 preterm infants randomly chosen from either a BC group (n = 60) or a control group (n = 60) revealed that preterm infants in the BC group presented a lower level of feeding intolerance, earlier full enteral intake, a shorter period of parenteral nutrition, and a shorter period of hospital requirement, resulting in high statistical and remarkable significance. The complete results indicated a reduction in NEC development among the BC group. None of the preterm infants in either the BC group or the control group developed severe NEC. Additionally, this study revealed sufficient differences between the two groups in terms of the mean hospitalization period. The mean duration of hospitalization was 23.8 days in the BC group and 31.95 days in the control group. However, the mortality rate between both groups was insignificant, with two deaths (3.3%) in the BC groups and three deaths (5%) in the control group. The findings of this study suggest that the use of bovine colostrum in place of infant formulations during the first week after birth may decrease the incidence of NEC in preterm infants. The time needed to achieve full enteral intake, the period of parenteral nutrition, and the period of hospitalization were also reduced [128]. All of the results of this study may be promising indicators that BC can be exploited and adapted to infant feeding more comprehensively.

Recent studies on the interaction between colostrum and NEC have revealed persistent and expected results in this disease. However, previous studies have indicated that colostrum and NEC are either not correlated or that low levels of correlation are observed. A study by Balachandran et al. (2017) reported no significant differences in the incidence rates of NEC and other related diseases upon the administration of BC compared with a placebo. The study was designed as a blinded, parallel-group, block-randomized, and placebo-controlled trial including infants with a birth weight of 1.5 kg, a gestational age of 32 completed weeks, and a chronological age of 96 h. Notably, there was a limitation in this study, as its sample size was too small to verify the obtained results [129]. In a complete set of studies, it was reported that infants who were administered colostrum were able to establish full enteral feeding earlier than those who were administered a placebo or no intervention. Although early development stemming from colostrum administration was proven clinically in preterm infants, the included studies did not show consistent evidence of an effect on the length of hospitalization [130]. Tao et al. (2020) reviewed related studies regarding the effects of colostrum on a set of diseases, including NEC, via a meta-analysis of randomized controlled trials (RCTs). Nine studies, with a total of 689 preterm infants, compared the incidence of NEC. The NEC incidence rate was determined to be 4.7% in the colostrum group compared with 7.7% in the control group. The pooled results indicated no statistically significant difference between the colostrum group and the control group. The development of NEC in the colostrum group was 41% lower than that in the control group [131]. Similarly, a meta-analysis by Sadeghirad et al. (2018) revealed that eight studies (n = 385) were eligible in demonstrating the prevention of NEC. Compared with a placebo, human or bovine colostrum had no effect on severe NEC infants. The only significant difference was in the reduction in the mean days for full enteral feeds (mean difference: −3.55 days). This analysis revealed that the indirect comparison of BC vs. HC showed no effect on any outcome [132]. Until the 2020s, trials and meta-analyses have shown no direct influence of BC on NEC infants. The most common limitation in these trials was the number of patients, where a modest or insignificant number of subjects hindered certain indications for the use of BC in NEC incidence. Future clinical trials are needed to elucidate the effects of BC more clearly.

4.2. Infectious Diarrhea

Diarrhea and related diseases are the main causes of more than half a million deaths in children under 5 years of age worldwide, especially in developing countries [133,134]. In developed countries such as those within Europe and the USA, this disease rarely causes death; nevertheless, it is a significant leading cause of hospitalization and emergency requirements [135]. Acute diarrhea, according to the definition by the World Health Organization (WHO), is the passage of three or more loose or liquid stools per day for 3 or more days and less than 14 days [136]. "Acute diarrhea" or "diarrheal disease" is the preferred definition of this disease in developing countries and the current literature; developed countries define this disease as "acute gastroenteritis", indicating that the effects and consequences of diarrhea have an impact on the classification and point of view [137]. The dynamics of diarrhea lead to a certain definition in which diarrhea is a gastrointestinal infection caused by certain microorganisms, such as rotavirus, norovirus, *Salmonella*, *E. coli*, and *Campylobacter* [138].

Since the prevalence of acute diarrhea is high worldwide, a sufficient number of clinical trials and studies have been designed to evaluate the interventions and overall effects of this disease. In the context of pediatrics, several studies have focused mostly on BC and other components that are high in immunoglobulins and have positive effects on the symptoms of diarrhea. In a study performed in Guatemala, the effects of BC on 301 Guatemalan child patients (154 BC and 147 placeboes) aged 6–35 months with acute non-bloody diarrhea were studied in a randomized, double-blind, and placebo-controlled trial by using PTM202, a derivative product from BC containing specific immunoglobulins eliminating rotavirus, enterotoxigenic *E. coli*, Shiga toxin-producing *E. coli*, and *Salmonella*. The results revealed no significant difference in the duration of diarrhea between the groups. However, a significant reduction in at least one targeted pathogen in the stool in the treatment group was observed. As a result, the duration of acute diarrhea among urban Guatemalan children with specific pathogens in the stool was shortened by PTM202 over a 3-day course. These results suggest that PTM202 may be an additional therapeutic agent for the intervention of infectious diarrhea in pediatric populations with similar stool pathogen distributions [139]. In a meta-analysis aimed at investigating the protective effects of BC against infectious diarrhea in children, a systematic search was performed via the literature, and among 166 research articles, only 5 were selected for the final analysis. A total of 324 children were analyzed to investigate the effects of BC (or related byproducts) on infectious diarrhea in the context of stool frequency, the incidence rate of diarrhea, and the presence of the pathogen in the stool. Consequently, this systematic review concluded that BC or its byproducts were indeed effective in diminishing the frequency rate of stool, the incidence rate at the end of the intervention, and positive detection of rotavirus, in which approximately 30% of children with diarrhea were rotavirus positive and had E. coli in stool, in comparison with the placebo [140]. All the data were pooled, and the collective results demonstrated that BC was associated with a significant reduction in the frequency of infectious diarrhea in the stool, with a value of approximately 1.42 times per day. BC intervention was also associated with an incidence rate of disease of 71%. The final evaluation revealed that BC and its byproducts have a significant positive effect on reducing the frequency and relieving the symptoms of infectious diarrhea in children [141].

These positive results are promising since children with severe diarrhea generally have recurring and/or persistent diarrhea symptoms and continuous problems in developing countries [142]. The inexpensive and safe conditions of BC make it a superior alternative in such situations. In Egypt, which is considered a developing country, a clinical trial aiming to evaluate the efficiency and tolerability of BC administration for the prevention of recurrent upper respiratory tract infections (URTIs) and diarrhea in 160 children (aged between 1 and 6 years) with previously mentioned diseases was conducted, with BC administered for 4 weeks. The number of episodes of the mentioned diseases and the frequency of hospitalization required for diseases during the study were assessed at weeks 8 and 24. The results indicated that after the administration of BC, the mean ($\pm$) SD number of episodes of diarrhea decreased from 6.1 ± 2.0 at baseline to 3.7 ± 2.5 at the end of 2 months. It has also been reported that BC is effective in the prevention of recurrent URTIs and diarrhea, as it causes a reduction in the number of episodes and hospitalizations. These results suggest that BC could be a novel therapeutic option for children with recurrent URTIs and diarrhea [143]. In general, BC is considered an alternative and curative source for treating GI tract diseases, and diarrhea is one of the most investigated diseases in BC. The limitations of BC use are affected by several factors, including its inability to target specific pathogens, the potential for allergic reactions in infants with milk protein sensitivities (discussed in Section 5), and the lack of a standardized dose for treating diarrhea. Further studies are advised to understand this more clearly.

4.3. *Inflammatory Bowel Disease*

Inflammatory bowel disease (IDB) is a chronic, relapsing inflammatory disease affecting the gastrointestinal compartments. There are two main IDB diseases, namely Crohn's disease (CD) and ulcerative colitis (UC) [144]. The pathogenesis and causes of IDB are due primarily to genetic and environmental factors, microbiota alterations, and strong immune responses [145–147]. The dysregulated immune response in IDB patients is linked to T helper (Th) 1 cells in CD patients and Th2 cells in UC patients [148]. The main mechanism of IDB pathogenesis is the activation of Th17 cells, which release IL-17, and the altered cross-regulation between Th17 and regulatory T cells in the GI tract of IDB patients [149]. If the intestinal epithelium, covered by the mucosal layer and in contact with extrinsic factors such as food antigens and bacteria, is damaged, intestinal inflammation may occur, in which dysfunction of the intestinal epithelium is also associated with nutrient malabsorption [150]. The treatment options for IDB patients include anti-inflammatory drugs (aminosalicylates and corticosteroids), immunosuppressive agents (methotrexate and azathioprine), antibiotics, and biological agents (infliximab and vedolizumab) [147,151,152]. Alternative therapeutic applications, such as a healthy lifestyle, personalized diets, and avoiding stress, are also possible for IDB patients [153,154]. Even if these approaches are used for IDB, they are insufficient, and more effective therapies are essential. In this regard, BC may be a potential therapeutic approach, and several related investigations have validated that BC ingredients may have an impact on the clinical course of the GI tract, including the prevalence of IDB [155].

The ingredients of BC have been investigated for IBD treatment in a few studies. These studies were conducted mainly in vitro and occasionally in mouse models, along with a few human clinical trials. One of the studies by Lee et al. (2019) indicated that both whole and whey BC fractions might suppress lipopolysaccharide-induced NF-κB activation in mouse adipocytes. The anti-inflammatory and antioxidative effects of whole BC were much greater than those of whey BC. In mice with DSS-induced colitis, the administration of BC aided in epithelial regeneration [156]. In the same mouse model, BC supplementation also contributed to clinical recovery from colitis [155]. Current studies on BC supplementation have focused on healthy subjects, primarily athletes and children [157]. Another study on BC revealed a correlation between BC supplementation and cytokine secretion in the peripheral blood mononuclear cells (PBMCs) of four male endurance athletes. The concentration of BC led to the increased secretion of IL-2, IL-10, and IFN-γ [158]. Aside from the indirect studies mentioned, there are currently no direct studies specifically investigating the effects of BC in patients with IDB. The sole study by Khan et al. (2002)

was a randomized, double-blind, and controlled trial which examined the efficiency of colostrum enemas in the treatment of distal colitis. Fourteen patients (eight females) with a mean age of 45 years (17–75 years range) and mild to moderate severe distal colitis were administered colostrum enemas (100 mL of a 10% solution) or a placebo (albumin solution) for 4 weeks. The activity of the disease was monitored at 0, 2, and 4 weeks. The study concluded that at the end of the fourth week, the colostrum group presented a mean reduction in symptom scores and disease remission in most patients with active left-sided colitis, whereas patients administered mesalazine with placebo enemas presented minimal levels of recurrence [159]. In the context of pediatric and child health, no clinical trials are currently available, and studies indicate that the activity of IBD has been significantly reduced. Common limitations such as sufficient evidence and potential allergic reactions are also present in IBD trials. Further studies regarding child health and pediatry are necessary to optimize and visualize the potential and proven effects of BC.

4.4. Short Bowel Syndrome

Short bowel syndrome (SBS) is a complication of extensive intestinal resection or atresia that commonly occurs in infants and children. This disease may occur in two periods: after birth or in older childhood. In newborns, this complication may arise most commonly from necrotizing enterocolitis (NEC), midgut volvulus, and gastroschisis but more commonly from trauma, intestinal thrombosis, and surgical failure in older children [160]. The progression of the disease can be used to classify SBS patients into two subgroups. According to the functional capability of the remaining gut, the disease is categorized as intestinal insufficiency (II) or intestinal failure (IF). II has been defined as a reduction in the functional gut with preserved ability, resulting in the digestion and absorption of a sufficient amount of nutrients along with fluids from a conventional diet to preserve growth. IF has been defined as a reduction in the functional gut without preserved ability, resulting in the inability to digest and absorb enough nutrients and fluids in a conventional diet, maintaining growth and preventing parenteral nutrition (PN) [161–164]. It can be concluded that II patients are non-PN-dependent, whereas IF patients are PN-dependent [165].

For other GI tract diseases, the effects of BC in SBS have been investigated. Since the beneficial ingredients and effects of BC are well known, a certain number of animal trials and studies are present in the current literature. A clinical study was conducted to examine the effectiveness of BC in improving intestinal function in children with short bowel syndrome (SBS) through metabolic balance assessments. The study involved nine children with SBS in a randomized crossover design, where 20% of their enteral fluid intake was replaced with either BC or a mixed milk diet for four weeks. Energy and wet weight absorption were measured to evaluate the impact of BC on intestinal function. The results revealed that, compared with a mixed milk diet, a BC diet did not increase energy or wet weight absorption. There were also no significant differences in growth or development, as measured by weight and knemometry, between the two diets. Additionally, less than 150% of enteral energy absorption met the basal metabolic rate, and only 50% of enteral fluid absorption met the basal fluid requirements, indicating intestinal failure and the continued necessity for PN. In summary, the study concluded that a diet supplemented with BC did not improve intestinal functions [165]. Another study, similar to the previous one, hypothesized that minimal enteral nutrition (MEN) with BC would stimulate the adaptation of the intestine, rather than formula, and would be sufficiently tolerated in SBS patients because of the growth factors in BC. In two distinct experiments involving 3-day-old piglets and five infants, BC was added to the determined diets. In experiment 2, the tolerance and feasibility of BC supplementation were monitored in a pilot study with five infants suffering from intestinal resection, and the results were compared with those of five previously resected infants as controls. After experiment 2, it was concluded that enteral BC supplementation was well tolerated, as expected, and that no infants experienced clinical symptoms of cow milk allergy [166]. As mentioned, colostrum was well tolerated by newly resected infants. Nevertheless, the clinical outcomes of BC supplementation in infants subjected to intestinal resection are still unclear and require further study. Even if the number of infant studies is limited compared with that of animal studies (especially piglets), further and more comprehensive studies are necessary for preterm infants to acquire more persistent and certain results and trustworthy data. Some piglet studies have investigated the effects of BC on short bowel disease [166–169]. To date, all the collected data imply that the efficiency of BC in developing SBS patients is mostly dependent on the maturation rate, along with other related factors [6]. It should be considered that individuals with SBS consult their healthcare providers before administering BC into their diets to ensure optimization for their specific conditions.

4.5. Neonatal Sepsis

Neonatal sepsis is a systemic disease that originates from bacteria, viruses, or fungi and is associated with circulatory alterations and other clinical manifestations. Although various definitions yet no consensus exists for neonatal sepsis, this condition is traditionally characterized as the isolation of a pathogen from a sterile body fluid such as blood. These alterations ultimately lead to morbidity and mortality [170]. According to the age of onset and timing of the sepsis episode, neonatal sepsis can be classified as early-onset sepsis (EOS) or late-onset sepsis (LOS). Clinical manifestations of early-onset infections generally emerge within the first 72 h [171]. Early-onset infections usually occur before or during birth and are due to vertical mother-to-infant transmission. However, late-onset infections occur after birth (usually between 3 and 7 days) and are linked to harmful organisms present in the hospital environment or society [170]. Even though the basis for this disease has several distinct factors, the effects on the body and the systemic consequences of neonatal sepsis involve common pathways that may be evaluated during investigations.

According to the current literature, few clinical trials or studies have been conducted on human infants with BC, although some preterm pig studies and related studies are available. In 2009, Manzoni et al. (2009) and colleagues conducted a trial on 11 tertiary neonatal intensive care infants by using BLF, where its peak levels were encountered in day 1 colostrum, to determine whether BLF alone or in combination with LGG reduces the incidence of LOS in a double-blind, placebo-controlled, and randomized trial. The trial concluded that the incidence of LOS was lower in both the BLF and BLF with LGG groups (5.9% and 4.6%, respectively) than in the control group (17.3%). Additionally, bacterial or fungal-originated sepsis levels decreased [172]. BLF or BLF with LGG could reduce the incidence of the first episode of LOS. Similarly, Alanwary Abdel et al., 2022 [128], conducted a series of experiments regarding the beneficial influences of BC on preterm infants. The results reported that the incidence rates of culture-proven LOS groups and clinically suspected LOS groups were not significantly different. Moreover, fewer sepsis episodes were observed in the BC group than in the control group [128]. Undoubtedly, these trials have elucidated the effects of colostrum on LOS, but it should be remembered that there is no direct and appropriate application of colostrum for LOS, and further studies should be designed, performed, and evaluated to extend the collection of data and all aspects of incidence effects. As previously mentioned, some preterm pig studies exist. Studies have reported that BC supplementation provides blood bacterial disinfection and supports hemodynamics, resulting in the prevention of septic shock [173].

4.6. Gastrointestinal and Respiratory Infections

Because of premature birth and inappropriate development, preterm infants are susceptible to certain diseases related to harmful microorganisms as well as insufficient systems. One of the most common diseases in these infants is gastrointestinal disease, which causes several types of disease, such as feeding intolerance and short bowel syndrome. Feeding intolerance, which is the most common GI disease in preterm infants, causes the malfunction of the intestines and the inability to digest enteral nutritional intake [174]. For previously examined diseases, BC is also able to promote the maturation of the intestine as well as GI digestion and absorption [175–177]. In a recent study, feeding intolerance was reduced in the BC group compared with the control group. The results also indicate that gut maturation involves both intestinal differentiation and proliferation and that these developments might be attributed to growth factors in BC, such as IGF (which has improved effects on feeding tolerance) [178]. All of these results suggest that BC can decrease the incidence of feeding intolerance [174].

In bacterial and pathogenic GI disorders caused by bacterial strains such as *E. coli*, *Staphylococcus aureus*, *Enterobacter aerogenes*, *Salmonella typhi*, *H. pylori*, and *Proteus vulgaris*, BC is mostly and commonly used to control and treat all infections caused by exposure to the preceding strains. Studies investigating various aspects of BC have concluded that the development of bacterial strains such as *E. coli*, *S. aureus*, *P. vulgaris*, *E. aerogenes*, and *S. typhi* has been hindered by BC, and the adult Wistar rats used in a particular study presented antimicrobial resistance [114]. Among all these bacteria, the most common species is *H. pylori*, which causes the most prevalent bacterial gastrointestinal infections in humans worldwide. The systemic intake of this bacterium is mostly due to oral entry, resulting in GI infections from the stomach to the later compartments. Owing to the viability of this bacterium in a highly acidic stomach environment, a series of diseases, namely, chronic gastritis, peptic and duodenal ulcers, and gastric adenocarcinoma, occur in the stomach [179]. Since the target of *H. pylori* is the receptor found in the mucosal layer of the stomach, the interaction between these receptors and bacteria was investigated in an in vitro study using BC concentrate (BCC) as an intervention agent. The study concluded that BCC was able to hinder the microbial adhesion of *H. pylori* bacteria to the lipid receptors of the mucosal layer, namely, gangliotetraosylceramide (Gg4), gangliotriaosylceramide (Gg3), and phosphatidylethanolamine (PE). The study also included *Helicobacter mustelae* strains, with similar results [180]. In addition, related studies on animal models regarding the effects of BC on *Helicobacter* strains have shown that BC and its components (i.e., lactoferrin and immunoglobulins) are capable of hindering bacterial viability and binding to receptors along with their antigens [181–184]. BLF was examined in this respect. Megahed et al. (2017) designed an experiment in which 50 patients were selected and divided into two groups; namely, group 1 was treated with traditional therapy (including clarithromycin, omeprazole, amoxicillin, or metronidazole), and group 2 was treated with BLF supplemented with traditional therapy for a 1-week period. Finally, they reported that the elimination of *H. pylori* infection was greater with BLF-supplemented treatment than with traditional treatment (92% and 68%, respectively) [185]. These results emphasize the importance of BC in the treatment of GI diseases caused by bacterial strains and suggest that the specific components of BC can diminish infections or their downstream effects. Undoubtedly, BC contributes to the GI tract by providing prebiotic components to the microbiota [186]. Nevertheless, more specific studies regarding different mechanisms and their interventions by BC components are necessary to comprehend the extent of BC in GI diseases.

4.7. Other Conditions

The inclusive and versatile nature of BC results in a rich component pool, and newborns are susceptible to various external factors, such as bacterial infections from several bodily compartments. Owing to the undeveloped systems of the body, specifically digestion and respiration, BC provides the first shield through its components and prepares the body for its first encounter against these external factors. In this context, BC supplementation has been used to recover additional harmful situations for preterm infants. URTIs include the most common tract infections caused by respiratory viruses. Studies regarding URTI and its symptoms indicate that BC can be an effective agent because of its incidence and severity [68]. A clinical study aiming to evaluate the effectiveness and tolerability of BC in the prevention of URTIs was performed in children. For this purpose, 160 children aged 1–6 years with repetitive URTIs were given BC for 4 weeks. According to the results, the mean total number of URTIs decreased radically after BC supplementation ($p < 0.001$). The study also concluded that BC is efficient in the prevention of repetitive URTIs by reducing the number of episodes and the hospitalization time [143]. In URTIs, other studies also claim the same effects for these episodes [187,188].

BC-supported trials have been conducted in the context of cancer and its complications. Childhood leukemia, the most prevalent cancer in children, causes gastrointestinal mucositis, which promotes morbidity and mortality through adverse effects due to cytotoxic anticancer treatment. This effect leads to a disease called chemotherapy-induced mucositis (CIM), which is defined as an inflammatory effect affecting mucosal surfaces and submucosal layers [6]. In an attributed randomized and placebo-controlled clinical study, newly diagnosed children were subjected to BC or placebo administration for 4 weeks. The results indicated that no alterations were observed in fever, infectious morbidity, or inflammatory responses. However, the results and data might reduce the peak severity levels of oral mucositis [189]. Since these studies are limited to patients with chemotherapy-induced GI toxicity, more comprehensive and inclusive studies are needed to verify these data and make these findings more comparable. BC undoubtedly has favorable effects on certain complications of acute lymphoblastic leukemia (ALL) induction treatment, but further trials will ensure the optimization and more accurate effects of BC in CIM.

5. Bovine Colostrum and Pediatric Health: Safety Concerns

BC is commonly used and applied in pediatric studies for its beneficial effects on several diseases and deficiencies, but dietary supplements for infants and children must be well examined in terms of short- and long-term safety. The determinants for BC to be used in pediatrics vary widely in terms of product supply, quality, purity, and microbiological safety; harmful microorganisms may develop in BC, resulting in contamination, severe child allergy risks, excessive supplies of components such as proteins and growth factors, a lack of certain BC components, and the inhibition of drug absorption [6]. Unfortunately, these factors have not been investigated sufficiently to interpret the risks of BC in pediatric patients since the current literature only partially mentions the risks of BC in a study-related manner. Bovine milk is the most preferred infant diet alternative worldwide [190]. Unfortunately, the major and most common reasons for food allergy reactions during early childhood are also triggered by milk along with bovine milk [191]. The most studied and defined risk is cow milk allergy, which can be triggered by the presence of IgE, which adversely affects reactions with milk proteins. The subsequent ingestion of these altered proteins might cause sensitivity or allergy. This allergic reaction is the most prevalent condition; therefore, approximately 2–3% of infants suffer from this disease, even in developed countries, which may indicate that developing countries have a greater rate of CMA in infants [19]. The current studies do not indicate any direct correlation between BC and CMA development other than bovine milk or infant formula. However, various milk products, such as bovine colostrum and yogurt, can induce similar allergic reactions due to their common ingredients in comparison with milk [192,193]. In addition to IgG, which is known to be nonallergenic and found only in BC, α-lactalbumin and β-lactoglobulin, which are allergenic factors that trigger allergies in bovine milk, can also be found in BC [6,193,194]. Because all ruminant mammalian milks share homologous proteins with the same structural and biological properties, cross-reactivity is likely possible in individuals and infants with allergies [192]. BC may lead to similar allergic reactions; thus, the prevalence, diagnosis, and treatment of CMA can be followed by milk approaches at this point. However, BC can be considered effective against allergic reactions based on its well-known rich components [29]. More BC-specific studies are essential in the future to evaluate the potential risk of BC in infant feed.

In a general sense, milk allergy is evaluated as a nontreatable disorder. Therefore, CMA can also be classified specifically as nontreatable. After diagnosis, patients with allergic reactions must avoid allergy-inducing food and nutrients to avoid allergic complications. Most of the time, CMA infants can overcome allergic reactions in adulthood, even though 15% of patients continue to suffer throughout adulthood [193]. In addition to this natural tolerance to milk components, there may be a diminishing portion of IgE due to the lack of milk consumption at the beginning or early stages of life [191]. When this tolerance and its symptoms are observed, the diagnosis of CMA can be commenced, followed by in vitro and in vivo tests, and finished with an oral food challenge (OFC) and a double-blind placebo-controlled food challenge (DBPCFC) by a specialist. The in vitro diagnostic test involves the detection of milk allergen-specific IgE in blood serum. After the diagnosis, the results are interpreted, and the OFC test results determine the conclusion. The detailed diagnostic procedure is described in this section [195]. The only treatment for CMA is a tolerable diet, but in the case of accidental consumption, medical applications, such as oral antihistamines for mild reactions or epinephrine for systemic and respiratory reactions, are possible [191,193,196]. If BC causes CMA, the same approach can be followed for the prevalence, diagnosis, and therapy of this disease.

BC has critical physiological and protective functions in neonates, such as immune-boosting, growth-promoting, and antimicrobial properties that aid in tissue development and the maturation of the digestive system and other essential organs in both neonatal mammals and humans. The immunoglobulins and lactoferrin in BC are vital for building natural immunity in neonates, aiding in the reduction in mortality rates in this age group. Importantly, unlike mature milk, BC has a lower lactose content, which makes it a better substitute for lactose intolerance in humans [197]. The composition of BC also includes glycans, which are crucial for immune defense. In the presence of glycans, pathogenic pathogens such as *E. coli*, *S. aureus*, *H. pylori*, rotavirus, and respiratory viruses are inhibited. In addition to providing essential nutrients, HC glycans also aid in the prevention of pathogen adhesion, the modulation of mucosal immune functions, and the support of healthy gut microbiota [88]. Nonetheless, there is limited information on the safety and efficacy of using BC for healthy term infants who do not have access to their own mothers' milk immediately after birth in cases of adverse conditions such as maternal illness or the inability to breastfeed. In general, such infants are fed infant formula or donor human milk where available [6]. As a result, while BC offers an enormous level of developmental and health-related advantages, there is no strong rationality for using BC as a supplement for healthy-term infants in long-term periods, especially in developed countries.

6. Conclusions

In this review, we extensively reviewed colostrum and its effects on pediatric diseases and infant health. BC is an important nutrient source for infants of mammalian species and is secreted immediately after birth. Each component of colostrum offers significant benefits to health by providing essential elements for critical compartments of body systems. It possesses anti-inflammatory, antioxidant, antibacterial, prebiotic, and antiviral effects, which are discussed separately in this review and provide a unique profile for colostrum. Bovine colostrum, which is the most consumed and prevalent colostrum worldwide, is frequently used in pediatric studies because of its shared homology with HC. The results of the composition and clinical studies of human and bovine colostrum show that BC can be the best alternative source for HC in infant feeding. The richer fat and protein ingredients of colostrum compared to milk provide essential immune protection. Remarkable components of colostrum contribute to infant health and regulate their systems. Lactoferrin promotes cellular proliferation and the growth of mutual bacteria, contributes to immune protection, and has potential therapeutic features. The multi-diverse nature of LF has also been investigated solely in dedicated studies. Lysozyme and α-lactalbumin also have protective effects by inhibiting harmful microorganisms and antibacterial effects, respectively. Immunoglobulins are essential for immune protection and prevent bacterial and viral infections as well as the activation of the immune system. The MFGM promotes healthy microbiota and reduces infections and related inflammation. The MFGM also affects neurodevelopment. Glycans, which are highly variable and versatile oligosaccharides, play crucial roles in immune functions and cell interactions. The colostrum contains high levels and variables of these glycans, supporting GI health and immune development in infants. Glycans are consumed by probiotics and shape the gut microbiota, resulting in improvements in the digestive system. However, alterations in glycosylation pathways are attributed to distinct autoimmune diseases, such as Crohn's disease, where altered glycan structures on antibodies correlate with disease severity. The potential therapeutic benefits of colostrum include the modulation of immune responses and the improvement of glycosylation pathways, although further research is needed. Additionally, milk oligosaccharides have shown promise in protecting against infections and NEC in preterm infants, indicating their importance in infant nutrition and health. All the components of colostrum have potential and determined benefits. Solely or altogether, studies of these components are necessary to optimize their dose-dependent use and compensate for their adverse effects.

These findings indicate that BC has diverse systemic effects in all parts of its life cycle. Considering the evolutionary mechanisms and timing of BC secretion, the primary role of BC is evaluated as an onset for immune promotion rather than nutritional support, since infants possess deficiencies in various systems. Premature birth makes this situation worse since crucial systems are inappropriately developed. To support preterm infants precisely, BC can be exploited solely or completely in infant formulas. It should also be remembered that there is no universally agreed-upon standard dosage for bovine colostrum in infants. Optimization, dose adjustments, and infant parameters must also be assessed to minimize adverse effects. BC has been proven to have beneficial effects on certain infant disorders, such as necrotizing enterocolitis, bowel syndrome, infectious diarrhea, and gastrointestinal tract (GI tract) disorders, by disrupting severe mechanisms, providing insufficient elements, and mediating reactions. However, ineffective or adverse effects of BC have been observed during clinical trials due to its elements, and these elements should be minimized when clinical experiments are designed. Since BC is a supplement and not a trustworthy treatment, its use should be guided by a healthcare professional, particularly in preterm infants or those with medical conditions. Additionally, more clinical studies with more subjects are needed to gather more data and assess the observed all-scale effects comprehensively. Future research on bovine colostrum should focus on determining optimal dosages, formulations, and safety profiles, particularly for allergic reactions in infants with cow's milk protein allergies or lactose intolerance. Additionally, studies are needed to address quality control and ensure product safety. Long-term studies should investigate the ongoing effects of colostrum supplementation on immune function and gut health in infants. Comparative studies should also be designed and examined to investigate the benefits of BC in relation to HC. Versatile and unique patient profiles also need to be obtained to assess the diversity of BC effects on infant diseases. Ultimately, the use of BC, often in pediatric conditions and neonatal health, is highly recommended.

Author Contributions: Conceptualization, S.K.; writing—original draft preparation, A.A.C., M.L., J.M.M.L., A.d.C.M. and M.B.; writing—review and editing, A.A.C.; visualization, A.A.C.; supervision, S.K. All authors have read and agreed to the published version of the manuscript.

Funding: This research received no external funding.

Conflicts of Interest: The authors declare no conflicts of interest.

Abbreviations

BC, bovine colostrum; HC, human colostrum; NEC, necrotizing enterocolitis; IBD, inflammatory bowel disease; LOS, late-onset sepsis; FI, food intolerance; CMA, cow's milk allergy; Ig, immunoglobulin; LF, lactoferrin; EGF, epidermal growth factor; TGF-β, transforming growth factor β; PDGF, platelet-derived growth factor; IGF, insulin-like growth factor; GI, gastrointestinal; LFR, lactoferrin receptor; BLF, bovine lactoferrin; HLF, human lactoferrin; SARS-CoV-1, severe acute respiratory syndrome coronavirus 1; ROS, reactive oxygen species; MGFM, milk fat globule membrane; FABP fatty acid-binding protein; RNS, reactive nitrogen species; HIV, human immunodeficiency; Glc, glucose; GAG, glycosaminoglycan, HS, heparan sulfate; Gal, galactose; *O*-GalNAc, *O*-linked *N*-acetylgalactosamine; Fuc, fucose; CTLF, *C*-type lectin family; RA, rheumatoid arthritis; IVIg, high-dose intravenous immunoglobulin; HMO, human milk oligosaccharide; SCFA, short-chain fatty acid; DC, dentritic cell; RCT, randomized controlled trial; WHO; World Health Organization; URTI, upper respiratory tract infection; CD, Crohn's disease; UC, ulcerative colitis; PBMC, peripheral blood mononuclear cell; SBS, short bowel syndrome; II, intestinal insufficiency; IF, intestinal failure; PN, parenteral nutrition; MEN, minimal enteral nutrition; EOS, early-onset sepsis; BCC, bovine colostrum concentrate (BCC); CIM, chemotherapy-induced mucositis; ALL, acute lymphoblastic leukemia; OFC, oral food challenge; DBPCFC, double-blind placebo-controlled food challenge.

References

1. Hammon, H.M.; Liermann, W.; Frieten, D.; Koch, C. Review: Importance of colostrum supply and milk feeding intensity on gastrointestinal and systemic development in calves. *Animal* **2020**, *14*, s133–s143. [CrossRef] [PubMed]
2. Playford, R.J.; Weiser, M.J. Bovine Colostrum: Its Constituents and Uses. *Nutrients* **2021**, *13*, 265. [CrossRef] [PubMed]
3. Arslan, A.; Duman, H.; Kaplan, M.; Uzkuç, H.; Bayraktar, A.; Ertürk, M.; Alkan, M.; Frese, S.A.; Duar, R.M.; Henrick, B.M.; et al. Determining Total Protein and Bioactive Protein Concentrations in Bovine Colostrum. *J. Vis. Exp.* **2021**, *10*, e63001. [CrossRef] [PubMed]
4. Li, Y.; Juhl, S.M.; Ye, X.; Shen, R.L.; Iyore, E.O.; Dai, Y.; Sangild, P.T.; Greisen, G.O. A Stepwise, Pilot Study of Bovine Colostrum to Supplement the First Enteral Feeding in Preterm Infants (Precolos): Study Protocol and Initial Results. *Front. Pediatr.* **2017**, *5*, 42. [CrossRef]
5. Goldman, A.S. Evolution of the Mammary Gland Defense System and the Ontogeny of the Immune System. *J. Mammary Gland. Biol. Neoplasia* **2002**, *7*, 277–289. [CrossRef]
6. Sangild, P.T.; Vonderohe, C.; Hebib, V.M.; Burrin, D.G. Potential benefits of bovine colostrum in pediatric nutrition and health. *Nutrients* **2021**, *13*, 2551. [CrossRef]
7. Karav, S.; Le Parc, A.; de Moura Bell, J.M.L.N.; Frese, S.A.; Kirmiz, N.; Block, D.E.; Barile, D.; Mills, D.A. Oligosaccharides Released from milk glycoproteins are selective growth substrates for infant-associated bifidobacteria. *Appl. Environ. Microbiol.* **2016**, *82*, 3622–3630. [CrossRef]
8. Blum, J.; Hammon, H. Colostrum effects on the gastrointestinal tract, and on nutritional, endocrine and metabolic parameters in neonatal calves. *Livest. Prod. Sci.* **2000**, *66*, 151–159. [CrossRef]
9. Blum, J.W.; Hammon, H.M. Bovine colostrum: More than just an immunoglobulin supplier. *Schweiz. Arch. Tierheilkd.* **2000**, *142*, 221–228.
10. Guilloteau, P.; Le Huërou-Luron, I.; Chayvialle, J.A.; Toullec, R.; Zabielski, R.; Blum, J.W. Gut Regulatory Peptides in Young Cattle and Sheep. *J. Vet. Med. Ser. A* **1997**, *44*, 1–23. [CrossRef]
11. Korhonen, H.J. Production and properties of health-promoting proteins and peptides from bovine colostrum and milk. *Cell. Mol. Biol.* **2013**, *59*, 12–24. [PubMed]
12. Yalçıntaş, Y.M.; Baydemir, B.; Duman, H.; Eker, F.; Biçen, A.B.; Ertürk, M.; Karav, S. Ay Exploring the impact of colostrum supplementation on athletes: A comprehensive analysis of clinical trials and diverse properties. *Front. Immunol.* **2024**, *15*, 1395437. [CrossRef] [PubMed]
13. Bagwe, S.; Tharappel, L.J.; Kaur, G.; Buttar, H.S. Bovine colostrum: An emerging nutraceutical. *J. Complement. Integr. Med.* **2015**, *12*, 175–185. [CrossRef] [PubMed]
14. Chae, A.; Aitchison, A.; Day, A.S.; Keenan, J.I. Bovine colostrum demonstrates anti-inflammatory and antibacterial activity in in vitro models of intestinal inflammation and infection. *J. Funct. Foods* **2017**, *28*, 293–298. [CrossRef]
15. Civra, A.; Francese, R.; Donalisio, M.; Tonetto, P.; Coscia, A.; Sottemano, S.; Balestrini, R.; Faccio, A.; Cavallarin, L.; Moro, G.E.; et al. Human Colostrum and Derived Extracellular Vesicles Prevent Infection by Human Rotavirus and Respiratory Syncytial Virus in Vitro. *J. Hum. Lact.* **2021**, *37*, 122–134. [CrossRef]
16. Stevens, E.E.; Patrick, T.E.; Pickler, R. A History of Infant Feeding. *J. Périnat. Educ.* **2009**, *18*, 32–39. [CrossRef]
17. Ananthan, A.; Balasubramanian, H.; Rao, S.; Patole, S. Human Milk–Derived Fortifiers Compared with Bovine Milk–Derived Fortifiers in Preterm Infants: A Systematic Review and Meta-Analysis. *Adv. Nutr. Int. Rev. J.* **2020**, *11*, 1325–1333. [CrossRef]
18. Burris, A.D.; Burris, J.; Järvinen, K.M. Cow's Milk Protein Allergy in Term and Preterm Infants: Clinical Manifestations, Immunologic Pathophysiology, and Management Strategies. *NeoReviews* **2020**, *21*, e795–e808. [CrossRef]
19. Host, A.; Halken, S. Cow's Milk Allergy: Where have we Come from and where are we Going? *Endocrine Metab. Immune Disord.-Drug Targets* **2014**, *14*, 2–8. [CrossRef]
20. Maffei, D.; Schanler, R.J. Human milk is the feeding strategy to prevent necrotizing enterocolitis! *Semin. Perinatol.* **2017**, *41*, 36–40. [CrossRef]
21. Michelet, M.; Schluckebier, D.; Petit, L.-M.; Caubet, J.-C. Food protein-induced enterocolitis syndrome—A review of the literature with focus on clinical management. *J. Asthma Allergy* **2017**, *10*, 197–207. [CrossRef] [PubMed]
22. Golkar, A.; Milani, J.M.; Vasiljevic, T. Altering allergenicity of cow's milk by food processing for applications in infant formula. *Crit. Rev. Food Sci. Nutr.* **2019**, *59*, 159–172. [CrossRef] [PubMed]

23. McGrath, B.A.; Fox, P.F.; McSweeney, P.L.H.; Kelly, A.L. Composition and properties of bovine colostrum: A review. *Dairy Sci. Technol.* **2016**, *96*, 133–158. [CrossRef]
24. Puppel, K.; Gołębiewski, M.; Grodkowski, G.; Slósarz, J.; Kunowska-Slósarz, M.; Solarczyk, P.; Łukasiewicz, M.; Balcerak, M.; Przysucha, T. Composition and Factors Affecting Quality of Bovine Colostrum: A Review. *Animals* **2019**, *9*, 1070. [CrossRef] [PubMed]
25. Ballard, O.; Morrow, A.L. Human milk composition: Nutrients and bioactive factors. *Pediatr. Clin. N. Am.* **2013**, *60*, 49–74. [CrossRef] [PubMed]
26. Bolino, M.; Duman, H.; Avcı, İ.; Kayili, H.M.; Petereit, J.; Zundel, C.; Salih, B.; Karav, S.; Frese, S.A. Proteomic and *N*-glycomic comparison of synthetic and bovine whey proteins and their effect on human gut microbiomes. *bioRxiv* **2024**. [CrossRef]
27. West, D.W.; Mitchell, C.J. Tracking the Fate of Milk Proteins: Better in Whole or in Part? *J. Nutr.* **2020**, *150*, 2001–2002. [CrossRef]
28. Martin, C.R.; Ling, P.-R.; Blackburn, G.L. Review of Infant Feeding: Key Features of Breast Milk and Infant Formula. *Nutrients* **2016**, *8*, 279. [CrossRef]
29. Yalçıntaş, Y.M.; Duman, H.; López, J.M.M.; Portocarrero, A.C.M.; Lombardo, M.; Khallouki, F.; Koch, W.; Bordiga, M.; El-Seedi, H.; Raposo, A.; et al. Revealing the Potency of Growth Factors in Bovine Colostrum. *Nutrients* **2024**, *16*, 2359. [CrossRef]
30. Dupont, D.; Tomé, D. Milk proteins: Digestion and absorption in the gastrointestinal tract. In *Milk Proteins*; Elsevier: Amsterdam, The Netherlands, 2020; pp. 701–714. [CrossRef]
31. Arslan, A.; Kaplan, M.; Duman, H.; Bayraktar, A.; Ertürk, M.; Henrick, B.M.; Frese, S.A.; Karav, S. Bovine Colostrum and Its Potential for Human Health and Nutrition. *Front. Nutr.* **2021**, *8*, 651721. [CrossRef]
32. Montagne, P.; Cuillière, M.L.; Molé, C.; Béné, M.C.; Faure, G. Changes in Lactoferrin and Lysozyme Levels in Human Milk During the First Twelve Weeks of Lactation. In *Bioactive Components of Human Milk*; Springer: Boston, MA, USA, 2001; pp. 241–247. [CrossRef]
33. Donovan, S.M.; Odle, J. Growth Factors in Milk as Mediators of Infant Development. *Annu. Rev. Nutr.* **1994**, *14*, 147–167. [CrossRef] [PubMed]
34. Eker, F.; Duman, H.; Ertürk, M.; Karav, S. The potential of lactoferrin as antiviral and immune-modulating agent in viral infectious diseases. *Front. Immunol.* **2024**, *15*, 1402135. [CrossRef] [PubMed]
35. Kaplan, M.; Baktıroğlu, M.; Kalkan, A.E.; Canbolat, A.A.; Lombardo, M.; Raposo, A.; Alves, J.L.d.B.; Witkowska, A.M.; Karav, S. Lactoferrin: A Promising Therapeutic Molecule against Human Papillomavirus. *Nutrients* **2024**, *16*, 3073. [CrossRef] [PubMed]
36. Gíslason, J.; Iyer, S.; Hutchens, T.; Lönnerdal, B. Lactoferrin receptors in piglet small intestine: Lactoferrin binding properties, ontogeny, and regional distribution in the gastrointestinal tract. *J. Nutr. Biochem.* **1993**, *4*, 528–533. [CrossRef]
37. Donovan, S.M. The Role of Lactoferrin in Gastrointestinal and Immune Development and Function: A Preclinical Perspective. *J. Pediatr.* **2016**, *173*, S16–S28. [CrossRef] [PubMed]
38. Karav, S.; German, J.B.; Rouquié, C.; Le Parc, A.; Barile, D. Studying lactoferrin *N*-glycosylation. *Int. J. Mol. Sci.* **2017**, *18*, 870. [CrossRef]
39. Karav, S. Selective deglycosylation of lactoferrin to understand glycans' contribution to antimicrobial activity of lactoferrin. *Cell. Mol. Biol.* **2018**, *64*, 52–57. [CrossRef]
40. Petschow, B.W.; Talbott, R.D.; Batema, R.P. Ability of lactoferrin to promote the growth of *Bifidobacterium* spp. in vitro is independent of receptor binding capacity and iron saturation level. *J. Med. Microbiol.* **1999**, *48*, 541–549. [CrossRef]
41. Zhang, J.; Han, X.; Shan, Y.; Zhang, L.; Du, M.; Liu, M.; Yi, H.; Ma, Y. Effect of bovine lactoferrin and human lactoferrin on the proliferative activity of the osteoblast cell line MC3T3-E1 in vitro. *J. Dairy Sci.* **2018**, *101*, 1827–1833. [CrossRef]
42. Embleton, N.D.; Berrington, J.E. Clinical Trials of Lactoferrin in the Newborn: Effects on Infection and the Gut Microbiome. In *Milk, Mucosal Immunity and the Microbiome: Impact on the Neonate*; Karger Publishers: Basel, Switzerland, 2020; pp. 141–151. [CrossRef]
43. Dall'Agnola, A.; Tomé, D.; Kaufman, D.A.; Tavella, E.; Pieretto, M.; Messina, A.; De Luca, D.; Bellaiche, M.; Mosca, A.; Piloquet, H.; et al. Role of Lactoferrin in Neonates and Infants: An Update. *Am. J. Perinatol.* **2018**, *35*, 561–565. [CrossRef]
44. Pammi, M.; Gautham, K.S. Enteral lactoferrin supplementation for prevention of sepsis and necrotizing enterocolitis in preterm infants. *Cochrane Database Syst. Rev.* **2020**, *3*, CD007137. [CrossRef] [PubMed]
45. Bolat, E.; Eker, F.; Kaplan, M.; Duman, H.; Arslan, A.; Saritaş, S.; Şahutoğlu, A.S.; Karav, S. Lactoferrin for COVID-19 prevention, treatment, and recovery. *Front. Nutr.* **2022**, *9*, 992733. [CrossRef] [PubMed]
46. Eker, F.; Bolat, E.; Pekdemir, B.; Duman, H.; Karav, S. Lactoferrin: Neuroprotection against Parkinson's disease and secondary molecule for potential treatment. *Front. Aging Neurosci.* **2023**, *15*, 1204149. [CrossRef] [PubMed]
47. Brandtzaeg, P.; Mann, W.V. A Comparative Study of the Lysozyme Activity of Human Gingival Pocket Fluid, Serum, and Saliva. *Acta Odontol. Scand.* **1964**, *22*, 441–455. [CrossRef] [PubMed]
48. Ibrahim, H.R.; Kato, A.; Kobayashi, K. Antimicrobial effects of lysozyme against gram-negative bacteria due to covalent binding of palmitic acid. *J. Agric. Food Chem.* **1991**, *39*, 2077–2082. [CrossRef]
49. Ferraboschi, P.; Ciceri, S.; Grisenti, P. Applications of Lysozyme, an Innate Immune Defense Factor, as an Alternative Antibiotic. *Antibiotics* **2021**, *10*, 1534. [CrossRef]
50. Morrin, S.T.; Buck, R.H.; Farrow, M.; Hickey, R.M. Milk-derived anti-infectives and their potential to combat bacterial and viral infection. *J. Funct. Foods* **2021**, *81*, 104442. [CrossRef]

51. Krissansen, G.W. Emerging Health Properties of Whey Proteins and Their Clinical Implications. *J. Am. Coll. Nutr.* **2007**, *26*, 713S–723S. [CrossRef]
52. Eker, F.; Akdaşçi, E.; Duman, H.; Yalçıntaş, Y.M.; Canbolat, A.A.; Kalkan, A.E.; Karav, S.; Šamec, D. Antimicrobial Properties of Colostrum and Milk. *Antibiotics* **2024**, *13*, 251. [CrossRef]
53. Lajnaf, R.; Gharsallah, H.; Jridi, M.; Attia, H.; Ayadi, M. Antioxidant and antibacterial activities, interfacial and emulsifying properties of the apo and holo forms of purified camel and bovine α-lactalbumin. *Int. J. Biol. Macromol.* **2020**, *165*, 205–213. [CrossRef]
54. Diao, M.; Yan, M.; Wang, Y.; Yan, X.; Dong, S.; Lu, Y.; Zhang, T. Characterization and antibacterial activity study of α-Lactalbumin-carvacrol complex. *Food Chem.* **2022**, *397*, 133820. [CrossRef] [PubMed]
55. Ahmad, S.; Anjum, F.M.; Huma, N.; Sameen, A.; Zahoor, T. Composition and Physico-chemical Characteristics of Buffalo Milk with Particular Emphasis on Lipids, Proteins, Minerals, Enzymes and Vitamins. *J. Anim. Plant Sci.* **2013**, *23*, 62–74.
56. Barrington, G.; Besser, T.; Davis, W.; Gay, C.; Reeves, J.; McFadden, T. Expression of Immunoglobulin G1 Receptors by Bovine Mammary Epithelial Cells and Mammary Leukocytes. *J. Dairy Sci.* **1997**, *80*, 86–93. [CrossRef] [PubMed]
57. Jensen, A.R.; Elnif, J.; Sangild, P.T.; Burrin, D.G. Development of Intestinal Immunoglobulin Absorption and Enzyme Activities in Neonatal Pigs Is Diet Dependent. *J. Nutr.* **2001**, *131*, 3259–3265. [CrossRef] [PubMed]
58. Sangild, P. Uptake of Colostral Immunoglobulins by the Compromised Newborn Farm Animal. *Acta Vet. Scand.* **2003**, *44*, S105. [CrossRef]
59. Marnila, P.; Korhonen, H. Milk | Colostrum. In *Encyclopedia of Dairy Sciences*; Elsevier: Amsterdam, The Netherlands, 2011; pp. 591–597. [CrossRef]
60. Rajala, P.; Castrén, H. Serum Immunoglobulin Concentrations and Health of Dairy Calves in Two Management Systems from Birth to 12 Weeks of Age. *J. Dairy Sci.* **1995**, *78*, 2737–2744. [CrossRef]
61. Baumrucker, C.R.; Bruckmaier, R.M. Colostrogenesis: IgG1 Transcytosis Mechanisms. *J. Mammary Gland. Biol. Neoplasia* **2014**, *19*, 103–117. [CrossRef]
62. Kaskous, S.; Fadlelmoula, A.A.; Kaskous, S.; Fadlelmoula, A. Immunoglobulin in Colostrum and Health of Newborn Calves (Review) Immunoglobulin in colostrum and health of newborn Calves. *Sci. J. Rev.* **2015**, *4*, 242–249.
63. Lee, H.; Padhi, E.; Hasegawa, Y.; Larke, J.; Parenti, M.; Wang, A.; Hernell, O.; Lönnerdal, B.; Slupsky, C. Compositional Dynamics of the Milk Fat Globule and Its Role in Infant Development. *Front. Pediatr.* **2018**, *6*, 313. [CrossRef]
64. Koletzko, B. Human Milk Lipids. *Ann. Nutr. Metab.* **2016**, *69* (Suppl. S2), 27–40. [CrossRef]
65. Manoni, M.; Di Lorenzo, C.; Ottoboni, M.; Tretola, M.; Pinotti, L. Comparative Proteomics of Milk Fat Globule Membrane (MFGM) Proteome across Species and Lactation Stages and the Potentials of MFGM Fractions in Infant Formula Preparation. *Foods* **2020**, *9*, 1251. [CrossRef] [PubMed]
66. Bhinder, G.; Allaire, J.M.; Garcia, C.; Lau, J.T.; Chan, J.M.; Ryz, N.R.; Bosman, E.S.; Graef, F.A.; Crowley, S.M.; Celiberto, L.S.; et al. Milk Fat Globule Membrane Supplementation in Formula Modulates the Neonatal Gut Microbiome and Normalizes Intestinal Development. *Sci. Rep.* **2017**, *7*, 45274. [CrossRef] [PubMed]
67. Salcedo, J.; Karav, S.; Le Parc, A.; Cohen, J.L.; de Moura Bell, J.M.; Sun, A.; Lange, M.C.; Barile, D. Application of industrial treatments to donor human milk: Influence of pasteurization treatments, storage temperature, and time on human milk gangliosides. *npj Sci. Food* **2018**, *2*, 5. [CrossRef] [PubMed]
68. Duman, H.; Karav, S. Bovine colostrum and its potential contributions for treatment and prevention of COVID-19. *Front. Immunol.* **2023**, *14*, 1214514. [CrossRef] [PubMed]
69. Hernell, O.; Lönnerdal, B.; Timby, N. Milk Fat Globule Membranes: Effects on Microbiome, Metabolome, and Infections in Infants and Children. In *Milk, Mucosal Immunity and the Microbiome: Impact on the Neonate*; Karger Publishers: Basel, Switzerland, 2020; pp. 133–140. [CrossRef]
70. Honan, M.C.; Fahey, M.J.; Fischer-Tlustos, A.J.; Steele, M.A.; Greenwood, S.L. Shifts in the Holstein dairy cow milk fat globule membrane proteome that occur during the first week of lactation are affected by parity. *J. Anim. Sci. Biotechnol.* **2020**, *11*, 81. [CrossRef]
71. Tanaka, K.; Hosozawa, M.; Kudo, N.; Yoshikawa, N.; Hisata, K.; Shoji, H.; Shinohara, K.; Shimizu, T. The pilot study: Sphingomyelin-fortified milk has a positive association with the neurobehavioural development of very low birth weight infants during infancy, randomized control trial. *Brain Dev.* **2013**, *35*, 45–52. [CrossRef]
72. Palmano, K.; Rowan, A.; Guillermo, R.; Guan, J.; Mc Jarrow, P. The Role of Gangliosides in Neurodevelopment. *Nutrients* **2015**, *7*, 3891–3913. [CrossRef]
73. Rueda, R.; Maldonado, J.; Narbona, E.; Gil, A. Neonatal dietary gangliosides. *Early Hum. Dev.* **1998**, *53*, S135–S147. [CrossRef]
74. Hernell, O.; Timby, N.; Domellöf, M.; Lönnerdal, B. Clinical Benefits of Milk Fat Globule Membranes for Infants and Children. *J. Pediatr.* **2016**, *173*, S60–S65. [CrossRef]
75. Spitsberg, V. Invited Review: Bovine Milk Fat Globule Membrane as a Potential Nutraceutical. *J. Dairy Sci.* **2005**, *88*, 2289–2294. [CrossRef]
76. Kaplan, M.; Şahutoğlu, A.S.; Sarıtaş, S.; Duman, H.; Arslan, A.; Pekdemir, B.; Karav, S. Role of milk glycome in prevention, treatment, and recovery of COVID-19. *Front. Nutr.* **2022**, *9*, 1033779. [CrossRef] [PubMed]
77. Abeler-Dörner, L.; Swamy, M.; Williams, G.; Hayday, A.C.; Bas, A. Butyrophilins: An emerging family of immune regulators. *Trends Immunol.* **2012**, *33*, 34–41. [CrossRef] [PubMed]

78. Arnett, H.A.; Viney, J.L. Immune modulation by butyrophilins. *Nat. Rev. Immunol.* **2014**, *14*, 559–569. [CrossRef] [PubMed]
79. Timby, N.; Domellöf, M.; Holgerson, P.L.; West, C.E.; Lönnerdal, B.; Hernell, O.; Johansson, I. Oral Microbiota in Infants Fed a Formula Supplemented with Bovine Milk Fat Globule Membranes—A Randomized Controlled Trial. *PLoS ONE* **2017**, *12*, e0169831. [CrossRef] [PubMed]
80. Urashima, T.; Taufik, E.; Fukuda, K.; Asakuma, S. Recent Advances in Studies on Milk Oligosaccharides of Cows and Other Domestic Farm Animals. *Biosci. Biotechnol. Biochem.* **2013**, *77*, 455–466. [CrossRef]
81. Duman, H.; Kaplan, M.; Arslan, A.; Sahutoglu, A.S.; Kayili, H.M.; Frese, S.A.; Karav, S. Potential Applications of Endo-β-*N*-Acetylglucosaminidases from *Bifidobacterium longum* Subspecies *infantis* in Designing Value-Added, Next-Generation Infant Formulas. *Front. Nutr.* **2021**, *8*, 646275. [CrossRef]
82. Albrecht, S.; Lane, J.A.; Mariño, K.; Al Busadah, K.A.; Carrington, S.D.; Hickey, R.M.; Rudd, P.M. A comparative study of free oligosaccharides in the milk of domestic animals. *Br. J. Nutr.* **2014**, *111*, 1313–1328. [CrossRef]
83. Gopal, P.K.; Gill, H.S. Oligosaccharides and glycoconjugates in bovine milk and colostrum. *Br. J. Nutr.* **2000**, *84*, 69–74. [CrossRef]
84. Tao, N.; DePeters, E.; Freeman, S.; German, J.; Grimm, R.; Lebrilla, C. Bovine Milk Glycome. *J. Dairy Sci.* **2008**, *91*, 3768–3778. [CrossRef]
85. Varki, A. Biological roles of glycans. *Glycobiology* **2017**, *27*, 3–49. [CrossRef]
86. Varki, A.; Cummings, R.D.; Esko, J.D.; Stanley, P.; Hart, G.W.; Aebi, M.; Mohnen, D.; Kinoshita, T.; Packer, N.H.; Prestegard, J.J. (Eds.) *Essentials of Glycobiology*, 4th ed.; Cold Spring Harbor Laboratory Press: Cold Spring Harbor, NY, USA, 2015.
87. Zhou, J.Y.; Cobb, B.A. Glycans in Immunologic Health and Disease. *Annu. Rev. Immunol.* **2021**, *39*, 511–536. [CrossRef] [PubMed]
88. Newburg, D.S. Neonatal protection by an innate immune system of human milk consisting of oligosaccharides and glycans1. *J. Anim. Sci.* **2009**, *87* (Suppl. S13), 26–34. [CrossRef] [PubMed]
89. Bunyatratchata, A.; Le Parc, A.; de Moura, J.M.; Cohen, J.L.; Duman, H.; Arslan, A.; Kaplan, M.; Barile, D.; Karav, S. Release of bifidogenic *N*-glycans from native bovine colostrum proteins by an endo-β-*N*-acetylglucosaminidase. *Enzym. Microb. Technol.* **2023**, *162*, 110138. [CrossRef] [PubMed]
90. Pekdemir, B.; Karav, S. Exploring the diverse biological significance and roles of fucosylated oligosaccharides. *Front. Mol. Biosci.* **2024**, *11*, 1403727. [CrossRef] [PubMed]
91. Parekh, R.B.; Dwek, R.A.; Sutton, B.J.; Fernandes, D.L.; Leung, A.; Stanworth, D.; Rademacher, T.W.; Mizuochi, T.; Taniguchi, T.; Matsuta, K.; et al. Association of rheumatoid arthritis and primary osteoarthritis with changes in the glycosylation pattern of total serum IgG. *Nature* **1985**, *316*, 452–457. [CrossRef]
92. Pekelharing, J.M.; Hepp, E.; Kamerling, J.P.; Gerwig, G.J.; Leijnse, B. Alterations in carbohydrate composition of serum IgG from patients with rheumatoid arthritis and from pregnant women. *Ann. Rheum. Dis.* **1988**, *47*, 91–95. [CrossRef]
93. van de Geijn, F.E.; Wuhrer, M.; Selman, M.H.; Willemsen, S.P.; de Man, Y.A.; Deelder, A.M.; Hazes, J.M.; Dolhain, R.J. Immunoglobulin G galactosylation and sialylation are associated with pregnancy-induced improvement of rheumatoid arthritis and the postpartum flare: Results from a large prospective cohort study. *Arthritis Res. Ther.* **2009**, *11*, R193. [CrossRef]
94. Konno, N.; Sugimoto, M.; Takagi, T.; Furuya, M.; Asano, T.; Sato, S.; Kobayashi, H.; Migita, K.; Miura, Y.; Aihara, T.; et al. Changes in *N*-glycans of IgG4 and its relationship with the existence of hypocomplementemia and individual organ involvement in patients with IgG4-related disease. *PLoS ONE* **2018**, *13*, e0196163. [CrossRef]
95. Zhang, J.; Zhao, L.; Gao, Y.; Liu, M.; Li, T.; Huang, Y.; Lu, G.; Gao, Y.; Guo, X.; Shi, B. A Classification of Hashimoto's Thyroiditis Based on Immunohistochemistry for IgG4 and IgG. *Thyroid®* **2014**, *24*, 364–370. [CrossRef]
96. Šimurina, M.; de Haan, N.; Vučković, F.; Kennedy, N.A.; Štambuk, J.; Falck, D.; Trbojević-Akmačić, I.; Clerc, F.; Razdorov, G.; Khon, A.; et al. Glycosylation of Immunoglobulin G Associates With Clinical Features of Inflammatory Bowel Diseases. *Gastroenterology* **2018**, *154*, 1320–1333.e10. [CrossRef]
97. Mestecky, J.; Tomana, M.; Moldoveanu, Z.; Julian, B.; Suzuki, H.; Matousovic, K.; Renfrow, M.; Novak, L.; Wyatt, R.; Novak, J. Role of Aberrant Glycosylation of IgA1 Molecules in the Pathogenesis of IgA Nephropathy. *Kidney Blood Press. Res.* **2008**, *31*, 29–37. [CrossRef] [PubMed]
98. Youinou, P.; Pennec, Y.-L.; Casburn-Budd, R.; Dueymes, M.; Letoux, G.; Lamour, A. Galactose terminating oligosaccharides of IgG in patients with primary Sjögren's syndrome. *J. Autoimmun.* **1992**, *5*, 393–400. [CrossRef] [PubMed]
99. Shade, K.-T.C.; Conroy, M.E.; Washburn, N.; Kitaoka, M.; Huynh, D.J.; Laprise, E.; Patil, S.U.; Shreffler, W.G.; Anthony, R.M. Sialylation of immunoglobulin E is a determinant of allergic pathogenicity. *Nature* **2020**, *582*, 265–270. [CrossRef] [PubMed]
100. Cobb, B.A. The history of IgG glycosylation and where we are now. *Glycobiology* **2020**, *30*, 202–213. [CrossRef]
101. Anthony, R.M.; Wermeling, F.; Ravetch, J.V. Novel roles for the IgG Fc glycan. *Ann. N. Y. Acad. Sci.* **2012**, *1253*, 170–180. [CrossRef]
102. Kaneko, Y.; Nimmerjahn, F.; Ravetch, J.V. Anti-Inflammatory Activity of Immunoglobulin G Resulting from Fc Sialylation. *Science* **2006**, *313*, 670–673. [CrossRef]
103. Maverakis, E.; Kim, K.; Shimoda, M.; Gershwin, M.E.; Patel, F.; Wilken, R.; Raychaudhuri, S.; Ruhaak, L.R.; Lebrilla, C.B. Glycans in the immune system and The Altered Glycan Theory of Autoimmunity: A critical review. *J. Autoimmun.* **2015**, *57*, 1–13. [CrossRef]
104. Oswald, D.M.; Sim, E.S.; Baker, C.; Farhan, O.; Debanne, S.M.; Morris, N.J.; Rodriguez, B.G.; Jones, M.B.; Cobb, B.A. Plasma glycomics predict cardiovascular disease in patients with ART-controlled HIV infections. *FASEB J.* **2019**, *33*, 1852–1859. [CrossRef]

105. Karav, S.; Mills, D.A. Selective Prebiotic Activity of *N*-Glycans Released from Milk Glycoproteins by Novel En-do-β-*N*-acetylglucosaminidase. United States—California. 2015. Available online: https://www.proquest.com/dissertations-theses/selective-prebiotic-activity-i-n-glycans-released/docview/1774020008/se-2?accountid=15572 (accessed on 28 July 2024).
106. Karav, S.; Bell, J.M.L.N.D.M.; Le Parc, A.; Liu, Y.; Mills, D.A.; Block, D.E.; Barile, D. Characterizing the release of bioactive *N*-glycans from dairy products by a novel endo-β-*N*-acetylglucosaminidase. *Biotechnol. Prog.* **2015**, *31*, 1331–1339. [CrossRef]
107. Lane, J.A.; Mariño, K.; Naughton, J.; Kavanaugh, D.; Clyne, M.; Carrington, S.D.; Hickey, R.M. Anti-infective bovine colostrum oligosaccharides: Campylobacter jejuni as a case study. *Int. J. Food Microbiol.* **2012**, *157*, 182–188. [CrossRef]
108. Bode, L. Human Milk Oligosaccharides in the Prevention of Necrotizing Enterocolitis: A Journey From in vitro and in vivo Models to Mother-Infant Cohort Studies. *Front. Pediatr.* **2018**, *6*, 385. [CrossRef] [PubMed]
109. Sarıtaş, S.; Portocarrero, A.C.M.; López, J.M.M.; Lombardo, M.; Koch, W.; Raposo, A.; El-Seedi, H.R.; Alves, J.L.d.B.; Esatbeyoglu, T.; Karav, S.; et al. The Impact of Fermentation on the Antioxidant Activity of Food Products. *Molecules* **2024**, *29*, 3941. [CrossRef] [PubMed]
110. Ahern, G.J.; Hennessy, A.; Ryan, C.A.; Ross, R.P.; Stanton, C. Advances in Infant Formula Science. *Annu. Rev. Food Sci. Technol.* **2019**, *10*, 75–102. [CrossRef] [PubMed]
111. Bagwe-Parab, S.; Yadav, P.; Kaur, G.; Tuli, H.S.; Buttar, H.S. Therapeutic Applications of Human and Bovine Colostrum in the Treatment of Gastrointestinal Diseases and Distinctive Cancer Types: The Current Evidence. *Front. Pharmacol.* **2020**, *11*, 01100. [CrossRef]
112. Hurley, W.L.; Theil, P.K. Perspectives on Immunoglobulins in Colostrum and Milk. *Nutrients* **2011**, *3*, 442–474. [CrossRef]
113. Ulfman, L.H.; Leusen, J.H.W.; Savelkoul, H.F.J.; Warner, J.O.; van Neerven, R.J.J. Effects of Bovine Immunoglobulins on Immune Function, Allergy, and Infection. *Front. Nutr.* **2018**, *5*, 52. [CrossRef]
114. Gomes, R.D.; Anaya, K.; Galdino, A.B.; Oliveira, J.P.; Gama, M.A.; Medeiros, C.A.; Gavioli, E.C.; Porto, A.L.F.; Rangel, A.H. Bovine colostrum: A source of bioactive compounds for prevention and treatment of gastrointestinal disorders. *NFS J.* **2021**, *25*, 1–11. [CrossRef]
115. Kaplan, M.; Arslan, A.; Duman, H.; Karyelioğlu, M.; Baydemir, B.; Günar, B.B.; Alkan, M.; Bayraktar, A.; Tosun, H.I.; Ertürk, M.; et al. Production of Bovine Colostrum for Human Consumption to Improve Health. *Front. Pharmacol.* **2022**, *12*, 796824. [CrossRef]
116. Kirkden, R.D.; Broom, D.M.; Andersen, I.L. INVITED REVIEW: Piglet mortality: Management solutions. *J. Anim. Sci.* **2013**, *91*, 3361–3389. [CrossRef]
117. Gomez, G.G.; Phillips, O.; A Goforth, R. Effect of immunoglobulin source on survival, growth, and hematological and immunological variables in pigs. *J. Anim. Sci.* **1998**, *76*, 1–7. [CrossRef]
118. Juhl, S.M.; Ye, X.; Zhou, P.; Li, Y.; Iyore, E.O.; Zhang, L.; Jiang, P.; van Goudoever, J.B.; Greisen, G.; Sangild, P.T. Bovine Colostrum for Preterm Infants in the First Days of Life. *J. Pediatr. Gastroenterol. Nutr.* **2018**, *66*, 471–478. [CrossRef] [PubMed]
119. Mehra, R.; Garhwal, R.; Sangwan, K.; Guiné, R.P.F.; Lemos, E.T.; Buttar, H.S.; Visen, P.K.S.; Kumar, N.; Bhardwaj, A.; Kumar, H. Insights into the Research Trends on Bovine Colostrum: Beneficial Health Perspectives with Special Reference to Manufacturing of Functional Foods and Feed Supplements. *Nutrients* **2022**, *14*, 659. [CrossRef] [PubMed]
120. Gao, X.; Li, Y.; Olin, A.B.; Nguyen, D.N. Fortification with Bovine Colostrum Enhances Antibacterial Activity of Human Milk. *J. Parenter. Enter. Nutr.* **2021**, *45*, 1417–1424. [CrossRef]
121. Burrin, D.; Sangild, P.T.; Stoll, B.; Thymann, T.; Buddington, R.; Marini, J.; Olutoye, O.; Shulman, R.J. Translational Advances in Pediatric Nutrition and Gastroenterology: New Insights from Pig Models. *Annu. Rev. Anim. Biosci.* **2020**, *8*, 321–354. [CrossRef] [PubMed]
122. Neu, J.; Walker, W.A. Necrotizing Enterocolitis. *N. Engl. J. Med.* **2011**, *364*, 255–264. [CrossRef] [PubMed]
123. Niño, D.F.; Sodhi, C.P.; Hackam, D.J. Necrotizing enterocolitis: New insights into pathogenesis and mechanisms. *Nat. Rev. Gastroenterol. Hepatol.* **2016**, *13*, 590–600. [CrossRef] [PubMed]
124. Lin, P.W.; Stoll, B.J. Necrotising enterocolitis. *Lancet* **2006**, *368*, 1271–1283. [CrossRef]
125. Schmid, K.O. A specially severe form of enteritis in newborn, enterocolitis ulcerosa necroticans. I. Pathological anatomy. *Osterr Z Kinderheilkd Kinderfuersorge* **1952**, *8*, 114–135.
126. Stiennon, O.A. Pneumatosis intestinalis in the newborn. *AMA Am. J. Dis. Child.* **1951**, *81*, 651–663. [CrossRef] [PubMed]
127. Duchon, J.; Barbian, M.E.; Denning, P.W. Necrotizing Enterocolitis. *Clin. Perinatol.* **2021**, *48*, 229–250. [CrossRef]
128. Abdel, S.A.; Monem, S.A.A.; Ezzeldin, Z.M.; Said, H.M.; Baris, S.S.H.; El Tatawy, S.S. Bovine Colostrum Supplementation for Prevention of Necrotizing Enterocolitis and Late-Onset Sepsis in Preterm Infants. *NeuroQuantology* **2022**, *20*, 1385–1392. [CrossRef]
129. Balachandran, B.; Dutta, S.; Singh, R.; Prasad, R.; Kumar, P. Bovine colostrum in prevention of necrotizing enterocolitis and sepsis in very low birth weight neonates: A randomized, double-blind, placebo-controlled pilot trial. *J. Trop. Pediatr.* **2017**, *63*, 10–17. [CrossRef] [PubMed]
130. Nasuf, A.W.A.; Ojha, S.; Dorling, J. Oropharyngeal colostrum in preventing mortality and morbidity in preterm infants. *Cochrane Database Syst. Rev.* **2018**, *2019*, CD011921. [CrossRef] [PubMed]
131. Tao, J.; Mao, J.; Yang, J.; Su, Y. Effects of oropharyngeal administration of colostrum on the incidence of necrotizing enterocolitis, late-onset sepsis, and death in preterm infants: A meta-analysis of RCTs. *Eur. J. Clin. Nutr.* **2020**, *74*, 1122–1131. [CrossRef] [PubMed]
132. Sadeghirad, B.; Morgan, R.L.; Zeraatkar, D.; Zea, A.M.; Couban, R.; Johnston, B.C.; Florez, I.D. Human and Bovine Colostrum for Prevention of Necrotizing Enterocolitis: A Meta-analysis. *Pediatrics* **2018**, *142*, e20180767. [CrossRef]

133. Black, R.E.; Morris, S.; Bryce, J. Where and why are 10 million children dying every year? *Lancet* **2003**, *361*, 2226–2234. [CrossRef]
134. Liu, L.; Oza, S.; Hogan, D.; Perin, J.; Rudan, I.; Lawn, J.E.; Cousens, S.; Mathers, C.; Black, R.E. Global, regional, and national causes of child mortality in 2000–13, with projections to inform post-2015 priorities: An updated systematic analysis. *Lancet* **2015**, *385*, 430–440. [CrossRef]
135. Schnadower, D.; Finkelstein, Y.; Freedman, S.B. Ondansetron and probiotics in the management of pediatric acute gastroenteritis in developed countries. *Curr. Opin. Gastroenterol.* **2015**, *31*, 1–6. [CrossRef]
136. World Health Organization. *The Treatment of Diarrhoea A Manual for Physicians and Other Senior Health Workers (4th Rev.)*; World Health Organization: Geneva, Switzerland, 2005.
137. Florez, I.D.; Niño-Serna, L.F.; Beltrán-Arroyave, C.P. Acute Infectious Diarrhea and Gastroenteritis in Children. *Curr. Infect. Dis. Rep.* **2020**, *22*, 4. [CrossRef]
138. Guerrant, R.L.; Hughes, J.M.; Lima, N.L.; Crane, J. Diarrhea in Developed and Developing Countries: Magnitude, Special Settings, and Etiologies. *Clin. Infect. Dis.* **1990**, *12* (Suppl. S1), S41–S50. [CrossRef]
139. Gaensbauer, J.T.; Melgar, M.A.; Calvimontes, D.M.; Lamb, M.M.; Asturias, E.J.; Contreras-Roldan, I.L.; Dominguez, S.R.; Robinson, C.C.; Berman, S. Efficacy of a bovine colostrum and egg-based intervention in acute childhood diarrhoea in Guatemala: A randomised, double-blind, placebo-controlled trial. *BMJ Glob. Health* **2017**, *2*, e000452. [CrossRef] [PubMed]
140. Yu, J.; Lai, S.; Geng, Q.; Ye, C.; Zhang, Z.; Zheng, Y.; Wang, L.; Duan, Z.; Zhang, J.; Wu, S.; et al. Prevalence of rotavirus and rapid changes in circulating rotavirus strains among children with acute diarrhea in China, 2009–2015. *J. Infect.* **2019**, *78*, 66–74. [CrossRef] [PubMed]
141. Li, J.; Xu, Y.-W.; Jiang, J.-J.; Song, Q.-K. Bovine colostrum and product intervention associated with relief of childhood infectious diarrhea. *Sci. Rep.* **2019**, *9*, 3093. [CrossRef] [PubMed]
142. Chandwe, K.; Kelly, P. Colostrum Therapy for Human Gastrointestinal Health and Disease. *Nutrients* **2021**, *13*, 1956. [CrossRef]
143. Saad, K.; Abo-Elela, M.G.M.; El-Baseer, K.A.A.; Ahmed, A.E.; Ahmad, F.-A.; Tawfeek, M.S.K.; Houfey, A.A.E.; Aboul_Khair, M.D.; Abdel-Salam, A.M.; Abo-Elgheit, A.; et al. Effects of bovine colostrum on recurrent respiratory tract infections and diarrhea in children. *Medicine* **2016**, *95*, e4560. [CrossRef]
144. Holtmann, G.J.; Ford, A.C.; Talley, N.J. Pathophysiology of irritable bowel syndrome. *Lancet Gastroenterol. Hepatol.* **2016**, *1*, 133–146. [CrossRef]
145. Bernstein, C.N.; Eliakim, A.; Fedail, S.; Fried, M.; Gearry, R.; Goh, K.-L.; Hamid, S.; Khan, A.G.; Khalif, I.; Ng, S.C.; et al. World Gastroenterology Organisation Global Guidelines Inflammatory Bowel Disease. *J. Clin. Gastroenterol.* **2016**, *50*, 803–818. [CrossRef]
146. Xu, H.; Liu, M.; Cao, J.; Li, X.; Fan, D.; Xia, Y.; Lu, X.; Li, J.; Ju, D.; Zhao, H. The Dynamic Interplay between the Gut Microbiota and Autoimmune Diseases. *J. Immunol. Res.* **2019**, *2019*, 7546047. [CrossRef]
147. Zhang, Y.-Z.; Li, Y.-Y. Inflammatory bowel disease: Pathogenesis. *World J. Gastroenterol.* **2014**, *20*, 91–99. [CrossRef]
148. Brand, S. Crohn's disease: Th1, Th17 or both? The change of a paradigm: New immunological and genetic insights implicate Th17 cells in the pathogenesis of Crohn's disease. *Gut* **2009**, *58*, 1152–1167. [CrossRef]
149. Geremia, A.; Jewell, D.P. The IL-23/IL-17 pathway in inflammatory bowel disease. *Expert Rev. Gastroenterol. Hepatol.* **2012**, *6*, 223–237. [CrossRef] [PubMed]
150. Salim, S.Y.; Söderholm, J.D. Importance of disrupted intestinal barrier in inflammatory bowel diseases. *Inflamm. Bowel Dis.* **2011**, *17*, 362–381. [CrossRef] [PubMed]
151. Fichna, J. Inflammatory bowel disease treatment. *Pharmacol. Rep.* **2016**, *68*, 787–788. [CrossRef] [PubMed]
152. Yamamoto-Furusho, J. Tratamiento de la enfermedad inflamatoria intestinal. *Rev. Gastroenterol. Mex.* **2012**, *77*, 39–41. [CrossRef] [PubMed]
153. Lee, D.; Albenberg, L.; Compher, C.; Baldassano, R.; Piccoli, D.; Lewis, J.D.; Wu, G.D. Diet in the Pathogenesis and Treatment of Inflammatory Bowel Diseases. *Gastroenterology* **2015**, *148*, 1087–1106. [CrossRef]
154. Sigall-Boneh, R.; Levine, A.; Lomer, M.; Wierdsma, N.; Allan, P.; Fiorino, G.; Gatti, S.; Jonkers, D.; Kierkuś, J.; Katsanos, K.H.; et al. Research Gaps in Diet and Nutrition in Inflammatory Bowel Disease. A Topical Review by D-ECCO Working Group [Dietitians of ECCO]. *J. Crohn's Colitis* **2017**, *11*, 1407–1419. [CrossRef]
155. Bodammer, P.; Maletzki, C.; Waitz, G.; Emmrich, J. Prophylactic Application of Bovine Colostrum Ameliorates Murine Colitis via Induction of Immunoregulatory Cells. *J. Nutr.* **2011**, *141*, 1056–1061. [CrossRef]
156. Lee, A.; Pontin, M.C.; Kosmerl, E.; Jimenez-Flores, R.; Moretti, D.B.; Ziouzenkova, O. Assessment of adipogenic, antioxidant, and anti-inflammatory properties of whole and whey bovine colostrum. *J. Dairy Sci.* **2019**, *102*, 8614–8621. [CrossRef]
157. Sienkiewicz, M.; Szymańska, P.; Fichna, J. Supplementation of Bovine Colostrum in Inflammatory Bowel Disease: Benefits and Contraindications. *Adv. Nutr. Int. Rev. J.* **2021**, *12*, 533–545. [CrossRef]
158. Shing, C.M.; Peake, J.M.; Suzuki, K.; Jenkins, D.G.; Coombes, J.S. Bovine Colostrum Modulates Cytokine Production in Human Peripheral Blood Mononuclear Cells Stimulated with Lipopolysaccharide and Phytohemagglutinin. *J. Interf. Cytokine Res.* **2009**, *29*, 37–44. [CrossRef]
159. Khan, Z.; Macdonald, C.; Wicks, A.C.; Holt, M.P.; Floyd, D.; Ghosh, S.; Wright, N.A.; Playford, R.J. Use of the 'nutriceutical', bovine colostrum, for the treatment of distal colitis: Results from an initial study. *Aliment. Pharmacol. Ther.* **2002**, *16*, 1917–1922. [CrossRef] [PubMed]
160. Sigalet, D. Short Bowel Syndrome in Infants and Children: An Overview. *Semin. Pediatr. Surg.* **2001**, *10*, 49–55. [CrossRef] [PubMed]

161. Goulet, O.; Ruemmele, F.; Lacaille, F.; Colomb, V. Irreversible Intestinal Failure. *J. Pediatr. Gastroenterol. Nutr.* **2004**, *38*, 250–269. [CrossRef] [PubMed]
162. Goulet, O.; Ruemmele, F. Causes and Management of Intestinal Failure in Children. *Gastroenterology* **2006**, *130*, S16–S28. [CrossRef]
163. Jeppesen, P.B.; Mortensen, P.B. Intestinal failure defined by measurements of intestinal energy and wet weight absorption. *Gut* **2000**, *46*, 701–706. [CrossRef]
164. O'keefe, S.J.; Buchman, A.L.; Fishbein, T.M.; Jeejeebhoy, K.N.; Jeppesen, P.B.; Shaffer, J. Short Bowel Syndrome and Intestinal Failure: Consensus Definitions and Overview. *Clin. Gastroenterol. Hepatol.* **2006**, *4*, 6–10. [CrossRef]
165. Aunsholt, L.; Jeppesen, P.B.; Lund, P.; Sangild, P.T.; Ifaoui, I.B.R.; Qvist, N.; Husby, S. Bovine colostrum to children with short bowel syndrome: A randomized, double-blind, crossover pilot study. *J. Parenter. Enter. Nutr.* **2014**, *38*, 99–106. [CrossRef]
166. Aunsholt, L.; Qvist, N.; Sangild, P.T.; Vegge, A.; Stoll, B.; Burrin, D.G.; Jeppesen, P.B.; Eriksen, T.; Husby, S.; Thymann, T. Minimal Enteral Nutrition to Improve Adaptation After Intestinal Resection in Piglets and Infants. *J. Parenter. Enter. Nutr.* **2018**, *42*, 446–454. [CrossRef]
167. Aunsholt, L.; Thymann, T.; Qvist, N.; Sigalet, D.; Husby, S.; Sangild, P.T. Prematurity Reduces Functional Adaptation to Intestinal Resection in Piglets. *J. Parenter. Enter. Nutr.* **2015**, *39*, 668–676. [CrossRef]
168. Pereira-Fantini, P.M.; Thomas, S.L.; Taylor, R.G.; Nagy, E.; Sourial, M.; Fuller, P.J.; Bines, J.E. Colostrum Supplementation Restores Insulin-like Growth Factor -1 Levels and Alters Muscle Morphology Following Massive Small Bowel Resection. *J. Parenter. Enter. Nutr.* **2008**, *32*, 266–275. [CrossRef]
169. Sangild, P.T.; Ney, D.M.; Sigalet, D.L.; Vegge, A.; Burrin, D. Animal models of gastrointestinal and liver diseases. Animal models of infant short bowel syndrome: Translational relevance and challenges. *Am. J. Physiol. Liver Physiol.* **2014**, *307*, G1147–G1168. [CrossRef] [PubMed]
170. Shane, A.L.; Sánchez, P.J.; Stoll, B.J. Neonatal sepsis. *Lancet* **2017**, *390*, 1770–1780. [CrossRef] [PubMed]
171. Wynn, J.L.; Wong, H.R.; Shanley, T.P.; Bizzarro, M.J.; Saiman, L.; Polin, R.A. Time for a Neonatal-Specific Consensus Definition for Sepsis. *Pediatr. Crit. Care Med.* **2014**, *15*, 523–528. [CrossRef] [PubMed]
172. Manzoni, P. Bovine Lactoferrin Supplementation for Prevention of Late-Onset Sepsis in Very Low-Birth-Weight NeonatesA Randomized Trial. *JAMA* **2009**, *302*, 1421–1428. [CrossRef] [PubMed]
173. Brunse, A.; Worsøe, P.; Pors, S.E.; Skovgaard, K.; Sangild, P.T. Oral Supplementation with Bovine Colostrum Prevents Septic Shock and Brain Barrier Disruption During Bloodstream Infection in Preterm Newborn Pigs. *Shock* **2019**, *51*, 337–347. [CrossRef]
174. Luo, F.; Zhang, M.; Zhang, L.; Zhou, P. Nutritional and health effects of bovine colostrum in neonates. *Nutr. Rev.* **2023**, *82*, 1631–1645. [CrossRef]
175. Jensen, M.L.; Sangild, P.T.; Lykke, M.; Schmidt, M.; Boye, M.; Jensen, B.B.; Thymann, T. Similar efficacy of human banked milk and bovine colostrum to decrease incidence of necrotizing enterocolitis in preterm piglets. *Am. J. Physiol. Integr. Comp. Physiol.* **2013**, *305*, R4–R12. [CrossRef]
176. Li, Y.; Jensen, M.L.; Chatterton, D.E.W.; Jensen, B.B.; Thymann, T.; Kvistgaard, A.S.; Sangild, P.T. Raw bovine milk improves gut responses to feeding relative to infant formula in preterm piglets. *Am. J. Physiol. Liver Physiol.* **2014**, *306*, G81–G90. [CrossRef]
177. Rasmussen, S.O.; Martin, L.; Østergaard, M.V.; Rudloff, S.; Li, Y.; Roggenbuck, M.; Bering, S.B.; Sangild, P.T. Bovine colostrum improves neonatal growth, digestive function, and gut immunity relative to donor human milk and infant formula in preterm pigs. *Am. J. Physiol. Liver Physiol.* **2016**, *311*, G480–G491. [CrossRef]
178. Ismail, R.I.H.; Awad, H.A.; Imam, S.S.; Gad, G.I.; Aboushady, N.M.; Abdou, R.M.; Eissa, D.S.; Azzam, N.T.; Barakat, M.M.; Yassin, M.M.; et al. Gut priming with bovine colostrum and T regulatory cells in preterm neonates: A randomized controlled trial. *Pediatr. Res.* **2021**, *90*, 650–656. [CrossRef]
179. Kao, C.-Y.; Sheu, B.-S.; Wu, J.-J. Helicobacter pylori infection: An overview of bacterial virulence factors and pathogenesis. *Biomed. J.* **2016**, *39*, 14–23. [CrossRef] [PubMed]
180. Bitzan, M.M.; Gold, B.D.; Philpott, D.J.; Huesca, M.; Sherman, P.M.; Karch, H.; Lissner, R.; Lingwood, C.A.; Karmali, M.A. Inhibition of Helicobacter pylori and Helicobacter mustelae Binding to Lipid Receptors by Bovine Colostrum. *J. Infect. Dis.* **1998**, *177*, 955–961. [CrossRef] [PubMed]
181. Baltierra-Uribe, S.L.; Montañez-Barragán, A.; Romero-Ramírez, H.; Klimov-Kravtchenko, K.; Martínez-Pedro, K.I.; Sánchez-Salguero, E.; Camorlinga-Ponce, M.; Torres, J.; Santos-Argumedo, L. Colostrum IgA1 antibodies recognize antigens from *Helicobacter pylori* and prevent cytoskeletal changes in human epithelial cells. *Eur. J. Immunol.* **2021**, *51*, 2641–2650. [CrossRef] [PubMed]
182. Casswall, T.H.; Nilsson, H.-O.; Björck, L.; Sjöstedt, S.; Xu, L.; Nord, C.-E.; Borén, T.; Wadström, T.; Hammarström, L. Bovine Anti-Helicobacter pylori Antibodies for Oral Immunotherapy. *Scand. J. Gastroenterol.* **2002**, *37*, 1380–1385. [CrossRef] [PubMed]
183. Marnila, P.; Rokka, S.; Rehnberg-Laiho, L.; Karkkainen, P.; Kosunen, T.U.; Rautelin, H.; Hanninen, M.-L.; Syvaoja, E.-L.; Korhonen, H. Prevention and Suppression of Helicobacter felis Infection in Mice Using Colostral Preparation with Specific Antibodies. *Helicobacter* **2003**, *8*, 192–201. [CrossRef]
184. Tran, C.D.; Kritas, S.; Campbell, M.A.F.; Huynh, H.Q.; Lee, S.-S.; Butler, R.N. Novel combination therapy for the eradication of *Helicobacter pylori* infection in a mouse model. *Scand. J. Gastroenterol.* **2010**, *45*, 1424–1430. [CrossRef]
185. Megahed, F.; El-Assal, M.; Dabour, A.S.; Samy, R.; Rizk, M.; Al Adhm, S.H. Lactoferrin as an added therapy in the treatment of Helicobacter pylori. *Benha Med. J.* **2017**, *34*, 119. [CrossRef]

186. Yalçıntaş, Y.M.; Duman, H.; Rocha, J.M.; Bartkiene, E.; Karav, S.; Ozogul, F. Role of bovine colostrum against various diseases. *Food Biosci.* **2024**, *61*, 104818. [CrossRef]
187. Brinkworth, G.D.; Buckley, J.D. Concentrated bovine colostrum protein supplementation reduces the incidence of self-reported symptoms of upper respiratory tract infection in adult males. *Eur. J. Nutr.* **2003**, *42*, 228–232. [CrossRef]
188. Patel, K.; Rana, R. Pedimune in recurrent respiratory infection and diarrhoea—The Indian experience—The PRIDE study. *Indian J. Pediatr.* **2006**, *73*, 585–591. [CrossRef]
189. Rathe, M.; De Pietri, S.; Wehner, P.S.; Frandsen, T.L.; Grell, K.; Schmiegelow, K.; Sangild, P.T.; Husby, S.; Müller, K. Bovine Colostrum Against Chemotherapy-Induced Gastrointestinal Toxicity in Children with Acute Lymphoblastic Leukemia: A Randomized, Double-Blind, Placebo-Controlled Trial. *J. Parenter. Enter. Nutr.* **2020**, *44*, 337–347. [CrossRef] [PubMed]
190. Do, A.B.; Williams, K.; Toomer, O.T. In vitro digestibility and immunoreactivity of bovine milk proteins. *Food Chem.* **2016**, *190*, 581–587. [CrossRef] [PubMed]
191. Hochwallner, H.; Schulmeister, U.; Swoboda, I.; Spitzauer, S.; Valenta, R. Cow's milk allergy: From allergens to new forms of diagnosis, therapy and prevention. *Methods* **2014**, *66*, 22–33. [CrossRef] [PubMed]
192. Monaci, L.; Tregoat, V.; Van Hengel, A.J.; Anklam, E. Milk allergens, their characteristics and their detection in food: A review. *Eur. Food Res. Technol.* **2006**, *223*, 149–179. [CrossRef]
193. Villa, C.; Costa, J.; Oliveira, M.B.P.; Mafra, I. Bovine Milk Allergens: A Comprehensive Review. *Compr. Rev. Food Sci. Food Saf.* **2018**, *17*, 137–164. [CrossRef]
194. Matsumoto, N.; Okochi, M.; Matsushima, M.; Kato, R.; Takase, T.; Yoshida, Y.; Kawase, M.; Isobe, K.-I.; Kawabe, T.; Honda, H. Peptide array-based analysis of the specific IgE and IgG4 in cow's milk allergens and its use in allergy evaluation. *Peptides* **2009**, *30*, 1840–1847. [CrossRef]
195. Fiocchi, A.; Brozek, J.; Schünemann, H.; Bahna, S.L.; von Berg, A.; Beyer, K.; Bozzola, M.; Bradsher, J.; Compalati, E.; Ebisawa, M.; et al. World allergy organization (WAO) diagnosis and rationale for action against cow's milk allergy (DRACMA) guidelines. *World Allergy Organ. J.* **2010**, *3*, 57–161. [CrossRef]
196. Martorell-Aragonés, A.; Echeverría-Zudaire, L.; Alonso-Lebrero, E.; Boné-Calvo, J.; Martín-Muñoz, M.; Nevot-Falcó, S.; Piquer-Gibert, M.; Valdesoiro-Navarrete, L. Position document: IgE-mediated cow's milk allergy. *Allergol. Immunopathol.* **2015**, *43*, 507–526. [CrossRef]
197. Buttar, H.S.; Bagwe, S.M.; Bhullar, S.K.; Kaur, G. Health Benefits of Bovine Colostrum in Children and Adults. In *Dairy in Human Health and Disease Across the Lifespan*; Elsevier: Amsterdam, The Netherlands, 2017; pp. 3–20. [CrossRef]

nutrients MDPI

Review

Breastfeeding Beyond Six Months: Evidence of Child Health Benefits

Anita Froń * and Magdalena Orczyk-Pawiłowicz

Division of Chemistry and Immunochemistry, Department of Biochemistry and Immunochemistry, Wroclaw Medical University, M. Skłodowskiej-Curie 48/50, 50-369 Wroclaw, Poland; magdalena.orczyk-pawilowicz@umw.edu.pl
* Correspondence: anita.fron@student.umw.edu.pl; Tel.: +48-660-083-243

Abstract: Breastfeeding is globally recognized as the optimal method of infant nutrition, offering health benefits for both the child and the mother, making it a public health priority. However, the potential advantages of breastfeeding extend well beyond initial months. Breast milk adapts to the evolving needs of the growing infant, and its immunological, microbiological, and biochemical properties have been associated with enhanced protection against infections and chronic diseases, improved growth and development, and lower rates of hospitalization and mortality. This review explores the evidence supporting the continuation of breastfeeding beyond six months. More meticulous studies employing consistent methodologies and addressing confounders are essential. This will enable a more accurate determination of the extent and mechanisms of the positive impact of prolonged breastfeeding and allow for the implementation of effective public health strategies.

Keywords: prolonged breastfeeding; physiological nutrition; biochemical composition of breast milk; immune properties; mother–breastmilk–infant triad; health outcomes

1. Introduction

The initial 1000 days of life is the most important period in shaping an individual's health trajectory. During this crucial window, various physiological, immunological, and neurological developments occur, laying the foundation for long-term well-being [1–6]. Among the myriad of factors influencing these developmental processes, nutrition stands out as a pivotal element. Breastfeeding, in particular, has been extensively studied and lauded for its profound impact on both immediate and future health outcomes.

Breast milk serves as a critical link between maternal and offspring health, representing a unique biological system known as the 'connected triad'. This triad, formed by the interactions among the mother, breast milk, and infant, creates a dynamic and interdependent relationship. Each variation within this triad can significantly influence the trajectory of both infant development and maternal health, highlighting the extensive impact of breastfeeding on overall well-being [7–9].

Breastfeeding provides a unique blend of nutrients and bioactive components tailored to meet infants' developmental needs [10]. Children breastfed for extended periods experience lower rates of infectious morbidity and mortality. Growing evidence suggests that longer breastfeeding durations may also protect against overweight, diabetes, allergies, and other chronic illnesses later in life, and contribute to fewer dental malocclusions and higher intelligence scores compared to shorter breastfeeding durations or no breastfeeding at all. These benefits persist into later stages of life [1,11–15]. As previously established, breastfeeding not only benefits infants but also offers considerable advantages for maternal health. It can lower the risk of breast, ovarian, and endometrial cancers, and potentially reduce the risk of diabetes, hypertension, and hyperlipidemia [16–18]. The act of breastfeeding not only provides essential nutrition but also fosters emotional closeness through intimate skin-to-skin contact. This physical proximity during breastfeeding has been shown to positively influence infants' vital signs, indicating a calming effect and enhancing the overall bonding experience between mother and child [19]. Research indicates that mothers who encounter breastfeeding challenges may experience difficulties in forming strong attachments with their infants during this period. Conversely, longer durations of breastfeeding have been found to correlate significantly with higher levels of attachment security [20,21].

In recent years, there has been growing evidence of the substantial health benefits of prolonged breastfeeding, defined as breastfeeding beyond six months [22]. Despite recommendations from organizations like the World Health Organization (WHO), the Association of Women's Health, Obstetric and Neonatal Nurses, and the US National Academy of Sciences, which advocate exclusive breastfeeding for the first six months and continued breastfeeding for at least one year, actual breastfeeding practices often fall short [19,23,24].

The CDC's Breastfeeding Report Card for 2022 indicates that among infants born in 2019 in the territory of the United States, a significant majority (83.2%) began breastfeeding, with 78.6% still receiving some breast milk at one month. At six months, 55.8% of infants continued to receive breast milk, while only 24.9% received it exclusively [25]. The data from Europe present a less encouraging picture. A 2021 study, which included data from six European countries (Belgium, Bulgaria, Germany, Greece, Poland, and Spain), revealed that although 85% of children were breastfed at some point, only 6.3% were exclusively breastfed for the first six months. Factors such as lower maternal education, smoking during pregnancy, pre-pregnancy overweight, and younger maternal age were associated with shorter durations of exclusive breastfeeding [26]. If all children were breastfed within an hour of birth, exclusively fed breast milk for the first six months, and continued breastfeeding until the age of two, approximately 800,000 child lives could be saved annually. However, worldwide, less than 40% of infants under six months old are exclusively breastfed [27].

Human milk continues to provide significant nutritional and immunological value beyond 6 months. Studies indicate that the macronutrient content of milk changes to meet the growing child's energy demands [28,29]. This milk retains high concentrations of immunoglobulins and other bioactive components, highlighting its continued importance for infant health. Promoting extended breastfeeding, even after introducing solid foods, should be a public health priority to prevent infections in infancy [30].

This paper aims to consolidate and present the current evidence on the health benefits of breastfeeding beyond six months.

2. Changes in Immune Factors in Breast Milk During Prolonged Lactation

Prolonged lactation is associated with significant changes in the concentrations of various immune factors in breast milk. In the later stages of lactation, especially as complementary foods that provide nutritional value are introduced, breast milk primarily supplies bioactive factors [10,28,31]. These changes are crucial for maintaining the health and development of the infant, offering continued immune protection as breastfeeding extends beyond the initial postpartum months.

2.1. Secretory IgA (sIgA)

The concentration of sIgA in breast milk generally remains stable throughout the first 18 months of lactation, averaging around 1.8 g/L [32–34]. However, Ongprasert et al. [35] found a positive correlation between the duration of lactation and sIgA concentration. Their study showed that mean total IgA levels were lowest in the first 6 months (1.11 ± 0.14 g/L) and increased in subsequent periods, reaching up to 1.27 ± 0.15 g/L at 18–24 months. According to Goldman et al. [36], both total and secretory IgA concentrations show a slight increase from 0.8 ± 0.3 g/L at 12 months to 1.1 ± 0.3 g/L at 13–15 months, maintaining this level up to 16–24 months (1.1 ± 0.3 g/L for total IgA and 1.1 ± 0.2 g/L for secretory IgA). Additionally, Perrin and colleagues [37] found that sIgA concentrations increase between 11 and 17 months, with a monthly change magnitude of +6.0%. As per the most recent analysis [30], the lowest concentration of sIgA was observed in the first year of lactation, averaging at 2.12 ± 0.62 g/L. After the second year, sIgA levels peaked at 7.55 ± 7.16 g/L. Over prolonged lactation, sIgA levels also positively correlated with IgG concentrations. The ratio of sIgA to protein remained stable for the first two years but significantly increased in the third year [30].

2.2. Lysozyme

The concentration of lysozyme in colostrum starts high at 87 mg/L, drops to its lowest point of 24 mg/L at 2–4 weeks postpartum, and then rises progressively over the next five months to reach 245 mg/L [34]. However, from 5 months to 12 months, there is a decrease in lysozyme levels, which are recorded to be 196 ± 41 mg/L at 12 months [34]. Subsequently, lysozyme levels increase to 244 ± 34 mg/L at 13–15 months [36,38]. Nevertheless, there is a slight decrease to 187 ± 33 mg/L by 16–24 month [36,37]. According to the data collected by Perrin et al. [37], between 11 and 17 months, lysozyme shows a monthly change magnitude of +10.2%, indicating a consistent increase during this period. The progressive increase in lysozyme concentration compensates for the decreasing milk volume, resulting in a significant rise in the amount of lysozyme ingested by the infant over time [32].

2.3. Lactoferrin

During the first year of lactation, lactoferrin (Lf) concentrations experience a pronounced decrease. Despite this reduction, the infant's daily intake of Lf remains substantial. By the end of the first year, lactoferrin levels stabilize, continuing to provide significant antimicrobial activity [38]. The mean Lf concentration is lowest during the first 12 months, at 3.39 ± 1.43 g/L, and increases significantly to 5.55 ± 4.00 g/L during the 13–18-month period ($p < 0.006$). Concentrations then remain relatively stable, at approximately 5.02 ± 2.97 g/L for the 19–24-month lactation group and 4.90 ± 3.18 g/L for those lactating beyond 24 months [39]. Lactoferrin concentration in breast milk is positively correlated with protein concentration over the course of lactation ($r = 0.3374$; $p = 0.0002$) [39]. According to Goldman et al. [36], from 12 to 24 months, Lf concentrations in breast milk increase steadily, starting at 1.0 ± 0.2 g/L at 12 months, rising to 1.1 ± 0.1 g/L between 13 and 15 months, and reaching 1.2 ± 0.1 g/L from 16 to 24 months, while Perrin et al. [37] found that between 11 and 17 months, lactoferrin concentrations rise by 9.7% per month. In light of the analyzed studies, the differences in Lf concentrations in human milk can be attributed to the various measurement methods employed by researchers. Methodological differences, including collection frequency, time of day, and storage conditions, likely contribute to the variations in reported lactoferrin concentrations.

2.4. Other Immune Factors

IgG concentrations are lowest during the first year of lactation, averaging at 14.71 ± 6.18 mg/L, and increase after the second year to 18.95 ± 6.76 mg/L. The ratio of IgG to protein decreases progressively from the 1st to the 48th month of lactation [30]. In contrast, the concentration of IgM remains relatively stable during the first two years of lactation, averaging at 2.81 ± 2.74 mg/L. Unlike sIgA and IgG, the ratio of IgM to protein does not show significant changes across different lactation periods [30]. Additionally, the concentrations of other immune proteins, such as C3 and C4, decrease during the first 12 months of lactation [38].

These compositional changes in breast milk ensure that it consistently meets the evolving nutritional and immunological needs of the infant throughout extended lactation. This adaptability indicates that as lactation progresses, the immunoprotective properties of breast milk are not only preserved but may also be enhanced, thereby supporting and promoting the health of the breastfeeding child. No infant formula can fully replicate the complex immunological qualities of breast milk. From an economic perspective, prolonged breastfeeding presents a cost-effective solution, providing ongoing immune protection without the need for expensive supplements or fortified formulas [11,40,41]. This highlights the superiority of extended lactation as a protective measure, ensuring optimal immune support for children in a way that artificial products cannot match.

3. Materials and Methods

For this narrative review, we conducted comprehensive English-language literature research for original and review articles published until August 2024 in the PUBMED/Scopus databases. We searched for the following terms, alone or in combination: human milk, breast milk, breastfeeding, breast-feeding, breast feeding, lactation, nutrition, infant, childhood, prolonged, duration, beyond 6 months, 12 months, macronutrients, benefits, advantages, and well-being. We found 486 related articles. The relevant studies were identified by evaluating the abstracts, and complete articles were obtained in cases where abstracts were unavailable. Duplicate papers were removed, and the data were screened to exclude irrelevant works. Case reports, comments, conference papers, commentaries, surveys, and animal studies were all excluded from the full-text publications. Additional manual searches were conducted on the indicated bibliographies, taking into consideration the articles' novelty, quality, and clinical significance. After applying the exclusion criteria, 179 full-text manuscripts were assessed for eligibility with the consensus of the authors.

4. Limitations and Gaps in the Current Research

The current literature on the benefits of prolonged breastfeeding reveals a nuanced and sometimes contradictory picture. While numerous studies suggest various positive effects, the quality and reliability of these findings are often compromised by methodological limitations and insufficient control for confounding variables. A significant issue with existing research is the lack of adequate control for confounding factors such as socioeconomic status, maternal education, and pre-existing health conditions. Furthermore, much of the data available come from studies conducted several years ago, with some articles dating back over 40 years. These older studies may not reflect current breastfeeding practices or advancements in research methodologies. As a result, there is a need for updated and comprehensive studies to validate and extend these earlier findings.

To provide a clearer overview of the current state of evidence, Figure 1 illustrates the strength of scientific evidence on various health conditions that may benefit from prolonged breastfeeding. This illustration serves a conceptual purpose, representing the "strength" as a reflection of the quantity of studies available on each topic.

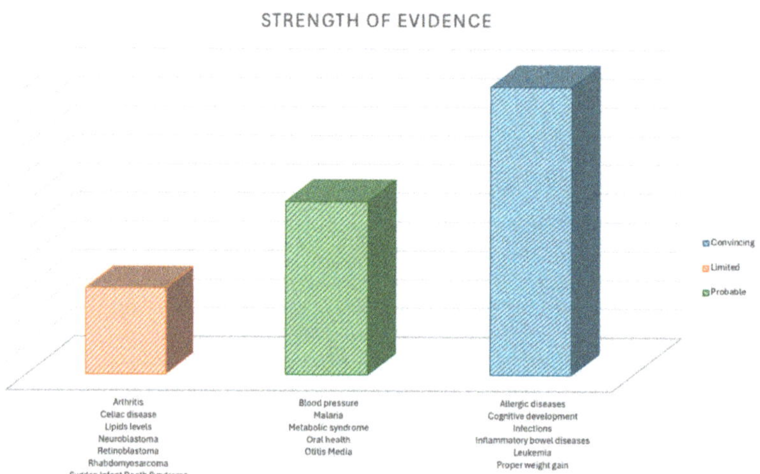

Figure 1. Strength of scientific evidence on health conditions which may benefit from prolonged breastfeeding.

5. Prolonged Breastfeeding's Effect on Health Outcomes

Research indicates that extended breastfeeding can positively impact a range of conditions, from infectious diseases to chronic illnesses. By examining these conditions, we aim to provide a comprehensive understanding of how prolonged breastfeeding contributes to better health outcomes. This exploration will draw attention to the potential protective effects of breastfeeding throughout infancy and show the importance of continued breastfeeding in the broader context of child well-being and development.

5.1. Allergic Diseases

The rising prevalence of allergic diseases in children has become a significant public health challenge globally. This trend is particularly alarming in pediatric populations. Recent data highlight a dramatic increase in allergic conditions, with asthma affecting between 1% and 20% of children, allergic rhinitis ranging from 1% to 18%, and skin allergies between 2% and 10% across various populations [42]. This escalation in allergy rates has been linked to several elements, including improved sanitary conditions, changes in delivery methods, increased antibiotic use, and shifts toward a Western-style diet. These factors not only influence the immune system directly but also impact the gut microbiota, potentially leading to dysbiosis—a microbial imbalance that may play a crucial role in the development of allergic diseases [43–46].

Bener et al. [47] observed that children breastfed for more than 6 months had a lower risk of allergic diseases than those breastfed for less than 6 months. Specifically, the prevalence rates of asthma, ear infections, wheezing, allergic rhinitis, and eczema were generally lower in children with prolonged breastfeeding. The prevalence of asthma was 15.1% in children with a short breastfeeding duration compared to 14.5% in those breastfed for longer periods. Similarly, rates were lower for ear infections (28.1% vs. 21.8%), wheezing (10.7% vs. 8.4%), allergic rhinitis (21.5% vs. 21.2%), and eczema (18.6% vs. 13.4%). These findings suggest that breastfeeding for more than 6 months may offer protective benefits against various allergic conditions during childhood.

Building on earlier research, Ehlaye et al. [48] found that infants breastfed for more than 6 months had lower prevalence rates of eczema (19.4%), allergic rhinitis (22.6%), and wheezing (12.7%) compared to those breastfed for shorter durations. This suggests that prolonged breastfeeding and exclusive breastfeeding (EBF) reduce the incidence of eczema and allergic diseases in children, even when there is a maternal history of allergy.

Furthermore, Saarinen et al. [49] followed infants with varying breastfeeding durations to assess the incidence of atopic diseases over the first 3 years of life. They found that infants breastfed for more than 6 months had a lower incidence of severe atopic dermatitis and food allergies compared to those breastfed for shorter durations or fed cow's milk-based formulas early. This protective effect was especially pronounced in children with a family history of atopy. Then, Saarinen et al. [50] conducted a long-term follow-up study of these 236 infants to investigate the impact of breastfeeding on atopic diseases from infancy through adolescence. They found that prolonged breastfeeding (>6 months) was associated with a lowest prevalence of eczema at ages 1 and 3 years compared to shorter durations of breastfeeding. This protective effect extended into adolescence, with the prolonged breastfeeding group showing a lower prevalence of overall atopy and substantial atopy at age 17 compared to the groups with intermediate (1–6 months) or minimal (<1 month) breastfeeding. These studies suggest that breastfeeding for over 6 months may help prevent atopic diseases throughout childhood and adolescence. Additionally, breastfeeding duration has a greater impact on reducing atopy than family history alone, especially in children consuming cow's milk, highlighting the role of dietary and other factors in promoting breastfeeding's protective effects.

Complementing previous findings, the study by van Ginkel et al. [51] examined how breastfeeding duration relates to the risk of clinical food allergies. The study included 492 participants, with breastfeeding durations ranging widely from less than 1 month to 42 months. Participants were categorized into quartiles based on breastfeeding duration, showing that longer breastfeeding appeared to provide a protective effect against food allergies. They found that for each additional month of breastfeeding, there was a 4% decrease in the risk of developing clinical food allergies to any type of food. However, it is important to note that they reported no significant association between breastfeeding (versus bottle-feeding) and food allergies, even after correcting for confounding factors.

Obihara et al. [52] discovered that children who were breastfed for longer durations (≥6 months) had a significantly lower risk of allergic diseases overall, particularly hay fever. The study showed a clear inverse relationship between breastfeeding duration and the incidence of allergic diseases, with adjusted odds ratios of 0.50 (95% CI: 0.31–0.82) for allergic disease and 0.53 (95% CI: 0.29–0.99) for hay fever. However, this association was not statistically significant for asthma (adjusted OR: 0.67; 95% CI: 0.31–1.49) or eczema (OR: 0.56; 95% CI: 0.29–1.08). Similar conclusions were drawn by Huang et al., who found that exclusive breastfeeding for more than 6 months was significantly associated with a reduced risk of hay fever (0.93, 95% CI: 0.89–0.97) and eczema (0.96, 95% CI: 0.93–0.99). Overall, the longer the duration of breastfeeding and the more exclusive it was, the lower the prevalence of these diseases [53].

The KOALA study conducted in the Netherlands investigated the relationship between the age of first introduction of cow's milk and other food products and atopic manifestations in the first two years of life, considering breastfeeding duration as a confounder. They found that delayed introduction of food products was associated with a higher risk of recurrent wheeze. Nevertheless, a longer duration of breastfeeding (7–9 months) was linked to a reduced risk of recurrent wheeze, with a similar trend observed for breastfeeding durations longer than 9 months. The study observed a statistically significant trend, indicating that longer breastfeeding duration is associated with a reduced risk of recurrent wheeze [54].

While exclusive breastfeeding for at least the first six months of life is widely promoted and recommended, the relationship between breastfeeding and the prevention of food allergies presents a more nuanced picture [19,24]. In populations where peanut allergy prevalence is notably high, the European Academy of Allergy and Clinical Immunology (EAACI) Task Force suggests that the optimal age for introducing peanuts is between four and six months as part of complementary feeding. The same timeframe is recommended for introducing eggs into the diet. A critical aspect of this strategy is that the protective effects associated with the early introduction of allergenic foods are most pronounced when breastfeeding continues for at least eight months. This highlights the importance of combining prolonged breastfeeding with the timely introduction of allergenic foods to maximize potential benefits. Moreover, the EAACI guidelines advocate against the avoidance of dietary allergens during pregnancy and breastfeeding as a preventive measure for food allergies. This recommendation underscores the evolving understanding of food allergies and their relationship with infant feeding practices. However, the best way to prevent food allergies remains unknown, necessitating more thorough research with robust diagnostic standards [55].

5.1.1. Asthma

It has been established that longer durations of exclusive and any breastfeeding are significantly associated with reduced risks of adverse respiratory outcomes at 15 months. Adjusted analyses in Silvers et al.'s study [56] showed that each additional month of exclusive breastfeeding decreased the risk of diagnosed asthma by 20%, wheezing by 12%, inhaler use by 14%, 'wheeze AND diagnosed asthma AND inhaler' by 24%, and current asthma by 21%. Similar reductions were observed for each month of any breastfeeding, albeit at slightly lower percentages. Subsequent research on the same cohort revealed that the protective effect of each month of exclusive breastfeeding decreased over time. Initially observed to offer 21% protection at 15 months, this effect diminished to approximately 9% by 6 years of age [57]. Comparable conclusions were obtained by von Kobyletzki [58], who discovered that infants breastfed for up to 6 months have a 57% higher risk of developing asthma compared to those breastfed for longer durations. However, the confidence interval indicates that this result may not be statistically significant.

The study conducted by Wickman et al. [59] evaluated 4089 children for diagnosed asthma at 2 years of age. They observed a statistically significant advantage associated with breastfeeding exclusively for ≥6 months compared to <3 months (odds ratio 0.67, 95% confidence interval 0.5–0.91). Likewise, Borba et al. [60] confirmed that breastfeeding—whether partial or exclusive—for more than 6 months was significantly associated with a reduced risk of asthma.

In line with these observations, Watanabe and colleagues [61] found that longer durations of breastfeeding, particularly 10–14 months, 14–19 months, and over 19 months, were associated with reduced odds of asthma in a Japanese cohort compared to breastfeeding for less than 10 months. The adjusted odds ratios for asthma were 0.69 (95% CI: 0.52–0.91), 0.73 (95% CI: 0.56–0.97), and 0.67 (95% CI: 0.51–0.88), respectively, for these breastfeeding durations, indicating a protective effect regardless of exclusivity.

Furthermore, according to Al-Makoshi et al. [62], full breastfeeding is linked to a decreased incidence of childhood wheezing and potentially asthma. Extended periods of full breastfeeding, particularly lasting 6 to 12 months or more, were associated with lower likelihoods of mothers reporting that their child had ever wheezed or experienced wheezing within the past year. Furthermore, children breastfed for over 12 months had a lower prevalence of reported asthma.

5.1.2. Allergic Rhinitis

In a large population study analyzing data from 1374 children participating in the Allergic Rhinitis Cohort Study for Kids (ARCO-kids study), long-term breastfeeding (≥12 months) was significantly associated with a lower prevalence of allergic rhinitis (AR). Specifically, compared to short-term breastfeeding (<6 months), long-term breastfeeding (≥12 months) was linked to a reduced prevalence of AR (aOR, 0.54; 95% CI, 0.34 to 0.88). However, the study found that breastfeeding for 6–11 months did not show a statistically significant relationship with the risk of AR [63].

Other studies also confirm that breastfeeding for more than 6 months significantly reduces the risk of AR [53,64]. Additionally, it was found that breastfeeding for less than 6 months increased the risk of developing asthma by 57%, and asthma, in turn, increased the odds of developing rhinitis nearly threefold [58].

5.2. Inflammatory Bowel Diseases

Over the past few years, inflammatory bowel diseases (IBDs), such as Crohn's disease (CD) and ulcerative colitis (UC), have emerged as global health concerns with rapidly increasing occurrence rates [65]. The incidence of pediatric-onset ulcerative colitis ranges from 1 to 4 per 100,000 per year in most regions of North America and Europe [66]. For Crohn's disease, the prevalence in the United States is estimated at 58 per 100,000 children [67]. Reports indicate that breastfeeding can reduce the prevalence of CD and UC. This protective effect is attributed to breast milk's ability to shield infants from gastrointestinal infections, as well as IBD, by promoting the development and growth of the gastrointestinal mucosal system along with enhancing the immune system's ability to remember and respond to pathogens [68–70].

Rigas et al. [71] conducted a study involving 68 patients with CD, 39 patients with UC, and 202 control subjects. Breastfeeding durations were as follows: ≤5 months, 6–11 months, and ≥12 months. Their findings indicated a negative association between breastfeeding and the incidence of both CD and UC, with a duration-dependent trend observed. The results showed that breastfeeding was negatively associated with Crohn's disease ($p < 0.04$) and ulcerative colitis ($p < 0.07$), with relative risk estimates around 0.5. There was also evidence of duration-dependent trends in both conditions, with the greatest reduction in the risk of Crohn's disease observed with breastfeeding for at least 12 months. Similar conclusions were drawn by Gearry and colleagues [72] based on research involving 638 CD patients, 653 UC patients, and 600 matched controls. The study found that being breastfed was associated with a reduced risk of developing both CD (adjusted odds ratio [OR] 0.55, 95% confidence interval [CI] 0.41–0.74) and UC (adjusted OR 0.71, 95% CI 0.52–0.96). There was a duration–response effect observed for both diseases, indicating that breastfeeding for more than 3 months was protective. However, the lowest risk of developing both diseases was noted when children were breastfed for more than 12 months. Other articles emphasizing the protective effects of breastfeeding for more than 12 months on IBDs include Ng et al. [73] and Xu et al. [74].

A different research project that supports these findings is paper by Ko et al. [75], which reported a reduced risk of CD with breastfeeding for ≥3 months and a decreased risk of UC with breastfeeding for ≥6 months. The study showed a clear duration–response effect, indicating that longer periods of breastfeeding were strongly associated with lower risks of developing IBDs. Another study indicating that a longer breastfeeding duration might be associated with a reduced risk of developing CD is the study by Bergstrand et al. [76]. Additionally, articles by Decker et al. [77], Hansen et al. [78], and Hlavaty et al. [79] suggest a similar protective effect for both IBDs. Lee et al. [80], on the other hand, highlights the protective effect of breastfeeding for ≥6 months specifically for UC.

5.3. Otitis Media

Shaaban et al. [81] found that children with acute otitis media (AOM) had been breastfed for a significantly shorter period (8.6 months) compared to healthy controls (13.7 months). Notably, 25% of children with ear infections had been breastfed for less than 6 months, while only 10% of the control group had a similar breastfeeding duration, resulting in an odds ratio of 3. This indicates that children with acute otitis media were three times more likely to have been breastfed for less than 6 months. The study suggests that shorter breastfeeding durations are a major risk factor for developing acute otitis media in early childhood.

Moreover, breastfeeding for up to 11 months significantly prevents AOM, with the strongest protective effects seen within the first 4 months, dropping in the 5th month, and then rising again from the 6th to 8th month. The protective effect decreases but remains statistically significant up to 11 months and positive, though not statistically significant, until 18 months. Furthermore, in their research, Vogazianos et al. [82] concluded that to achieve optimal prevention of AOM, breastfeeding should continue for at least the first 11 months, with some additional benefit extending up to 18 months. The varying importance of breastfeeding corresponds to the child's developmental stages and changing immunological needs.

In addition to this, Ardc et al. [83] discovered that infants breastfed for longer than 12 months had a lower incidence of acute otitis media compared to those breastfed for less than 12 months ($p < 0.05$). Additionally, exclusive breastfeeding during the first 6 months significantly reduced the occurrence of this condition. Similarly, Weiss [84] noted that breastfeeding for 6 months or longer was most effective in reducing the risk of otitis media (OM), although no continued benefits were observed beyond 2 years of age.

5.4. Metabolic Health

The global prevalence of excessive weight gain is an escalating public health concern. Alarmingly, in 2022, over 390 million children and adolescents aged 5–19 years were overweight, including 160 million of them being obese [85]. This rising trend is particularly troubling due to its strong association with a heightened susceptibility to various chronic health conditions, such as cardiovascular disease (CVD), type 2 diabetes (T2DM), and metabolic syndrome (MetS) [86].

MetS, in particular, poses significant health risks, as it consists of a cluster of interrelated metabolic abnormalities. Individuals with MetS typically present with at least three of the following conditions: abdominal obesity, hyperglycemia, hypertension, hypertriglyceridemia, and low levels of HDL cholesterol (HDL-C). The presence of these risk factors, especially when obesity is concentrated in the abdominal area and originates in childhood, shows the critical need for early intervention and preventive measures to combat the growing incidence of MetS and its associated health complications [86–88].

5.4.1. Weight Gain

Liu et al. [89] conducted a comprehensive study to evaluate the relationship between breastfeeding duration and body mass index (BMI) in children and adolescents aged 6 to 16 years. The study found a significant negative correlation between breastfeeding duration and BMI after adjusting for various covariates. Specifically, children who were breastfed for more than 12 months had significantly lower BMIs compared to those breastfed for less than 12 months ($\beta = -0.274$; 95% CI: -0.422, -0.127; $p < 0.01$). This inverse relationship was consistent across different age groups and genders, though it was particularly pronounced in boys. The study further highlighted that children and adolescents breastfed for more than 12 months had a significantly lower prevalence of obesity compared to those breastfed for shorter durations. Specifically, the adjusted odds ratio (OR) for obesity among participants breastfed for more than 12 months was 0.853 (95% CI: 0.748, 0.974, $p < 0.05$).

Similar findings were reached by Gewa et al. [90], who found that longer breastfeeding durations, particularly beyond 18 months, are significantly associated with lower risks of childhood overweight/obesity ($p < 0.05$). Children breastfed for more than 24 months had a 45% decrease in the odds of being overweight compared to those breastfed for less than 12 months. Nascimento Simon et al. [91] also found comparable results. Their hierarchical multiple analysis revealed that longer breastfeeding durations provide greater protection against overweight and obesity. Specifically, exclusive breastfeeding for six months or more was associated with a significantly lower risk of overweight and obesity, and breastfeeding for more than 24 months further reduced the risk (OR = 0.13; 95% CI [0.05, 0.37]; $p = 0.00$). What is more, similar conclusions were drawn by Fallahzadeh et al. [92], Liese et al. [93], and Von Kries et al. [94].

Grummer-Strawn and colleagues [95] came up with interesting conclusions. They found that longer breastfeeding is not associated with a decrease in mean BMI but rather with a decrease in the standard deviation of BMI, leading to simultaneously lower rates of underweight and overweight. Breastfeeding seems to protect against overweight not by uniformly reducing BMI in all children but by reducing the variability in BMI. However, this study was conducted in 2004, which is relatively dated, and there is a lack of more recent data to corroborate these findings.

5.4.2. Blood Pressure

The study by Hosaka et al. [96] examined how breastfeeding duration influences blood pressure in 7-year-old Japanese children. It categorized mother–offspring pairs into short-term (mean 5.1 months) and long-term (mean 11.3 months) breastfeeding groups, measuring both self-measured home blood pressure (HBP) and conventional blood pressure (CBP). Children in the long-term breastfeeding group exhibited significantly lower HBP compared to those in the short-term group, whereas CBP did not differ significantly between the groups. Breastfeeding for more than 8 months, regardless of birth weight, was strongly linked with lower HBP, underscoring breastfeeding's protective role against elevated blood pressure in young children. Similar conclusions were drawn by Lin and colleagues [97], who found that the duration of breastfeeding had an inverse relationship with blood pressure values in children entering the first grade. For each additional month of breastfeeding, systolic blood pressure decreased by 0.07 mmHg and diastolic blood pressure decreased by 0.05 mmHg. These differences were statistically significant. Furthermore, breastfeeding for more than 12 months was associated with a reduced risk of hypertension, with an adjusted risk ratio of 0.83 (95% CI: 0.70 to 0.98, $p = 0.03$).

An interesting relationship was discovered in the study by Liang et al. [98]. Children who were breastfed for 4 to 10 months exhibited the lowest prevalence of hypertension.

Conversely, those breastfed for more than 10 months showed an increased risk of hypertension, particularly among rural children. This elevated risk in the rural cohort may be partly due to the fact that 33.86% of these children were breastfed for more than 10 months, which could help explain the higher prevalence of hypertension observed in these areas.

5.4.3. Metabolic Syndrome

Breastfeeding has a universal protective effect. The study by Wang et al. [99] compared two sample populations of young people in Spain and China, highlighting significant differences in metabolic health markers. Spanish children generally exhibited higher mean values for height, weight, BMI, waist circumference, triglycerides (TGs), and systolic blood pressure (SBP) compared to their Chinese counterparts. This disparity was reflected in an elevated prevalence of metabolic risk factors, leading to a higher overall prevalence of MetS (2.5%) compared to Chinese adolescents (0.5%). Breastfeeding duration appeared to be an important factor influencing these outcomes. The Spanish cohort, which was breastfed for a longer duration (9 months on average), showed a significantly more pronounced protective effect of breastfeeding against metabolic risk factors. This included a reduced likelihood of low HDL-C, hyperglycemia, and hypertriglyceridemia, and ultimately, a lower risk of MetS. In contrast, the correlation between breastfeeding duration and these metabolic markers was weaker in the Chinese cohort, suggesting that the benefits of breastfeeding may be significantly modulated by cultural or environmental factors.

Also, Gonzales-Jimenez et al. [100] found that longer breastfeeding durations, especially beyond 6 months, were associated with a reduced likelihood of MetS diagnosis in both males and females. Additional risk factors for MetS included maternal smoking during pregnancy, along with maternal overweight and obesity. The same conclusions were reached by Esfarjani et al. [101] and Wang et al. [102].

5.5. *Oral Health*

The relationship between prolonged breastfeeding and oral health, specifically its impact on childhood dental caries (ECC) and severe early childhood caries (S-ECC), has been the subject of several studies with varying findings. These studies collectively suggest that while breastfeeding offers numerous health benefits, extended breastfeeding durations may be associated with an increased risk of dental caries, particularly in specific contexts.

Chaffee et al. [103] investigated the association between breastfeeding for 24 months or longer and the prevalence of S-ECC. They found that breastfeeding for 24 months or beyond, especially when done frequently, was associated with the highest adjusted prevalence of S-ECC (0.45; 95% CI, 0.36 to 0.54). In contrast, breastfeeding durations of less than 6 months, 6–11 months, and 12–23 months had lower prevalence rates of S-ECC (0.22, 95% CI: 0.15 to 0.28; 0.38, 95% CI: 0.25 to 0.53; and 0.39, 95% CI: 0.20 to 0.56, respectively). However, the prevalence ratio for ECC with breastfeeding for $\geq$24 months was 1.17 (95% CI, 0.85 to 1.78), which did not reach statistical significance.

Similarly, Tanaka et al. [104] found a relationship between breastfeeding duration and dental caries prevalence. Compared to breastfeeding for less than 6 months, breastfeeding for 18 months or longer was significantly associated with a higher prevalence of dental caries (adjusted prevalence ratio of 1.66; 95% CI, 1.33–2.06). In contrast, breastfeeding for 6 to 17 months did not show a significant association with caries prevalence, indicating that the risk associated with breastfeeding may increase after 18 months.

Conversely, Nirunsittirat et al. [105] reported that full breastfeeding for 6–11 months was significantly associated with a lower risk of dental caries, evidenced by a lower decayed, missing, and filled surface (DMFS) score (adjusted RR 0.77; 95% CI, 0.63–0.93) and lower caries prevalence (adjusted RR 0.45; 95% CI, 0.22–0.90).

Adding to the body of evidence, Peres et al. [106] observed that children breastfed for 24 months or more had a higher prevalence of dental caries and a 2.4 times greater risk of S-ECC compared to those breastfed for up to 12 months. The risk of dental caries among children who were breastfed for 13 to 23 months was not significantly different from those breastfed for up to 12 months. Their study underscored the increased risk associated with prolonged breastfeeding and suggested that preventive dental interventions should be introduced early to mitigate caries risk.

Multiple meta-analyses and reviews [107–111] support these findings, indicating that breastfeeding for up to 12 months is associated with a reduced risk of caries. However, breastfeeding beyond 12 months has been reported to be linked to an increased risk of caries. It is essential to consider this relationship in the context of eating habits, feeding hours, and hygiene practices. Even with these considerations, the advantages of breastfeeding beyond six months outweigh the potential issues and harm associated with caries.

5.6. Infections

Given the numerous benefits of breast milk, including its potent anti-infective and immunological properties, exclusive breastfeeding has been shown to significantly reduce the risk of infectious diseases during infancy. Diarrheal diseases and acute respiratory infections remain the leading causes of morbidity and mortality among children under five years old globally [112–114]. While the protective effects of breastfeeding against infections are well established, it is important to note that there are specific, albeit rare, instances where breast milk feeding should be withheld. These include maternal infections such as HIV, HTLV, viral hemorrhagic fevers, and untreated brucellosis, where the risk of transmission outweighs the benefits of breastfeeding [114].

Extended breastfeeding has the potential to offer a protective effect against hospitalizations during infancy. In their study, Størdal et al. [115] underscore the beneficial impact of breastfeeding beyond 12 months of age. The research revealed that infants breastfed for shorter durations, specifically 6 months or less, had a higher risk of hospitalization (10.0%) compared to those breastfed for 12 months or more (7.6%). After adjusting for various factors, the adjusted relative risk (RR) was 1.22 (95% confidence interval: 1.14–1.31), indicating a significant difference in hospitalization rates. Interestingly, infants breastfed for 6 to 11 months showed similar risks of hospitalization compared to those breastfed for 12 months or longer.

5.6.1. Respiratory Tract Infections

One of the initial findings in this area was reported by Nafstad et al. [116], showing that children breastfed for more than 6 months had a lower incidence of lower respiratory tract infections (LRTIs) compared to those breastfed for less than 6 months and demonstrated that for each month of shorter breastfeeding duration, the odds of LRTIs increased by an average of 5%. The disparity in infection rates between these breastfeeding groups widened with higher levels of maternal smoking. Similar results were obtained by Tromp and colleagues [117], who found that breastfeeding for 6 months or more significantly reduced the risk of lower respiratory tract infections (LRTIs) up to the age of 4 years, with an adjusted odds ratio (aOR) of 0.71 (95% confidence interval [CI]: 0.51–0.98).

It is also worth noting that Li R. et al. [118] found significant health benefits associated with longer breastfeeding durations and higher breast milk intensity (proportion of milk feedings). Children breastfed for 9 months or longer had lower odds of throat (aOR: 0.68) and sinus infections (aOR: 0.47) compared to those breastfed for less than 3 months. Moreover, the likelihood of these infections was reduced by 34% to 50% compared to children who were breastfed for up to 6 months but received formula supplementation before reaching 6 months. Additionally, high breastfeeding intensity (>66.6%) during the first 6 months was linked to lower odds of sinus infections (aOR: 0.53) compared to low breastfeeding intensity (<33.3%).

In addition, Fisk et al. [119] conducted a birth cohort study in the UK and found that longer breastfeeding durations were associated with a reduced risk of respiratory infections in a dose-dependent manner. Breastfeeding for more than 6 months significantly decreased the risk of wheezing, lower respiratory infections, and general respiratory morbidity compared to never breastfeeding (adjusted RR 0.43; 95% CI 0.30–0.61). Each additional month of breastfeeding further reduced the risk of these conditions, with adjusted RRs of 0.88 (95% CI 0.83–0.92) for the first 6 months ($p < 0.001$) and 0.97 (95% CI 0.95–0.99) for 6–12 months ($p = 0.002$).

5.6.2. Gastrointestinal Infections and Diarrhea

Ardc et al. [83] discovered that the incidence of acute gastroenteritis was significantly lower in infants who were breastfed for longer durations. Specifically, infants who were breastfed for more than 12 months experienced fewer instances of acute gastroenteritis compared to those breastfed for less than 12 months ($p < 0.05$). Additionally, infants who were exclusively breastfed during the first 6 months also had a significantly reduced risk of acute gastroenteritis. This suggests that both exclusive breastfeeding in the early months and prolonged breastfeeding can provide protective benefits against gastroenteritis in infants. In line with these observations, Fisk et al. [119] noted that breastfeeding for more than 6 months significantly reduces the risk of gastrointestinal infections, with each additional month of breastfeeding further lowering this risk.

A different approach was taken by Rebhan et al. [120], who examined how breastfeeding duration influences gastrointestinal infections among infants, categorizing them into three groups based on breastfeeding practices: Group A (≥6 months of exclusive breastfeeding), Group B (≥4–6 months of breastfeeding with varying exclusivity), and Group C (no or <4 months of any breastfeeding). Their analysis found that infants exclusively breastfed for 6 months or more had a significantly lower risk of experiencing ≥1 episode of gastrointestinal infections during months 1–9 of life compared to those with shorter durations of breastfeeding (adjusted OR: 0.60; 95% CI: 0.44–0.82). The incidence rates of these infections were 20.4% in Group A, 28.0% in Group B, and 27.9% in Group C. These findings highlight the protective effect of exclusive breastfeeding for at least 6 months against early-life gastrointestinal infections.

To explore the benefits of prolonged breastfeeding, Mølbak et al. [121] assessed its impact on the risk and duration of diarrhea in 849 infants under three years of age. With a median weaning age of 22 months and 25% of children still breastfed at 27 months, the study found that children who had been weaned experienced significantly more diarrheal episodes compared to those who continued breastfeeding past one year. Specifically, weaned children had relative risks of 1.41 and 1.67 for diarrhea at one and two years of age, respectively. Additionally, the duration of diarrheal episodes was one day longer in weaned children compared to those still breastfed at 1 and 2 years of age. The incidence of diarrhea was higher in weaned children than in partially breastfed children, both in one-year-olds (relative risk 1.41; 95% CI 1.23 to 1.62) and in two-year-olds (1.67; 95% CI 1.29 to 2.15). The mean duration of a diarrheal episode was 5.3 days in breastfed children compared to 6.3 days in weaned children ($p = 0.001$). These findings suggest that the beneficial effects of breastfeeding are not restricted to infancy.

After adjusting for various maternal and infant factors, including smoking during pregnancy and age at introduction of solid foods, Fisk et al. [119] discovered that each additional month of breastfeeding reduced the risk of diarrhea. Specifically, the adjusted relative risks (RRs) were 0.88 (95% CI 0.83–0.92) for 0–6 months (p for trend < 0.001) and 0.97 (95% CI 0.95–0.99) for 6–12 months (p for trend = 0.002). The protective effect of breastfeeding was most pronounced in the first 6 months after birth; however, the study also showed significant benefits associated with extended breastfeeding into later infancy.

Moreover, Ruuska et al. [122] found that breastfeeding for over 6 months reduced the incidence of diarrhea during the first year of life in both atopic and nonatopic infants. However, they observed no significant effect on the overall incidence of diarrhea over the two-year follow-up period, as infants breastfed for longer durations experienced more diarrhea in the second year of life. Additionally, prolonged breastfeeding was associated with reduced severity of diarrhea, specifically among infants aged 7–12 months.

5.7. Cognitive Development

One of the first significant insights into this issue was provided by Daniels et al. [123], who conducted a study with 1984 participants and found strong associations between prolonged breastfeeding and improved intellectual growth. The research used a nonverbal intelligence test assessing fluid abilities at 8.5 and 11.5 years of age. At 8.5 years of age, among healthy and low-birthweight children, breastfeeding for 12–18 months was associated with increases in nonverbal intelligence test scores by 1.6 and 9.8 points, respectively. For low-birthweight children, breastfeeding for 18–24 months and $\geq$2 years led to a 6.6-point and 7.1-point increase in test scores, respectively. After 2 years, the beneficial association with prolonged breastfeeding persisted, albeit weaker. Improved cognitive development was primarily observed in healthy-birthweight children breastfed for 12 to 18 months.

In the study of Duazo and colleagues [124], mothers who breastfed their children for longer periods tended to have lower educational attainment and come from lower-income households. Despite these socioeconomic disparities, breastfeeding duration emerged as a significant predictor of future psychosocial development in late childhood, particularly after adjusting for socioeconomic and related factors. Compared to children breastfed for 5 months or less, those breastfed for longer durations showed higher psychosocial scores. Specifically, among 5-year-olds, children breastfed for 12 months or more scored 2 to 3 points higher on psychosocial assessments compared to those breastfed for less than 6 months. Interestingly, the study noted that the apparent protective effect of breastfeeding peaked during the second year of life and then gradually declined.

While breastfeeding duration did not significantly impact intelligence scores across the entire sample, Slykerman et al. [125] observed notable associations among children classified as small for gestational age (SGA). However, a trend suggested that longer breastfeeding periods correlated with higher intelligence scores overall. Among SGA children, breastfeeding for longer than 12 months was significantly associated with higher IQ scores at 3.5 years. Specifically, children breastfed for more than 12 months had adjusted scores that were 6.0 points higher than those who were not breastfed (p = 0.06). Exclusive breastfeeding for 5 months or longer within the SGA group was also significantly linked to higher intelligence scores, showing a 5.9-point increase compared to non-breastfed children. Additionally, the duration of predominant breastfeeding impacts language development. Whitehouse et al. [126] found that children predominantly breastfed for 4–6 months or more than 6 months had significantly higher language scores compared to those breastfed for 0–4 months or not breastfed at all. The study also revealed significant associations between the duration of predominant breastfeeding and language ability at 10 years. Specifically, children breastfed predominantly for 6 months showed a language score increase (β = 4.04).

Furthermore, Jedrychowski et al. [127] found that the duration of exclusive breastfeeding had a positive impact on children's intelligence quotients (IQs). Children exclusively breastfed for up to 3 months had an average IQ score that was 2.1 points higher compared to others (95% CI, 0.24–3.9). Those breastfed for 4–6 months had IQs higher by 2.6 points (95% CI, 0.87–4.27). Children breastfed for more than 6 months experienced an even greater benefit, with IQs increasing by 3.8 points (95% CI, 2.11–5.45). However, Sajjad [128] suggests that the association between breastfeeding duration and child IQ may largely stem from sociodemographic factors, parental lifestyle, and maternal IQ. In his study, initially, each additional month of breastfeeding conferred an advantage of 0.32 points (95% CI, 0.20–0.44). Yet, after adjusting for child-specific factors and various environmental influences, this association weakened considerably to 0.09 points (95% CI, −0.03 to 0.21).

5.8. Leukemia

The study by Shu and colleagues [129] suggests that primarily breastfed children have a reduced risk of childhood acute leukemia, including both acute myeloid leukemia (AML) and acute lymphoblastic leukemia (ALL). A stronger inverse association was observed for children breastfed for more than 6 months (AML: OR = 0.57, 95% CI: 0.39–0.84;

ALL: OR = 0.72, 95% CI: 0.60–0.87). Leukemia risk decreased with longer breastfeeding durations, particularly up to 12 months for ALL and 9 months for AML. Although the risk was lower for children breastfed beyond 12 months, this reduction was not statistically significant.

The relationship between the duration of breastfeeding and the risk of childhood leukemia appears to follow a non-linear dose–response pattern. Gong et al. [130] discovered that as the duration of breastfeeding increased, the odds of childhood cancer, including leukemia, significantly decreased. The study found that breastfeeding for a duration of 7–9 months was particularly protective against childhood leukemia, with a significant reduction in risk compared to other breastfeeding periods (OR: 0.498; 95% CI: 0.318–0.780; $p = 0.002$). This suggests that the protective effect of breastfeeding may peak at a specific duration, beyond which the benefits may plateau. This correlation is further supported by the results obtained by Gao et al. [131]. Interestingly, they found that a lower education level among mothers was associated with an increased risk of leukemia in children.

The findings from MacArthur et al. [132] suggest that breastfeeding, particularly for more than six months, provides significant protective benefits against childhood leukemia (OR = 0.78, 95% CI 0.71–0.85). However, introducing a significant amount of milk supplementation (more than 50% of the child's diet) after six months of age was associated with an increased risk of childhood leukemia, particularly when compared to exclusive breastfeeding. This indicates that while breastfeeding itself is protective, the benefits may diminish or be counteracted when a high proportion of milk supplements are introduced.

There are also other studies that confirm the beneficial impact of breastfeeding for more than 6 months, compared to not breastfeeding or breastfeeding for less than 6 months, in reducing the risk of leukemia. Among these are studies by Cheng et al. [133], Bener et al. [134], Rudant et al. [135], Altinkaynak et al. [136], and Bener et al. [137].

5.9. Malaria

Pincelli et al. [138] found that children who received breast milk for ≥12 months, irrespective of complementary feeding practices, were significantly less likely to develop antibodies to blood-stage *Plasmodium vivax*, indicating a lower risk of infection. Breastfeeding for this duration reduced the risk of *P. vivax* seropositivity by 79.8% during the first 2 years of life among children born to mothers who had experienced *P. vivax* infection during pregnancy. Also, Safeukui-Noubissi et al. [139] discovered that prolonged breastfeeding for at least 2 years was associated with a decreased risk of severe malaria in children (OR: 0.57; 95% CI [0.33–0.94]). An intriguing study by Vora et al. [140] revealed that breastfeeding was associated with a markedly lower incidence of malaria (1.36 vs. 2.44, $p = 0.008$) in HIV-exposed children aged 6–15 months who were still being breastfed and receiving TS prophylaxis.

5.10. Individual Reports

There are several conditions for which prolonged breastfeeding has shown beneficial effects. However, it is important to note that the existing literature lacks a robust body of reliable evidence, and many of the findings are based on relatively old studies that have not been consistently confirmed by more recent research. Therefore, while there are hints in the literature connecting prolonged breastfeeding with the prophylactic potential of certain conditions, these associations require further investigation. Continued research is essential to determine whether the protective effects of prolonged breastfeeding hold true across different populations and updated methodologies. Additionally, the existing data remain fragmentary and require further research to fully understand the extent of these protective effects.

5.10.1. Arthritis

Research indicates that shorter breastfeeding durations, particularly those of less than 4 months or ending by 6 months, are associated with an increased risk of developing juvenile idiopathic arthritis (JIA). In contrast, exclusive breastfeeding for at least 4 months, followed by continued partial breastfeeding while introducing other proteins, may help reduce the risk of JIA in childhood [141].

5.10.2. Celiac Disease

Breastfeeding during the introduction of dietary gluten has been associated with a reduced risk of celiac disease in children under 2 years old. Specifically, breastfeeding while introducing gluten reduced the risk (adjusted OR: 0.59), and continuing breastfeeding after gluten introduction provided an even greater protective effect (adjusted OR: 0.36). It is noteworthy that this study was conducted in a population where most infants were breastfed for at least six months [142].

5.10.3. Hand, Foot, and Mouth Disease

A study by Li et al. [143] investigating the relationship between breastfeeding duration and the risk of severe hand, foot, and mouth disease (HFMD) revealed that breastfeeding for more than 6 months was significantly associated with a reduced risk of severe HFMD. Specifically, durations of 6–12 months (OR 0.701, 95% CI 0.539–0.913) and over 12 months (OR 0.504, 95% CI 0.341–0.746) were independently linked to a lower risk of severe HFMD after adjusting for confounding factors.

5.10.4. Lipid Levels

Recent research has shown the association between breastfeeding duration and lipid profiles among 12,110 children and adolescents aged 5–19 years across China. They discovered that participants breastfed for more than 12 months exhibited significantly lower levels of total cholesterol (TC), LDL cholesterol (LDL-C), HDL cholesterol (HDL-C), and TC/HDL-C ratios compared to those who were not breastfed. Additionally, children breastfed for more than 12 months also experienced a 43% reduced risk of high TC. This protective effect was particularly notable in children and young adolescents aged 5–14 years, suggesting that a longer breastfeeding duration is linked to lower lipid levels and a decreased risk of abnormal lipids in this age group [144].

5.10.5. Neuroblastoma

Children with neuroblastoma were found to be less likely to have been breastfed compared to control children, with an OR of 0.6 (95% CI = 0.5–0.9). The potential protective effect of breastfeeding against neuroblastoma appeared to strengthen with longer breastfeeding durations, with children breastfed for 13 months or more showing the lowest likelihood (OR = 0.5, 95% CI = 0.3–0.9) [145].

5.10.6. Retinoblastoma

According to the research conducted by Heck and colleagues [146], breastfeeding is associated with a reduced risk of unilateral retinoblastoma, particularly when it lasts for 7–11 months. However, extending breastfeeding beyond 12 months does not appear to offer additional protective benefits, as no dose–response relationship was observed with longer breastfeeding durations.

5.10.7. Rhabdomyosarcoma

The findings by Lupo et al. [147] indicate that breastfeeding for 12 or more months is strongly associated with a reduced risk of childhood RMS (Rhabdomyosarcoma), as demonstrated by the odds ratio (OR = 0.36, 95% CI: 0.18–0.70). Additionally, the significant trend ($p = 0.01$) suggests that as the duration of breastfeeding increases, the risk of childhood RMS decreases further, highlighting a dose–response relationship between breastfeeding duration and reduced RMS risk.

5.10.8. Sudden Infant Death Syndrome

The study by Thompson et al. [148] suggests that a longer breastfeeding duration provides substantial protection against sudden infant death syndrome (SIDS). Both any breastfeeding and exclusive breastfeeding durations exceeding 2 months offer increased protection, with the most significant benefit observed for durations greater than 6 months, which is associated with a 64% reduction in the risk of SIDS.

5.10.9. Type 2 Diabetes

Kue Young et al. [149] explored prenatal and early-infancy risk factors for type 2 diabetes among native Canadians. Their findings indicate that being breastfed for more than 6 months (odds ratio = 0.36; 95% CI: 0.13–0.99) is significantly associated with a reduced risk of developing type 2 diabetes compared to being breastfed for less than 6 months.

6. Discussion

Breastfeeding is widely recognized for its numerous health benefits, particularly in protecting infants against infections and impacting the proper growth and development of children. The mechanisms through which breastfeeding imparts these benefits are multifaceted, involving immunological, microbiological, and biochemical processes, and they are depicted in Figure 2.

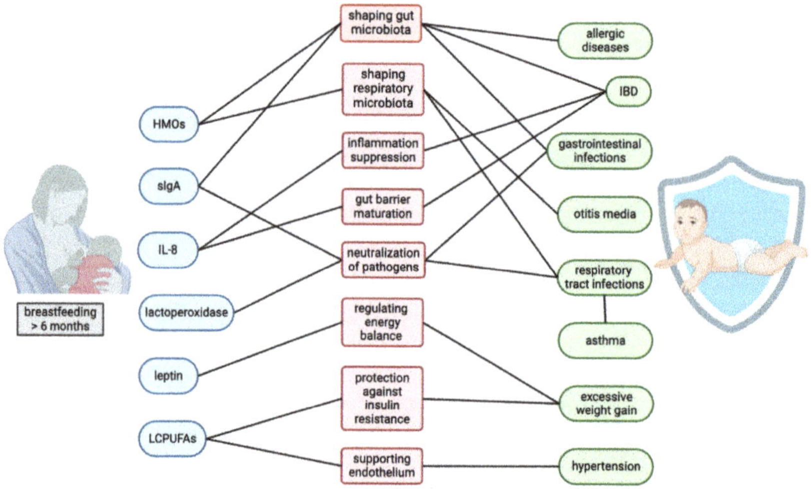

Figure 2. The mother–breastmilk–infant triad: how bioactive components in breast milk contribute to disease protection for infants. Legend: HMOs, human milk oligosaccharides; sIgA, secretory immunoglobulin A; IL-8, interleukin 8; LCPUFAs, long-chain polyunsaturated fatty acids; IBD, inflammatory bowel disease.

One of the primary protective mechanisms of breastfeeding is the transfer of sIgA from mother to infant through breast milk. sIgA is resistant to digestion, allowing it to accumulate in the infant's intestine where it binds to antigens on pathogens, rendering them less infective and protecting against infections [69,150]. This immunological defense is especially crucial during the early months of life when the infant's immune system is still developing [151]. Interestingly, the absence of passive sIgA in the gut is associated with the upregulation of Gram-negative *Pasteurellaceae* and Gram-positive *Lachnospiraceae*. These bacterial families are often found in higher abundance in the gut microbiota of pediatric patients with inflammatory bowel disease, suggesting a protective role of sIgA against such conditions [152]. Moreover, sIgA antibodies provide protection against gastrointestinal infections caused by microbes like Giardia, ETEC, and *Campylobacter* [153]. Additionally, non-breastfed children exhibit an increased abundance of *Clostridium difficile*, a pathogen linked to allergic sensitization and immune-mediated diseases, protecting against asthma, eczema, wheezing, etc. [68,154,155].

Breast milk plays a significant role in shaping the infant microbiota, promoting the colonization of beneficial bacteria and suppressing the growth of pathogenic bacteria [156,157]. The prebiotic effect of glycans and human milk oligosaccharides (HMOs) in breast milk supports the growth of beneficial bacteria while inhibiting the colonization of pathogens [69,158–161]. This modulation of the gut microbiota is essential for developing immunologic tolerance and preventing inappropriate immune responses [68,69,161–163]. Breastfeeding also shapes the composition of the respiratory microbiota in the nasopharynx [164–166].

For instance, the presence of *Lactobacilli* in breast milk contributes to distinct nasopharyngeal colonization, reducing the incidence of otitis media during breastfeeding. This effect is facilitated by the direct bacteriostatic properties of breast milk and the microbiota associated with it, which collectively help in reducing the pathogens responsible for OM [167]. Additionally, breast milk also forms a protective layer on the nasopharyngeal mucosa, shielding against the transmission of bacteria and viruses that cause respiratory illnesses [168]. This may also enhance the protective effect of breastfeeding against asthma development, as reduced respiratory tract infections—well-known risk factors for asthma—are associated with breastfeeding. Furthermore, breastfeeding has been demonstrated to support lung development and improve lung function. Children who were breastfed show increased lung volumes, with this benefit attributed to the mechanical stimulation of suckling at the breast during early infancy, which can prevent asthma [157].

Breast milk contains various bioactive components that contribute to its protective effects. Lactoperoxidase, an enzyme present in milk, catalyzes the formation of hypothiocyanate from saliva thiocyanate, which can kill the bacteria responsible for infections such as OM. This enzymatic activity provides a biochemical defense against pathogenic bacteria, complementing immunological and microbiological protections [167]. Breastfeeding also reduces the overall disease burden, which in turn allows for more resources to be allocated toward combating infections [169]. Moreover, prolonged breastfeeding has been shown to reduce the likelihood of hospital stays in early childhood [115].

Furthermore, breast milk factors can suppress the induction of inflammatory responses, such as IL-8 expression in cultured intestinal epithelial cells, thereby attenuating early inappropriate inflammatory reactions [69]. This anti-inflammatory property of breast milk is crucial in preventing conditions like IBD by promoting the maturation of the gut barrier and supporting the development of immunological memory to pathogens [68,69]. Another reason breastfeeding helps prevent chronic inflammation is that it promotes mother–child attachment, which positively affects cortisol regulation in breastfed infants [157].

Moreover, through its stimulation and modulation of the infant's immune system, breast milk leads to enhanced vaccine responses and increased thymus size [129]. Additionally, it is worth highlighting that breast milk contains soluble tumor necrosis factor (TNF)-related apoptosis-inducing ligand (TRAIL), which regulates apoptosis and cell proliferation in various tissues, as well as human alpha-lactalbumin made lethal to tumor cells (HAMLET), a substance with known anticancer properties [170]. Together, these components may influence leukemogenesis and reduce the risk of childhood leukemia [129,170].

Infant formulas typically contain higher levels of fats, proteins, and sodium compared to breast milk. This composition can lead to elevated levels of Insulin-like Growth Factor 1 (IGF-1) in the bloodstream. IGF-1 stimulates the proliferation of adipocytes, leading to increased fat accumulation and, consequently, higher risks of obesity. Moreover, breast milk contains bioactive compounds such as leptin, which is crucial in regulating energy balance and appetite. Breast milk's balance of proteins, fats, and carbohydrates promotes appropriate growth and satiety, preventing overfeeding. Unlike formula, which can lead to higher caloric intake, breast milk's tailored composition reduces the risk of excessive weight gain [89,171,172]. Additionally, breast milk helps maintain proper blood pressure levels by reducing sodium intake during infancy, providing long-chain unsaturated fatty acids (LCPUFAs) that support the health of tissue membranes and the coronary endothelial system, and protecting against hyperinsulinemia and insulin resistance throughout early life [171,173,174].

Moreover, breastfed infants often have a different trajectory of brain development compared to those who are never breastfed or those with shorter breastfeeding durations. Breastfeeding has been linked to increased gray matter, hippocampal volume, brain activation, and cortical thickness [175–177]. It is also important to highlight that HMOs act as prebiotics, supporting the developing gut microbiome, which can help reduce inflammation and promote the production of metabolites affecting brain function through the gut–brain axis. Additionally, HMOs may supply sialic acid, a crucial nutrient for brain tissue organization [178]. These combined effects contribute to enhanced cognitive and neurodevelopmental outcomes in children [175–178].

The multifaceted benefits of prolonged breastfeeding extend beyond basic nutrition, offering profound and long-lasting effects on an infant's health and development. The immunological, microbiological, and biochemical properties of breast milk work synergistically to protect against infections, support optimal growth, and enhance proper development.

However, the data regarding the beneficial impacts of prolonged breastfeeding present a complex picture, with many studies failing to adequately control for confounding variables. This underscores the necessity for more rigorous and comprehensive research efforts. There is a significant need for well-designed, prospective studies that employ mixed-method approaches to capture both quantitative and qualitative data. Additionally, cross-cultural research is essential to understand how different societal, environmental, and genetic factors may influence the outcomes of prolonged breastfeeding. Such studies should aim to control for potential confounders such as socioeconomic status, maternal education, and pre-existing health conditions to provide clearer insights. By addressing these gaps, future research can more accurately determine the extent and mechanisms of the protective effects of prolonged breastfeeding on various health outcomes in children.

7. Conclusions

Breastfeeding, especially when extended beyond the early months, provides substantial health benefits that significantly influence infant development and well-being. The immunological, microbiological, and biochemical properties of breast milk work synergistically to offer strong protection against infections, reducing rates of hospitalizations and even mortality, promote optimal growth, and support cognitive development and brain function. As breast milk adapts to the evolving needs of the growing infant, prolonged breastfeeding remains a cost-effective means of delivering comprehensive immune and developmental support, surpassing the advantages of costly formulas.

Key findings from the literature highlight that longer durations of breastfeeding are associated with numerous health benefits. These include a reduced risk of gastrointestinal and respiratory infections, better growth and cognitive development, and a lower likelihood of developing allergic diseases and obesity later in life. Additionally, breastfeeding positively impacts metabolic syndrome, blood pressure regulation, otitis media, and malaria. Although less common, there are also isolated reports suggesting the potential advantages of extended breastfeeding for conditions like arthritis, blastomas, celiac disease, and even sudden infant death syndrome. Therefore, it is essential to encourage mothers to breastfeed, particularly to continue breastfeeding for extended periods, as this practice offers significant health benefits for both the infant and the mother and addresses the growing need for effective preventive health measures amid declining breastfeeding rates and rising health issues.

More rigorous and controlled studies are needed to fully understand the complexities and mechanisms of extended breastfeeding. Future research should address potential confounders and include diverse populations to better assess its impact on long-term health outcomes, refine public health recommendations, and improve child health practices.

Author Contributions: Conceptualization, M.O.-P. and A.F.; methodology, A.F. and M.O.-P.; validation, M.O.-P. and A.F.; formal analysis, A.F.; investigation, A.F.; resources, A.F.; data curation, M.O.-P.; writing—original draft preparation, A.F.; writing—review and editing, M.O.-P.; visualization, A.F.; supervision, M.O.-P.; project administration, M.O.-P. All authors have read and agreed to the published version of the manuscript.

Funding: This research is funded by the Wroclaw Medical University, Poland (SUBZ.A410.24.017).

Institutional Review Board Statement: Not applicable.

Informed Consent Statement: Not applicable.

Data Availability Statement: The data can be shared upon request.

Conflicts of Interest: The authors declare no conflicts of interest.

References

1. Bertin, B.; Foligne, B.; Ley, D.; Lesage, J.; Beghin, L.; Morcel, J.; Gottrand, F.; Hermann, E. An Overview of the Influence of Breastfeeding on the Development of Inflammatory Bowel Disease. *Nutrients* **2023**, *15*, 5103. [CrossRef]
2. Agosti, M.; Tandoi, F.; Morlacchi, L.; Bossi, A. Nutritional and Metabolic Programming during the First Thousand Days of Life. *Pediatr. Med. Chir.* **2017**, *39*, 157. [CrossRef]
3. Williams, A.M.; Suchdev, P.S. Assessing and Improving Childhood Nutrition and Growth Globally. *Pediatr. Clin. N. Am.* **2017**, *64*, 755–768. [CrossRef]
4. Rodríguez-Mañas, L.; Murray, R.; Glencorse, C.; Sulo, S. Good Nutrition across the Lifespan Is Foundational for Healthy Aging and Sustainable Development. *Front. Nutr.* **2023**, *9*, 1113060. [CrossRef]
5. Pieri, M.; Nicolaidou, V.; Papaneophytou, C. Special Issue: The Impact of Early Life Nutrition on Gut Maturation and Later Life Gut Health. *Nutrients* **2023**, *15*, 1498. [CrossRef]
6. Schwarzenberg, S.J.; Georgieff, M.K. Advocacy for Improving Nutrition in the First 1000 Days to Support Childhood Development and Adult Health. *Pediatrics* **2018**, *141*, e20173716. [CrossRef]
7. Lynch, H.F.; Greiner, D.J.; Cohen, I.G. Understanding the Mother-Breastmilk-Infant "Triad". *Science* **2020**, *367*, 1078–1080. [CrossRef]
8. Christian, P.; Smith, E.R.; Lee, S.E.; Vargas, A.J.; Bremer, A.A.; Raiten, D.J. The Need to Study Human Milk as a Biological System. *Am. J. Clin. Nutr.* **2021**, *113*, 1063–1072. [CrossRef]
9. Verduci, E.; Giannì, M.L.; Vizzari, G.; Vizzuso, S.; Cerasani, J.; Mosca, F.; Zuccotti, G.V. The Triad Mother-Breast Milk-Infant as Predictor of Future Health: A Narrative Review. *Nutrients* **2021**, *13*, 486. [CrossRef]
10. Andreas, N.J.; Kampmann, B.; Mehring Le-Doare, K. Human Breast Milk: A Review on Its Composition and Bioactivity. *Early Hum. Dev.* **2015**, *91*, 629–635. [CrossRef]
11. Victora, C.G.; Bahl, R.; Barros, A.J.D.; França, G.V.A.; Horton, S.; Krasevec, J.; Murch, S.; Sankar, M.J.; Walker, N.; Rollins, N.C.; et al. Breastfeeding in the 21st Century: Epidemiology, Mechanisms, and Lifelong Effect. *Lancet* **2016**, *387*, 475–490. [CrossRef]
12. Kramer, M.S.; Kakuma, R. The Optimal Duration of Exclusive Breastfeeding: A Systematic Review. *Adv. Exp. Med. Biol.* **2004**, *554*, 63–77. [CrossRef]
13. Gila-Diaz, A.; Arribas, S.M.; Algara, A.; Martín-Cabrejas, M.A.; de Pablo, Á.L.L.; de Pipaón, M.S.; Ramiro-Cortijo, D. A Review of Bioactive Factors in Human Breastmilk: A Focus on Prematurity. *Nutrients* **2019**, *11*, 1307. [CrossRef]
14. Yi, D.Y.; Kim, S.Y. Human Breast Milk Composition and Function in Human Health: From Nutritional Components to Microbiome and MicroRNAs. *Nutrients* **2021**, *13*, 3094. [CrossRef]
15. Eidelman, A.I.; Schanler, R.J. Breastfeeding and the Use of Human Milk. *Pediatrics* **2012**, *129*, e827–e841. [CrossRef]
16. Chowdhury, R.; Sinha, B.; Sankar, M.J.; Taneja, S.; Bhandari, N.; Rollins, N.; Bahl, R.; Martines, J. Breastfeeding and Maternal Health Outcomes: A Systematic Review and Meta-Analysis. *Acta Paediatr.* **2015**, *104*, 96–113. [CrossRef]
17. Sattari, M.; Serwint, J.R.; Levine, D.M. Maternal Implications of Breastfeeding: A Review for the Internist. *Am. J. Med.* **2019**, *132*, 912–920. [CrossRef]
18. Del Ciampo, L.A.; del Ciampo, I.R.L. Breastfeeding and the Benefits of Lactation for Women's Health. *Rev. Bras. Ginecol. Obstet.* **2018**, *40*, 354–359. [CrossRef]
19. Breastfeeding. *J. Obstet. Gynecol. Neonatal Nurs.* **2015**, *44*, 145–150. [CrossRef]
20. Linde, K.; Lehnig, F.; Nagl, M.; Kersting, A. The Association between Breastfeeding and Attachment: A Systematic Review. *Midwifery* **2020**, *81*, 102592. [CrossRef]
21. Roth, M.C.; Humphreys, K.L.; King, L.S.; Gotlib, I.H.; Robakis, T.K. Breastfeeding Difficulties Predict Mothers' Bonding with Their Infants from Birth to Age Six Months. *Matern. Child. Health J.* **2021**, *25*, 777–785. [CrossRef]
22. Davisse-Paturet, C.; Adel-Patient, K.; Divaret-Chauveau, A.; Pierson, J.; Lioret, S.; Cheminat, M.; Dufourg, M.N.; Charles, M.A.; de Lauzon-Guillain, B. Breastfeeding Status and Duration and Infections, Hospitalizations for Infections, and Antibiotic Use in the First Two Years of Life in the ELFE Cohort. *Nutrients* **2019**, *11*, 1607. [CrossRef]

23. Birch, L.L.; Parker, L.; Burns, A. *Early Childhood Obesity Prevention Policies*; The National Academies Press: Washington, DC, USA, 2011; pp. 1–190. [CrossRef]
24. Lessen, R.; Kavanagh, K. Position of the Academy of Nutrition and Dietetics: Promoting and Supporting Breastfeeding. *J. Acad. Nutr. Diet.* **2015**, *115*, 444–449. [CrossRef]
25. Breastfeeding Report Card—Breastfeeding—CDC. Available online: https://www.cdc.gov/breastfeeding-data/breastfeeding-report-card/index.html (accessed on 14 August 2024).
26. Usheva, N.; Lateva, M.; Galcheva, S.; Koletzko, B.V.; Cardon, G.; De Craemer, M.; Androutsos, O.; Kotowska, A.; Socha, P.; Moreno, L.A.; et al. Breastfeeding and Overweight in European Preschoolers: The ToyBox Study. *Nutrients* **2021**, *13*, 2880. [CrossRef]
27. Gertosio, C.; Meazza, C.; Pagani, S.; Bozzola, M. Breastfeeding and Its Gamut of Benefits. *Minerva Pediatr.* **2016**, *68*, 201–212.
28. Czosnykowska-łukacka, M.; Królak-Olejnik, B.; Orczyk-Pawiłowicz, M. Breast Milk Macronutrient Components in Prolonged Lactation. *Nutrients* **2018**, *10*, 1893. [CrossRef]
29. Sinkiewicz-Darol, E.; Martysiak-Żurowska, D.; Puta, M.; Adamczyk, I.; Barbarska, O.; Wesołowska, A.; Bernatowicz-ŁOjko, U. Nutrients and Bioactive Components of Human Milk After One Year of Lactation: Implication for Human Milk Banks. *J. Pediatr. Gastroenterol. Nutr.* **2022**, *74*, 284–291. [CrossRef]
30. Czosnykowska-Łukacka, M.; Lis-Kuberka, J.; Królak-Olejnik, B.; Orczyk-Pawiłowicz, M. Changes in Human Milk Immunoglobulin Profile During Prolonged Lactation. *Front. Pediatr.* **2020**, *8*, 428. [CrossRef]
31. Perrin, M.T.; Fogleman, A.; Allen, J.C. The Nutritive and Immunoprotective Quality of Human Milk beyond 1 Year Postpartum: Are Lactation-Duration-Based Donor Exclusions Justified? *J. Hum. Lact.* **2013**, *29*, 341–349. [CrossRef]
32. Hennart, P.F.; Brasseur, D.J.; Delogne-Desnoeck, J.B.; Dramaix, M.M.; Robyn, C.E. Lysozyme, Lactoferrin, and Secretory Immunoglobulin A Content in Breast Milk: Influence of Duration of Lactation, Nutrition Status, Prolactin Status, and Parity of Mother. *Am. J. Clin. Nutr.* **1991**, *53*, 32–39. [CrossRef]
33. Weaver, L.T.; Arthur, H.M.L.; Bunn, J.E.G.; Thomas, J.E. Human Milk IgA Concentrations during the First Year of Lactation. *Arch. Dis. Child.* **1998**, *78*, 235–239. [CrossRef] [PubMed]
34. Goldman, A.S.; Garza, C.; Nichols, B.L.; Goldblum, R.M. Immunologic Factors in Human Milk during the First Year of Lactation. *J. Pediatr.* **1982**, *100*, 563–567. [CrossRef]
35. Ongprasert, K.; Ruangsuriya, J.; Malasao, R.; Sapbamrer, R.; Suppansan, P.; Ayood, P.; Kittisakmontri, K.; Siviroj, P. Macronutrient, Immunoglobulin a and Total Antioxidant Capacity Profiles of Human Milk from 1 to 24 Months: A Cross-Sectional Study in Thailand. *Int. Breastfeed. J.* **2020**, *15*, 90. [CrossRef]
36. Goldman, A.S.; Goldblum, R.M.; Garza, C. Immunologic Components in Human Milk during the Second Year of Lactation. *Acta Paediatr. Scand.* **1983**, *72*, 461–462. [CrossRef]
37. Perrin, M.T.; Fogleman, A.D.; Newburg, D.S.; Allen, J.C. A Longitudinal Study of Human Milk Composition in the Second Year Postpartum: Implications for Human Milk Banking. *Matern. Child. Nutr.* **2017**, *13*, e12239. [CrossRef]
38. Prentice, A.M.; Cole, T.J.; Paul, A.A.; Whitehead, R.G. Breast-Milk Antimicrobial Factors of Rural Gambian Mothers. I. Influence of Stage of Lactation and Maternal Plane of Nutrition. *Acta Paediatr. Scand.* **1984**, *73*, 796–802. [CrossRef]
39. Czosnykowska-Łukacka, M.; Orczyk-Pawiłowicz, M.; Broers, B.; Królak-Olejnik, B. Lactoferrin in Human Milk of Prolonged Lactation. *Nutrients* **2019**, *11*, 2350. [CrossRef]
40. Rollins, N.C.; Bhandari, N.; Hajeebhoy, N.; Horton, S.; Lutter, C.K.; Martines, J.C.; Piwoz, E.G.; Richter, L.M.; Victora, C.G. Why Invest, and What It Will Take to Improve Breastfeeding Practices? *Lancet* **2016**, *387*, 491–504. [CrossRef]
41. Smith, J.P.; Harvey, P.J. Chronic Disease and Infant Nutrition: Is It Significant to Public Health? *Public Health Nutr.* **2011**, *14*, 279–289. [CrossRef]
42. Gutowska-Ślesik, J.; Samoliński, B.; Krzych-Fałta, E. The Increase in Allergic Conditions Based on a Review of Literature. *Adv. Dermatol. Allergol.* **2023**, *40*, 1–7. [CrossRef]
43. Hu, T.; Dong, Y.; Yang, C.; Zhao, M.; He, Q. Pathogenesis of Children's Allergic Diseases: Refocusing the Role of the Gut Microbiota. *Front. Physiol.* **2021**, *12*, 749544. [CrossRef]
44. Aldakheel, F.M. Allergic Diseases: A Comprehensive Review on Risk Factors, Immunological Mechanisms, Link with COVID-19, Potential Treatments, and Role of Allergen Bioinformatics. *Int. J. Environ. Res. Public Health* **2021**, *18*, 12105. [CrossRef]
45. Akagawa, S.; Kaneko, K. Gut Microbiota and Allergic Diseases in Children. *Allergol. Int.* **2022**, *71*, 301–309. [CrossRef]
46. Davis, E.C.; Castagna, V.P.; Sela, D.A.; Hillard, M.A.; Lindberg, S.; Mantis, N.J.; Seppo, A.E.; Järvinen, K.M. Gut Microbiome and Breast-Feeding: Implications for Early Immune Development. *J. Allergy Clin. Immunol.* **2022**, *150*, 523–534. [CrossRef]
47. Bener, A.; Ehlayel, M.S.; Alsowaidi, S.; Sabbah, A. Role of Breast Feeding in Primary Prevention of Asthma and Allergic Diseases in a Traditional Society. *Eur. Ann. Allergy Clin. Immunol.* **2007**, *39*, 337–343.
48. Ehlaye, M.S.; Bener, A. Duration of Breast-Feeding and the Risk of Childhood Allergic Diseases in a Developing Country. *Allergy Asthma Proc.* **2008**, *29*, 386–391. [CrossRef]
49. Saarinen, U.M.; Backman, A.; Kajosaari, M.; Siimes, M.A. Prolonged Breast-Feeding as Prophylaxis for Atopic Disease. *Lancet* **1979**, *2*, 163–166. [CrossRef]
50. Saarinen, U.M.; Kajosaari, M. Breastfeeding as Prophylaxis against Atopic Disease: Prospective Follow-up Study until 17 Years Old. *Lancet* **1995**, *346*, 1065–1069. [CrossRef]

51. Van Ginkel, C.D.; Van Der Meulen, G.N.; Bak, E.; Flokstra-De Blok, B.M.J.; Kollen, B.J.; Koppelman, G.H.; Dubois, A.E.J. Retrospective Observational Cohort Study Regarding the Effect of Breastfeeding on Challenge-Proven Food Allergy. *Eur. J. Clin. Nutr.* **2018**, *72*, 557–563. [CrossRef]
52. Obihara, C.C.; Marais, B.J.; Gie, R.P.; Potter, P.; Bateman, E.D.; Lombard, C.J.; Beyers, N.; Kimpen, J.L.L. The Association of Prolonged Breastfeeding and Allergic Disease in Poor Urban Children. *Eur. Respir. J.* **2005**, *25*, 970–977. [CrossRef]
53. Huang, C.; Liu, W.; Cai, J.; Weschler, L.B.; Wang, X.; Hu, Y.; Zou, Z.; Shen, L.; Sundell, J. Breastfeeding and Timing of First Dietary Introduction in Relation to Childhood Asthma, Allergies, and Airway Diseases: A Cross-Sectional Study. *J. Asthma* **2017**, *54*, 488–497. [CrossRef]
54. Snijders, B.E.P.; Thijs, C.; Van Ree, R.; Van Den Brandt, P.A. Age at First Introduction of Cow Milk Products and Other Food Products in Relation to Infant Atopic Manifestations in the First 2 Years of Life: The KOALA Birth Cohort Study. *Pediatrics* **2008**, *122*, e115–e122. [CrossRef]
55. Halken, S.; Muraro, A.; de Silva, D.; Khaleva, E.; Angier, E.; Arasi, S.; Arshad, H.; Bahnson, H.T.; Beyer, K.; Boyle, R.; et al. EAACI Guideline: Preventing the Development of Food Allergy in Infants and Young Children (2020 Update). *Pediatr. Allergy Immunol.* **2021**, *32*, 843–858. [CrossRef]
56. Silvers, K.M.; Frampton, C.M.; Wickens, K.; Epton, M.J.; Pattemore, P.K.; Ingham, T.; Fishwick, D.; Crane, J.; Town, G.I.; Duignan, M.; et al. Breastfeeding Protects against Adverse Respiratory Outcomes at 15 Months of Age. *Matern. Child. Nutr.* **2009**, *5*, 243–250. [CrossRef]
57. Silvers, K.M.; Frampton, C.M.; Wickens, K.; Pattemore, P.K.; Ingham, T.; Fishwick, D.; Crane, J.; Town, G.I.; Epton, M.J. Breastfeeding Protects against Current Asthma up to 6 Years of Age. *J. Pediatr.* **2012**, *160*, 991–996.e1. [CrossRef]
58. von Kobyletzki, L.B.; Bornehag, C.G.; Hasselgren, M.; Larsson, M.; Lindström, C.B.; Svensson, Å. Eczema in Early Childhood Is Strongly Associated with the Development of Asthma and Rhinitis in a Prospective Cohort. *BMC Dermatol.* **2012**, *12*, 11. [CrossRef]
59. Wickman, M.; Melén, E.; Berglind, N.; Lennart Nordvall, S.; Almqvist, C.; Kull, I.; Svartengren, M.; Pershagen, G. Strategies for Preventing Wheezing and Asthma in Small Children. *Allergy* **2003**, *58*, 742–747. [CrossRef]
60. Vieira Borba, V.; Sharif, K.; Shoenfeld, Y. Breastfeeding and Autoimmunity: Programing Health from the Beginning. *Am. J. Reprod. Immunol.* **2018**, *79*, e12778. [CrossRef]
61. Watanabe, J.; Tanaka, K.; Nagata, C.; Furukawa, S.; Arakawa, M.; Miyake, Y. Breastfeeding Duration Is Inversely Associated with Asthma in Japanese Children Aged 3 Years. *J. Asthma* **2018**, *55*, 511–516. [CrossRef]
62. Al-Makoshi, A.; Al-Frayh, A.; Turner, S.; Devereux, G. Breastfeeding Practice and Its Association with Respiratory Symptoms and Atopic Disease in 1-3-Year-Old Children in the City of Riyadh, Central Saudi Arabia. *Breastfeed. Med.* **2013**, *8*, 127–133. [CrossRef]
63. Han, D.H.; Shin, J.M.; An, S.; Kim, J.S.; Kim, D.Y.; Moon, S.; Kim, J.S.; Cho, J.S.; Kim, S.W.; Kim, Y.H.; et al. Long-Term Breastfeeding in the Prevention of Allergic Rhinitis: Allergic Rhinitis Cohort Study for Kids (ARCO-Kids Study). *Clin. Exp. Otorhinolaryngol.* **2019**, *12*, 301. [CrossRef]
64. Tong, H.; Gao, L.; Deng, Y.; Kong, Y.; Xiang, R.; Tan, L.; Tao, Z.; Xu, Y. Prevalence of Allergic Rhinitis and Associated Risk Factors in 6 to 12 Years Schoolchildren from Wuhan in Central China: A Cross-Sectional Study. *Am. J. Rhinol. Allergy* **2020**, *34*, 632–641. [CrossRef] [PubMed]
65. Ng, S.C.; Shi, H.Y.; Hamidi, N.; Underwood, F.E.; Tang, W.; Benchimol, E.I.; Panaccione, R.; Ghosh, S.; Wu, J.C.Y.; Chan, F.K.L.; et al. Worldwide Incidence and Prevalence of Inflammatory Bowel Disease in the 21st Century: A Systematic Review of Population-Based Studies. *Lancet* **2017**, *390*, 2769–2778. [CrossRef]
66. Turner, D.; Ruemmele, F.M.; Orlanski-Meyer, E.; Griffiths, A.M.; De Carpi, J.M.; Bronsky, J.; Veres, G.; Aloi, M.; Strisciuglio, C.; Braegger, C.P.; et al. Management of Paediatric Ulcerative Colitis, Part 1: Ambulatory Care-An Evidence-Based Guideline from European Crohn's and Colitis Organization and European Society of Paediatric Gastroenterology, Hepatology and Nutrition. *J. Pediatr. Gastroenterol. Nutr.* **2018**, *67*, 257–291. [CrossRef] [PubMed]
67. Veauthier, B.; Hornecker, J.R. Crohn's Disease: Diagnosis and Management. *Am. Fam. Physician* **2018**, *98*, 661–669.
68. Iyengar, S.R.; Walker, W.A. Immune Factors in Breast Milk and the Development of Atopic Disease. *J. Pediatr. Gastroenterol. Nutr.* **2012**, *55*, 641–647. [CrossRef]
69. Newburg, D.S.; Walker, W.A. Protection of the Neonate by the Innate Immune System of Developing Gut and of Human Milk. *Pediatr. Res.* **2007**, *61*, 2–8. [CrossRef]
70. Seyedian, S.S.; Nokhostin, F.; Malamir, M.D. A Review of the Diagnosis, Prevention, and Treatment Methods of Inflammatory Bowel Disease. *J. Med. Life* **2019**, *12*, 113. [CrossRef]
71. Rigas, A.; Rigas, B.; Glassman, M.; Yen, Y.Y.; Lan, S.J.; Petridou, E.; Hsieh, C.C.; Trichopoulos, D. Breast-Feeding and Maternal Smoking in the Etiology of Crohn's Disease and Ulcerative Colitis in Childhood. *Ann. Epidemiol.* **1993**, *3*, 387–392. [CrossRef]
72. Gearry, R.B.; Richardson, A.K.; Frampton, C.M.; Dodgshun, A.J.; Barclay, M.L. Population-Based Cases Control Study of Inflammatory Bowel Disease Risk Factors. *J. Gastroenterol. Hepatol.* **2010**, *25*, 325–333. [CrossRef]
73. Ng, S.C.; Tang, W.; Leong, R.W.; Chen, M.; Ko, Y.; Studd, C.; Niewiadomski, O.; Bell, S.; Kamm, M.A.; De Silva, H.J.; et al. Environmental Risk Factors in Inflammatory Bowel Disease: A Population-Based Case-Control Study in Asia-Pacific. *Gut* **2015**, *64*, 1063–1071. [CrossRef]
74. Xu, L.; Lochhead, P.; Ko, Y.; Claggett, B.; Leong, R.W.; Ananthakrishnan, A.N. Systematic Review with Meta-Analysis: Breastfeeding and the Risk of Crohn's Disease and Ulcerative Colitis. *Aliment. Pharmacol. Ther.* **2017**, *46*, 780–789. [CrossRef]

75. Ko, Y.; Kariyawasam, V.; Karnib, M.; Butcher, R.; Samuel, D.; Alrubaie, A.; Rahme, N.; McDonald, C.; Cowlishaw, J.; Katelaris, P.; et al. Inflammatory Bowel Disease Environmental Risk Factors: A Population-Based Case-Control Study of Middle Eastern Migration to Australia. *Clin. Gastroenterol. Hepatol.* **2015**, *13*, 1453–1463.e1. [CrossRef] [PubMed]
76. Bergstrand, O.; Hellers, G. Breast-Feeding during Infancy in Patients Who Later Develop Crohn's Disease. *Scand. J. Gastroenterol.* **1983**, *18*, 903–906. [CrossRef]
77. Decker, E.; Engelmann, G.; Findeisen, A.; Gerner, P.; Laaß, M.; Ney, D.; Posovszky, C.; Hoy, L.; Hornef, M.W. Cesarean Delivery Is Associated with Celiac Disease but Not Inflammatory Bowel Disease in Children. *Pediatrics* **2010**, *125*, e1433–e1440. [CrossRef]
78. Hansen, T.S.; Jess, T.; Vind, I.; Elkjaer, M.; Nielsen, M.F.; Gamborg, M.; Munkholm, P. Environmental Factors in Inflammatory Bowel Disease: A Case-Control Study Based on a Danish Inception Cohort. *J. Crohns Colitis* **2011**, *5*, 577–584. [CrossRef]
79. Hlavaty, T.; Toth, J.; Koller, T.; Krajcovicova, A.; Oravcova, S.; Zelinkova, Z.; Huorka, M. Smoking, Breastfeeding, Physical Inactivity, Contact with Animals, and Size of the Family Influence the Risk of Inflammatory Bowel Disease: A Slovak Case-Control Study. *United Eur. Gastroenterol. J.* **2013**, *1*, 109–119. [CrossRef]
80. Lee, W.S.; Song, Z.L.; Wong, S.Y.; Gan, C.W.; Koay, Z.L.; Em, J.M.; Chong, S.Y.; Lim, C.B.; Wong, S.Y.; Chew, K.S.; et al. Environmental Risk Factors for Inflammatory Bowel Disease: A Case Control Study in Southeast Asian Children. *J. Paediatr. Child. Health* **2022**, *58*, 782–790. [CrossRef]
81. Shaaban, K.M.; Hamadnalla, I. The Effect of Duration of Breast Feeding on the Occurrence of Acute Otitis Media in Children under Three Years. *East. Afr. Med. J.* **1993**, *70*, 632–634.
82. Vogazianos, E.; Vogazianos, P.; Fiala, J.; Janeček, D.; Šlapák, I. The Effect of Breastfeeding and Its Duration on Acute Otitis Media in Children in Brno, Czech Republic. *Cent. Eur. J. Public. Health* **2007**, *15*, 143–146. [CrossRef]
83. Ardc, C.; Yavuz, E. Effect of Breastfeeding on Common Pediatric Infections: A 5-Year Prospective Cohort Study. *Arch. Argent. Pediatr.* **2018**, *116*, 126–132. [CrossRef]
84. Weiss, Y.T.; Tamir, S.O.; Globus, O.; Marom, T. Protective Characteristics of Human Breast Milk on Early Childhood Otitis Media: A Narrative Review. *Breastfeed. Med.* **2024**, *19*, 73–80. [CrossRef]
85. Obesity and Overweight. Available online: https://www.who.int/news-room/fact-sheets/detail/obesity-and-overweight (accessed on 21 August 2024).
86. Lourenço, L.P.; Viola, P.C.d.A.F.; Franceschini, S.d.C.C.; Rosa, C.d.O.B.; Ribeiro, S.A.V. Metabolic Syndrome and Risk Factors in Children: A Risk Score Proposal. *Eur. J. Clin. Nutr.* **2023**, *77*, 278–282. [CrossRef]
87. Weiss, R.; Bremer, A.A.; Lustig, R.H. What Is Metabolic Syndrome, and Why Are Children Getting It? *Ann. N. Y. Acad. Sci.* **2013**, *1281*, 123–140. [CrossRef]
88. Tropeano, A.; Corica, D.; Pomi, A.L.; Pepe, G.; Morabito, L.A.; Curatola, S.L.; Casto, C.; Aversa, T.; Wasniewska, M. The Metabolic Syndrome in Pediatrics: Do We Have a Reliable Definition? A Systematic Review. *Eur. J. Endocrinol.* **2021**, *185*, 265–278. [CrossRef]
89. Liu, F.; Lv, D.; Wang, L.; Feng, X.; Zhang, R.; Liu, W.; Han, W. Breastfeeding and Overweight/Obesity among Children and Adolescents: A Cross-Sectional Study. *BMC Pediatr.* **2022**, *22*, 347. [CrossRef]
90. Gewa, C.A. Childhood Overweight and Obesity among Kenyan Pre-School Children: Association with Maternal and Early Child Nutritional Factors. *Public Health Nutr.* **2010**, *13*, 496–503. [CrossRef]
91. Nascimento Simon, V.G.; Pacheco de Souza, J.M.; de Souza, S.B. Breastfeeding, Complementary Feeding, Overweight and Obesity in Pre-School Children. *Rev. Saude Publica* **2009**, *43*, 60–69. [CrossRef]
92. Fallahzadeh, H.; Golestan, M.; Rezvanian, T.; Ghasemian, Z. Breast-Feeding History and Overweight in 11 to 13-Year-Old Children in Iran. *World J. Pediatr.* **2009**, *5*, 36–41. [CrossRef]
93. Liese, A.D.; Hirsch, T.; Von Mutius, E.; Keil, U.; Leupold, W.; Weiland, S.K. Inverse Association of Overweight and Breast Feeding in 9 to 10-y-Old Children in Germany. *Int. J. Obes. Relat. Metab. Disord.* **2001**, *25*, 1644–1650. [CrossRef]
94. Von Kries, R.; Koletzko, B.; Sauerwald, T.; Von Mutius, E.; Barnert, D.; Grunert, V.; Von Voss, H. Breast Feeding and Obesity: Cross Sectional Study. *BMJ* **1999**, *319*, 147–150. [CrossRef] [PubMed]
95. Grummer-Strawn, L.M.; Mei, Z. Does Breastfeeding Protect against Pediatric Overweight? Analysis of Longitudinal Data from the Centers for Disease Control and Prevention Pediatric Nutrition Surveillance System. *Pediatrics* **2004**, *113*, e81–e86. [CrossRef] [PubMed]
96. Hosaka, M.; Asayama, K.; Staessen, J.A.; Ohkubo, T.; Hayashi, K.; Tatsuta, N.; Kurokawa, N.; Satoh, M.; Hashimoto, T.; Hirose, T.; et al. Breastfeeding Leads to Lower Blood Pressure in 7-Year-Old Japanese Children: Tohoku Study of Child Development. *Hypertens. Res.* **2013**, *36*, 117–122. [CrossRef]
97. Lin, D.; Chen, D.; Huang, J.; Li, Y.; Wen, X.; Ou, P.; Shi, H. Breastfeeding Is Associated with Reduced Risks of Central Obesity and Hypertension in Young School-Aged Children: A Large, Population-Based Study. *Int. Breastfeed. J.* **2023**, *18*, 52. [CrossRef]
98. Liang, X.; Xiao, L.; Luo, Y.; Xu, J. Prevalence and Risk Factors of Childhood Hypertension in Urban-Rural Areas of China: A Cross-Sectional Study. *Int. J. Hypertens.* **2020**, *2020*, 2374231. [CrossRef]
99. Wang, J.; Perona, J.S.; Schmidt-RioValle, J.; Chen, Y.; Jing, J.; González-Jiménez, E. Metabolic Syndrome and Its Associated Early-Life Factors among Chinese and Spanish Adolescents: A Pilot Study. *Nutrients* **2019**, *11*, 1568. [CrossRef]
100. González-Jiménez, E.; Montero-Alonso, M.A.; Schmidt-RioValle, J.; García-García, C.J.; Padez, C. Metabolic Syndrome in Spanish Adolescents and Its Association with Birth Weight, Breastfeeding Duration, Maternal Smoking, and Maternal Obesity: A Cross-Sectional Study. *Eur. J. Nutr.* **2015**, *54*, 589–597. [CrossRef]

101. Esfarjani, F.; Khalafi, M.; Mohammadi, F.; Zamani-Nour, N.; Kelishadi, R. Metabolic Syndrome and Its Determinants in a Sample of Young Iranian Children with Obesity. *Pak. J. Med. Sci. Old. Website* **2013**, *29*, 253–257. [CrossRef]
102. Wang, J.; Zhu, Y.; Cai, L.; Jing, J.; Chen, Y.; Mai, J.; Ma, L.; Ma, Y.; Ma, J. Metabolic Syndrome and Its Associated Early-Life Factors in Children and Adolescents: A Cross-Sectional Study in Guangzhou, China. *Public Health Nutr.* **2016**, *19*, 1147–1154. [CrossRef] [PubMed]
103. Chaffee, B.W.; Feldens, C.A.; Vítolo, M.R. Association of Long-Duration Breastfeeding and Dental Caries Estimated with Marginal Structural Models. *Ann. Epidemiol.* **2014**, *24*, 448–454. [CrossRef]
104. Tanaka, K.; Miyake, Y. Association between Breastfeeding and Dental Caries in Japanese Children. *J. Epidemiol.* **2012**, *22*, 72–77. [CrossRef]
105. Nirunsittirat, A.; Pitiphat, W.; McKinney, C.M.; Derouen, T.A.; Chansamak, N.; Angwaravong, O.; Patcharanuchat, P.; Pimpak, T. Breastfeeding Duration and Childhood Caries: A Cohort Study. *Caries Res.* **2016**, *50*, 498–507. [CrossRef]
106. Peres, K.G.; Nascimento, G.G.; Peres, M.A.; Mittinty, M.N.; Demarco, F.F.; Santos, I.S.; Matijasevich, A.; Barros, A.J.D. Impact of Prolonged Breastfeeding on Dental Caries: A Population-Based Birth Cohort Study. *Pediatrics* **2017**, *140*, e20162943. [CrossRef] [PubMed]
107. Shrestha, S.K.; Arora, A.; Manohar, N.; Ekanayake, K.; Foster, J. Association of Breastfeeding and Early Childhood Caries: A Systematic Review and Meta-Analysis. *Nutrients* **2024**, *16*, 1355. [CrossRef]
108. Cui, L.; Li, X.; Tian, Y.; Bao, J.; Wang, L.; Xu, D.; Zhao, B.; Li, W. Breastfeeding and Early Childhood Caries: A Meta-Analysis of Observational Studies. *Asia Pac. J. Clin. Nutr.* **2017**, *26*, 867–880. [CrossRef]
109. Tham, R.; Bowatte, G.; Dharmage, S.; Tan, D.; Lau, M.; Dai, X.; Allen, K.; Lodge, C. Breastfeeding and the Risk of Dental Caries: A Systematic Review and Meta-Analysis. *Acta Paediatr.* **2015**, *104*, 62–84. [CrossRef]
110. Panchanadikar, N.T.; Abirami, S.; Muthu, M.S.; Selvakumar, H.; Jayakumar, P.; Agarwal, A. Breastfeeding and Its Association with Early Childhood Caries-An Umbrella Review. *J. Clin. Pediatr. Dent.* **2022**, *46*, 75–85. [CrossRef]
111. Valaitis, R.; Hesch, R.; Passarelli, C.; Sheehan, D.; Sinton, J. A Systematic Review of the Relationship between Breastfeeding and Early Childhood Caries. *Can. J. Public Health* **2000**, *91*, 411–417. [CrossRef]
112. Hossain, S.; Mihrshahi, S. Exclusive Breastfeeding and Childhood Morbidity: A Narrative Review. *Int. J. Environ. Res. Public Health* **2022**, *19*, 14804. [CrossRef]
113. Duijts, L.; Jaddoe, V.W.V.; Hofman, A.; Moll, H.A. Prolonged and Exclusive Breastfeeding Reduces the Risk of Infectious Diseases in Infancy. *Pediatrics* **2010**, *126*, e18–e25. [CrossRef]
114. Madore, L.S.; Fisher, D.J. The Role of Breast Milk in Infectious Disease. *Clin. Perinatol.* **2021**, *48*, 359–378. [CrossRef] [PubMed]
115. Størdal, K.; Lundeby, K.M.; Brantsæter, A.L.; Haugen, M.; Nakstad, B.; Lund-Blix, N.A.; Stene, L.C. Breast-Feeding and Infant Hospitalization for Infections: Large Cohort and Sibling Analysis. *J. Pediatr. Gastroenterol. Nutr.* **2017**, *65*, 225–231. [CrossRef] [PubMed]
116. Nafstad, P.; Jaakkola, J.J.K.; Hagen, J.A.; Botten, G.; Kongerud, J. Breastfeeding, Maternal Smoking and Lower Respiratory Tract Infections. *Eur. Respir. J.* **1996**, *9*, 2623–2629. [CrossRef]
117. Tromp, I.; De Jong, J.K.; Raat, H.; Jaddoe, V.; Franco, O.; Hofman, A.; De Jongste, J.; Moll, H. Breastfeeding and the Risk of Respiratory Tract Infections after Infancy: The Generation R Study. *PLoS ONE* **2017**, *12*, e0172763. [CrossRef]
118. Li, R.; Dee, D.; Li, C.M.; Hoffman, H.J.; Grummer-Strawn, L.M. Breastfeeding and Risk of Infections at 6 Years. *Pediatrics* **2014**, *134* (Suppl. S1), S13–S20. [CrossRef]
119. Fisk, C.M.; Crozier, S.R.; Inskip, H.M.; Godfrey, K.M.; Cooper, C.; Roberts, G.C.; Robinson, S.M. Breastfeeding and Reported Morbidity during Infancy: Findings from the Southampton Women's Survey. *Matern. Child. Nutr.* **2011**, *7*, 61–70. [CrossRef]
120. Rebhan, B.; Kohlhuber, M.; Schwegler, U.; Fromme, H.; Abou-Dakn, M.; Koletzko, B.V. Breastfeeding Duration and Exclusivity Associated with Infants' Health and Growth: Data from a Prospective Cohort Study in Bavaria, Germany. *Acta Paediatr.* **2009**, *98*, 974–980. [CrossRef]
121. Molbak, K.; Gottschau, A.; Aaby, P.; Hojlyng, N.; Ingholt, L.; da Silva, A.P.J. Prolonged Breast Feeding, Diarrhoeal Disease, and Survival of Children in Guinea-Bissau. *BMJ* **1994**, *308*, 1403. [CrossRef]
122. Ruuska, T. Occurrence of Acute Diarrhea in Atopic and Nonatopic Infants: The Role of Prolonged Breast-Feeding. *J. Pediatr. Gastroenterol. Nutr.* **1992**, *14*, 27–33. [CrossRef]
123. Daniels, M.C.; Adair, L.S. Breast-Feeding Influences Cognitive Development in Filipino Children. *J. Nutr.* **2005**, *135*, 2589–2595. [CrossRef]
124. Duazo, P.; Avila, J.; Kuzawa, C.W. Breastfeeding and Later Psychosocial Development in the Philippines. *Am. J. Hum. Biol.* **2010**, *22*, 725–730. [CrossRef] [PubMed]
125. Slykerman, R.; Thompson, J.M.D.; Becroft, D.M.O.; Robinson, E.; Pryor, J.; Clark, P.; Wild, C.; Mitchell, E. Breastfeeding and Intelligence of Preschool Children. *Acta Paediatr.* **2005**, *94*, 832–837. [CrossRef]
126. Whitehouse, A.J.O.; Robinson, M.; Li, J.; Oddy, W.H. Duration of Breast Feeding and Language Ability in Middle Childhood. *Paediatr. Perinat. Epidemiol.* **2011**, *25*, 44–52. [CrossRef] [PubMed]
127. Jedrychowski, W.; Perera, F.; Jankowski, J.; Butscher, M.; Mroz, E.; Flak, E.; Kaim, I.; Lisowska-Miszczyk, I.; Skarupa, A.; Sowa, A. Effect of Exclusive Breastfeeding on the Development of Children's Cognitive Function in the Krakow Prospective Birth Cohort Study. *Eur. J. Pediatr.* **2012**, *171*, 151–158. [CrossRef]

128. Sajjad, A.; Tharner, A.; Kiefte-de Jong, J.C.; Jaddoe, V.V.W.; Hofman, A.; Verhulst, F.C.; Franco, O.H.; Tiemeier, H.; Roza, S.J. Breastfeeding Duration and Non-Verbal IQ in Children. *J. Epidemiol. Commun. Health* **2015**, *69*, 775–781. [CrossRef]
129. Shu, X.O.; Linet, M.S.; Steinbuch, M.; Wen, W.Q.; Buckley, J.D.; Neglia, J.P.; Potter, J.D.; Reaman, G.H.; Robison, L.L. Breast-Feeding and Risk of Childhood Acute Leukemia. *J. Natl. Cancer Inst.* **1999**, *91*, 1765–1772. [CrossRef]
130. Gong, Q.Q.; Quan, D.D.; Guo, C.; Zhang, C.; Zhang, Z.J. Association between Maternal Breastfeeding and Risk of Systemic Neoplasms of Offspring. *Ital. J. Pediatr.* **2022**, *48*, 98. [CrossRef]
131. Gao, Z.; Wang, R.; Qin, Z.X.; Dong, A.; Liu, C.B. Protective Effect of Breastfeeding against Childhood Leukemia in Zhejiang Province, P.R. China: A Retrospective Case-Control Study. *Libyan J. Med.* **2018**, *13*, 1508273. [CrossRef]
132. MacArthur, A.C.; McBride, M.L.; Spinelli, J.J.; Tamaro, S.; Gallagher, R.P.; Theriault, G.P. Risk of Childhood Leukemia Associated with Vaccination, Infection, and Medication Use in Childhood: The Cross-Canada Childhood Leukemia Study. *Am. J. Epidemiol.* **2008**, *167*, 598–606. [CrossRef]
133. Cheng, K.K.; Day, N.E.; Cartwright, R.; Craft, A.; Birch, J.M.; Eden, O.B.; McKinney, P.A.; Peto, J.; Beral, V.; Roman, E.; et al. Breastfeeding and Childhood Cancer. *Br. J. Cancer* **2001**, *85*, 1685. [CrossRef]
134. Bener, A.; Denic, S.; Galadari, S. Longer Breast-Feeding and Protection against Childhood Leukaemia and Lymphomas. *Eur. J. Cancer* **2001**, *37*, 234–238. [CrossRef] [PubMed]
135. Rudant, J.; Orsi, L.; Menegaux, F.; Petit, A.; Baruchel, A.; Bertrand, Y.; Lambilliotte, A.; Robert, A.; Michel, G.; Margueritte, G.; et al. Childhood Acute Leukemia, Early Common Infections, and Allergy: The ESCALE Study. *Am. J. Epidemiol.* **2010**, *172*, 1015–1027. [CrossRef]
136. Altinkaynak, S.; Selimoglu, M.A.; Turgut, A.; Kilicaslan, B.; Ertekin, V. Breast-Feeding Duration and Childhood Acute Leukemia and Lymphomas in a Sample of Turkish Children. *J. Pediatr. Gastroenterol. Nutr.* **2006**, *42*, 568–572. [CrossRef]
137. Bener, A.; Tokaç, M.; Tewfik, I.; Zughaier, S.M.; Ağan, A.F.; Day, A.S. Breastfeeding Duration Reduces the Risk of Childhood Leukemia and Modifies the Risk of Developing Functional Gastrointestinal Disorders. *Breastfeed. Med.* **2024**, *19*, 539–546. [CrossRef]
138. Pincelli, A.; Cardoso, M.A.; Malta, M.B.; Nicolete, V.C.; Soares, I.S.; Castro, M.C.; Ferreira, M.U. Prolonged Breastfeeding and the Risk of Plasmodium Vivax Infection and Clinical Malaria in Early Childhood: A Birth Cohort Study. *Pediatr. Infect. Dis. J.* **2022**, *41*, 793–799. [CrossRef]
139. Safeukui-Noubissi, I.; Ranque, S.; Poudiougou, B.; Keita, M.; Traoré, A.; Traoré, D.; Diakité, M.; Cissé, M.B.; Keita, M.M.; Dessein, A.; et al. Risk Factors for Severe Malaria in Bamako, Mali: A Matched Case-Control Study. *Microbes Infect.* **2004**, *6*, 572–578. [CrossRef]
140. Vora, N.; Homsy, J.; Kakuru, A.; Arinaitwe, E.; Wanzira, H.; Sandison, T.G.; Bigira, V.; Kamya, M.R.; Tappero, J.W.; Dorsey, G. Breastfeeding and the Risk of Malaria in Children Born to HIV-Infected and Uninfected Mothers in Rural Uganda. *J. Acquir. Immune Defic. Syndr.* **2010**, *55*, 253–261. [CrossRef]
141. Kindgren, E.; Fredrikson, M.; Ludvigsson, J. Early Feeding and Risk of Juvenile Idiopathic Arthritis: A Case Control Study in a Prospective Birth Cohort. *Pediatr. Rheumatol. Online J.* **2017**, *15*, 46. [CrossRef]
142. Ivarsson, A.; Hernell, O.; Stenlund, H.; Persson, L.Å. Breast-Feeding Protects against Celiac Disease. *Am. J. Clin. Nutr.* **2002**, *75*, 914–921. [CrossRef]
143. Li, Y.; Deng, H.; Li, M.; Wang, W.; Jia, X.; Gao, N.; Dang, S. Prolonged Breastfeeding Is Associated with Lower Risk of Severe Hand, Foot and Mouth Disease in Chinese Children. *Pediatr. Infect. Dis. J.* **2016**, *35*, 353–355. [CrossRef]
144. Li, Y.; Gao, D.; Chen, L.; Ma, T.; Ma, Y.; Chen, M.; Dong, B.; Dong, Y.; Ma, J.; Arnold, L. The Association between Breastfeeding Duration and Lipid Profile among Children and Adolescents. *Nutrients* **2021**, *13*, 2728. [CrossRef] [PubMed]
145. Daniels, J.L.; Olshan, A.F.; Pollock, B.H.; Shah, N.R.; Stram, D.O. Breast-Feeding and Neuroblastoma, USA and Canada. *Cancer Causes Control* **2002**, *13*, 401–405. [CrossRef] [PubMed]
146. Heck, J.E.; Omidakhsh, N.; Azary, S.; Ritz, B.; von Ehrenstein, O.S.; Bunin, G.R.; Ganguly, A. A Case-Control Study of Sporadic Retinoblastoma in Relation to Maternal Health Conditions and Reproductive Factors: A Report from the Children's Oncology Group. *BMC Cancer* **2015**, *15*, 735. [CrossRef] [PubMed]
147. Lupo, P.J.; Zhou, R.; Skapek, S.X.; Hawkins, D.S.; Spector, L.G.; Scheurer, M.E.; Fatih Okcu, M.; Melin, B.; Papworth, K.; Erhardt, E.B.; et al. Allergies, Atopy, Immune-Related Factors and Childhood Rhabdomyosarcoma: A Report from the Children's Oncology Group. *Int. J. Cancer* **2014**, *134*, 431–436. [CrossRef]
148. Thompson, J.M.D.; Tanabe, K.; Moon, R.Y.; Mitchell, E.A.; McGarvey, C.; Tappin, D.; Blair, P.S.; Hauck, F.R. Duration of Breastfeeding and Risk of SIDS: An Individual Participant Data Meta-Analysis. *Pediatrics* **2017**, *140*, e20171324. [CrossRef]
149. Kue Young, T.; Martens, P.J.; Taback, S.P.; Sellers, E.A.C.; Dean, H.J.; Cheang, M.; Flett, B. Type 2 Diabetes Mellitus in Children: Prenatal and Early Infancy Risk Factors among Native Canadians. *Arch. Pediatr. Adolesc. Med.* **2002**, *156*, 651–655. [CrossRef]
150. Donald, K.; Petersen, C.; Turvey, S.E.; Finlay, B.B.; Azad, M.B. Secretory IgA: Linking Microbes, Maternal Health, and Infant Health through Human Milk. *Cell Host Microbe* **2022**, *30*, 650–659. [CrossRef]
151. Reniker, L.N.; Frazer, L.C.; Good, M. Key Biologically Active Components of Breast Milk and Their Beneficial Effects. *Semin. Pediatr. Surg.* **2023**, *32*, 151306. [CrossRef]
152. Rogier, E.W.; Frantz, A.L.; Bruno, M.E.C.; Wedlund, L.; Cohen, D.A.; Stromberg, A.J.; Kaetzel, C.S. Lessons from Mother: Long-Term Impact of Antibodies in Breast Milk on the Gut Microbiota and Intestinal Immune System of Breastfed Offspring. *Gut Microbes* **2014**, *5*, 663. [CrossRef]

153. Story, L.; Perish, T. Breastfeeding Helps Prevent Two Major Infant Illnesses. *Internet J. Allied Health Sci. Pract.* **2008**, *6*, 10. [CrossRef]
154. Azad, M.B.; Konya, T.; Maughan, H.; Guttman, D.S.; Field, C.J.; Chari, R.S.; Sears, M.R.; Becker, A.B.; Scott, J.A.; Kozyrskyj, A.L. Gut Microbiota of Healthy Canadian Infants: Profiles by Mode of Delivery and Infant Diet at 4 Months. *CMAJ* **2013**, *185*, 385–394. [CrossRef] [PubMed]
155. Van Nimwegen, F.A.; Penders, J.; Stobberingh, E.E.; Postma, D.S.; Koppelman, G.H.; Kerkhof, M.; Reijmerink, N.E.; Dompeling, E.; Van Den Brandt, P.A.; Ferreira, I.; et al. Mode and Place of Delivery, Gastrointestinal Microbiota, and Their Influence on Asthma and Atopy. *J. Allergy Clin. Immunol.* **2011**, *128*, 948–955.e3. [CrossRef] [PubMed]
156. Masi, A.C.; Stewart, C.J. Untangling Human Milk Oligosaccharides and Infant Gut Microbiome. *iScience* **2021**, *25*, 103542. [CrossRef] [PubMed]
157. Miliku, K.; Azad, M.B. Breastfeeding and the Developmental Origins of Asthma: Current Evidence, Possible Mechanisms, and Future Research Priorities. *Nutrients* **2018**, *10*, 995. [CrossRef]
158. Cheema, A.S.; Trevenen, M.L.; Turlach, B.A.; Furst, A.J.; Roman, A.S.; Bode, L.; Gridneva, Z.; Lai, C.T.; Stinson, L.F.; Payne, M.S.; et al. Exclusively Breastfed Infant Microbiota Develops over Time and Is Associated with Human Milk Oligosaccharide Intakes. *Int. J. Mol. Sci.* **2022**, *23*, 2804. [CrossRef]
159. Bode, L. Human Milk Oligosaccharides: Every Baby Needs a Sugar Mama. *Glycobiology* **2012**, *22*, 1147–1162. [CrossRef]
160. Cheema, A.S.; Gridneva, Z.; Furst, A.J.; Roman, A.S.; Trevenen, M.L.; Turlach, B.A.; Lai, C.T.; Stinson, L.F.; Bode, L.; Payne, M.S.; et al. Human Milk Oligosaccharides and Bacterial Profile Modulate Infant Body Composition during Exclusive Breastfeeding. *Int. J. Mol. Sci.* **2022**, *23*, 2865. [CrossRef]
161. Zhou, P.; Chen, C.; Patil, S.; Dong, S. Unveiling the Therapeutic Symphony of Probiotics, Prebiotics, and Postbiotics in Gut-Immune Harmony. *Front. Nutr.* **2024**, *11*, 1355542. [CrossRef]
162. Gopalakrishna, K.P.; Hand, T.W. Influence of Maternal Milk on the Neonatal Intestinal Microbiome. *Nutrients* **2020**, *12*, 823. [CrossRef]
163. Kebbe, M.; Shankar, K.; Redman, L.M.; Andres, A. Human Milk Components and the Infant Gut Microbiome at 6 Months: Understanding the Interconnected Relationship. *J. Nutr.* **2024**, *154*, 1200–1208. [CrossRef]
164. Biesbroek, G.; Bosch, A.A.T.M.; Wang, X.; Keijser, B.J.F.; Veenhoven, R.H.; Sanders, E.A.M.; Bogaert, D. The Impact of Breastfeeding on Nasopharyngeal Microbial Communities in Infants. *Am. J. Respir. Crit. Care Med.* **2014**, *190*, 298–308. [CrossRef] [PubMed]
165. Notarbartolo, V.; Giuffre, M.; Montante, C.; Corsello, G.; Carta, M. Composition of Human Breast Milk Microbiota and Its Role in Children's Health. *Pediatr. Gastroenterol. Hepatol. Nutr.* **2022**, *25*, 194. [CrossRef] [PubMed]
166. Karampatsas, K.; Faal, A.; Jaiteh, M.; Garcia-Perez, I.; Aller, S.; Shaw, A.G.; Kopytek, A.; Witney, A.A.; Le Doare, K. Gastrointestinal, Vaginal, Nasopharyngeal, and Breast Milk Microbiota Profiles and Breast Milk Metabolomic Changes in Gambian Infants over the First Two Months of Lactation: A Prospective Cohort Study. *Medicine* **2022**, *101*, E31419. [CrossRef]
167. Kørvel-Hanquist, A.; Djurhuus, B.D.; Homøe, P. The Effect of Breastfeeding on Childhood Otitis Media. *Curr. Allergy Asthma Rep.* **2017**, *17*, 45. [CrossRef]
168. Schlaudecker, E.P.; Steinhoff, M.C.; Omer, S.B.; McNeal, M.M.; Roy, E.; Arifeen, S.E.; Dodd, C.N.; Raqib, R.; Breiman, R.F.; Zaman, K. IgA and Neutralizing Antibodies to Influenza a Virus in Human Milk: A Randomized Trial of Antenatal Influenza Immunization. *PLoS ONE* **2013**, *8*, e70867. [CrossRef]
169. Roberts, T.J.; Carnahan, E.; Gakidou, E. Can Breastfeeding Promote Child Health Equity? A Comprehensive Analysis of Breastfeeding Patterns across the Developing World and What We Can Learn from Them. *BMC Med.* **2013**, *11*, 254. [CrossRef]
170. Su, Q.; Sun, X.; Zhu, L.; Yan, Q.; Zheng, P.; Mao, Y.; Ye, D. Breastfeeding and the Risk of Childhood Cancer: A Systematic Review and Dose-Response Meta-Analysis. *BMC Med.* **2021**, *19*, 90. [CrossRef]
171. Kelishadi, R.; Farajian, S. The Protective Effects of Breastfeeding on Chronic Non-Communicable Diseases in Adulthood: A Review of Evidence. *Adv. Biomed. Res.* **2014**, *3*, 3. [CrossRef]
172. Juharji, H.; Albalawi, K.; Aldwaighri, M.; Almalki, A.; Alshiti, H.; Kattan, W.; Alqarni, M.; Alsulaimani, S.; AlShaikh, T.; Alsulaimani, F. Impact of Breastfeeding on Low Birthweight Infants, Weight Disorders in Infants, and Child Development. *Cureus* **2022**, *14*, e32894. [CrossRef]
173. Miliku, K.; Moraes, T.J.; Becker, A.B.; Mandhane, P.J.; Sears, M.R.; Turvey, S.E.; Subbarao, P.; Azad, M.B. Breastfeeding in the First Days of Life Is Associated with Lower Blood Pressure at 3 Years of Age. *J. Am. Heart Assoc.* **2021**, *10*, e019067. [CrossRef]
174. Hofman, A.; Hazebroek, A.; Valkenburg, H.A. A Randomized Trial of Sodium Intake and Blood Pressure in Newborn Infants. *JAMA* **1983**, *250*, 370–373. [CrossRef] [PubMed]
175. Ou, X.; Andres, A.; Pivik, R.T.; Cleves, M.A.; Snow, J.H.; Ding, Z.; Badger, T.M. Voxel-Based Morphometry and FMRI Revealed Differences in Brain Gray Matter in Breastfed and Milk Formula-Fed Children. *AJNR Am. J. Neuroradiol.* **2016**, *37*, 713–719. [CrossRef]
176. Grevet, L.T.; Teixeira, D.S.; Pan, P.M.; Jackowski, A.P.; Zugman, A.; Miguel, E.C.; Rohde, L.A.; Salum, G.A. The Association between Duration of Breastfeeding and the Trajectory of Brain Development from Childhood to Young Adulthood: An 8-Year Longitudinal Study. *Eur. Child. Adolesc. Psychiatry* **2024**, *33*, 1863–1873. [CrossRef]

177. Belfort, M.B.; Anderson, P.J.; Nowak, V.A.; Lee, K.J.; Molesworth, C.; Thompson, D.K.; Doyle, L.W.; Inder, T.E. Breast Milk Feeding, Brain Development, and Neurocognitive Outcomes: A 7-Year Longitudinal Study in Infants Born at Less Than 30 Weeks' Gestation. *J. Pediatr.* **2016**, *177*, 133–139.e1. [CrossRef]
178. Berger, P.K.; Ong, M.L.; Bode, L.; Belfort, M.B. Human Milk Oligosaccharides and Infant Neurodevelopment: A Narrative Review. *Nutrients* **2023**, *15*, 719. [CrossRef]

nutrients

MDPI

Review

Review on the Impact of Milk Oligosaccharides on the Brain and Neurocognitive Development in Early Life

Yuting Fan [1], Arden L. McMath [2] and Sharon M. Donovan [1,2,*]

1 Department of Food Science and Human Nutrition, University of Illinois Urbana-Champaign, Urbana, IL 61801, USA; yutingf2@illinois.edu
2 Division of Nutritional Sciences, University of Illinois Urbana-Champaign, Urbana, IL 61801, USA; amcmath2@illinois.edu
* Correspondence: sdonovan@illinois.edu

Abstract: Milk Oligosaccharides (MOS), a group of complex carbohydrates found in human and bovine milk, have emerged as potential modulators of optimal brain development for early life. This review provides a comprehensive investigation of the impact of milk oligosaccharides on brain and neurocognitive development of early life by synthesizing current literature from preclinical models and human observational studies. The literature search was conducted in the PubMed search engine, and the inclusion eligibility was evaluated by three reviewers. Overall, we identified 26 articles for analysis. While the literature supports the crucial roles of fucosylated and sialylated milk oligosaccharides in learning, memory, executive functioning, and brain structural development, limitations were identified. In preclinical models, the supplementation of only the most abundant MOS might overlook the complexity of naturally occurring MOS compositions. Similarly, accurately quantifying MOS intake in human studies is challenging due to potential confounding effects such as formula feeding. Mechanistically, MOS is thought to impact neurodevelopment through modulation of the microbiota and enhancement of neuronal signaling. However, further advancement in our understanding necessitates clinical randomized-controlled trials to elucidate the specific mechanisms and long-term implications of milk oligosaccharides exposure. Understanding the interplay between milk oligosaccharides and cognition may contribute to early nutrition strategies for optimal cognitive outcomes in children.

Keywords: narrative review; milk oligosaccharides; HMO; cognition; neurodevelopment; brain development; early life

1. Introduction

Cognition refers to complex mental functions, including memory, learning, thinking, and perception [1]. During infancy and early childhood, brain growth and the development of cognitive, behavioral, and social functions occurs rapidly [2] and influence later academic achievement [3]. Although cognitive development in this critical early life period is impacted by numerous factors [4], nutrition is at the forefront [4]. Previous research suggests that suboptimal nutrition early in life is associated with poorer cognitive development and functioning [5]. For example, nutritional supplementations for infants and young children led to a significant increase in cognition and school performance later in life [6].

Human milk is the optimal nutrition source for infants [7]. The American Academy of Pediatrics recommends exclusive breastfeeding for the first six months of life and 12 months or longer in combination with complementary foods [8]. Breastfeeding is associated with various benefits, such as preventing infectious disease, reducing all-cause mortality, and influencing both short-term and long-term infant development [9]. Specifically, feeding preterm and term infants human milk rather than formula has demonstrated benefits for neurodevelopment [10], an effect that may persist through adolescence [11–14]. The benefits of human milk for neurodevelopment have been attributed to components of its complex composition [15], including a group of complex carbohydrates known as human milk oligosaccharides (HMOs) [16]. While the milk of all mammals contains milk oligosaccharides (MOS), human milk is unique in its high concentration and structural complexity of oligosaccharides [16]. Infant formulas made from bovine milk have historically contained low concentrations of predominantly sialylated oligosaccharides compared to human milk [17–19], although one or two to up to five or six different synthetic MOS have been added to some infant formulas [20–22].

Numerous associations between HMOs and neurodevelopment and cognitive outcomes have been reported [23]. The gut microbiota has been shown to play an essential role in this interaction [24,25] through the gut-brain axis, defined as bidirectional communication between the enteric and central nervous systems [24]. HMOS exhibit physiological functions related to establishing healthy microbiota during early life [26] and may promote brain and cognitive development through the gut-brain axis. However, more than 200 unique HMOs structures have been identified [16], making it difficult to understand the unique function of individual HMOs with different structures on the neurocognitive development of infants from observational studies.

The benefits of HMOs for cognitive development may be due to their components, sialic acid and fucose, which have been implicated in brain development. Sialic acid (SA) is an essential nutrient for brain development as it is a component of gangliosides in the brain [27]. Also, SA has been reported to be an essential compound during neurodevelopment as it supports brain development, neuro transmission, and synapse formation [28].

SA rarely exist in free form in nature [29]; in milk, it is bound to lactose to form sialyllactose (SL) to more complex oligosaccharides or glycoproteins [30]. SL is the most abundant MOS in bovine milk, although its concentration is still lower than in human milk [31]. Accordingly, the SL concentration in bovine-milk-based infant formula is lower than that of human milk [32]. Fucosylated oligosaccharides predominate in human milk, such as fucosyllactose (FL) and HMOs, with more complex structures, whereas bovine milk contains very low fucosylated oligosaccharides [33]. Fucosylated glycans are implicated in neuronal processes that underpin neuronal development, learning and memory [34–37]. The composition of human milk differs by secretor genotypes, where secretor mothers have a functional *FUT2* gene that produces α1,2-fucosylated compounds, with 2′-FL being the most abundant [38]. However, preclinical studies suggested that intact 2′-FL does not cross the blood-brain barrier, although cleaved fucose or other gut microbial 2′-FL metabolites may be incorporated into the brain [39,40]. Thus, this raises the question of whether the effects of MOS were mediated directly via the incorporations of MOS components in the brain or indirectly via the mediation of microbiota and gut-brain axis.

The goals of this review are to critically appraise the current evidence from preclinical and human studies relating to MOS and neurocognitive outcomes, discuss potential mechanisms of action, identify key knowledge gaps, and highlight areas for future research. Although others have reviewed HMOS's role in infant cognitive development, they focused on interventions in animal models [41] or observational studies in human infants alone [42]. Since this field is rapidly evolving, we aim to synthesize and critically evaluate the current evidence on the role of MOS, both HMOs and bovine milk oligosaccharides (BMOS), in brain or cognitive development in early life.

2. Materials and Methods

2.1. Search Strategy

The literature search was performed in the PubMed database until April 2023. The search terms included * Infant(s), child, children, early childhood, toddler(s), early life, mice, mouse, murine, rat, rodent, piglet, monkey, animal, human milk oligosaccharide, HMO(s), bovine milk oligosaccharide, BMO(s), 2′-fucosyllactose, 3′-sialyllactose, 6′-sialyllactose, sialyllactose, sialylation, fucosylation, sialic acid, cognitive function, cognitive control, cognition, self-regulation, self-control, executive function, inhibition, inhibitory control, attention, fMRI, interference control, working memory, short-term memory, long-term memory, episodic memory, spatial memory, cognitive flexibility, task switching, social, emotion, temperament, negative affect, positive affect, mood, neural development, neural growth, neurogenesis, prefrontal cortex, dorsolateral prefrontal cortex, anterior cingulate cortex, cerebral cortex, hippocampus, amygdala, basal ganglia, striatum, brain, (gastro)intestinal microbiome, (gastro)intestinal microbiota, (gastro)intestinal microbes, gut microbiome, gut microbiota, gut microbes, fecal microbiome, fecal microbiota, fecal microbes, metagenome(s), metabolome(s), metabolite(s), short-chain-fatty acid(s), and volatile fatty acid(s).

2.2. Selection Criteria

To be included in the review, studies need to be related to MOS exposure in early life, any aspects of cognitive development, and were either interventions were conducted in animal models or observational studies in human subjects. Search terms related to gut microbiome were also included in the search strategy to identify potential studies about the gut-brain axis. Articles were excluded if there was no full version, no English version, or if it was conducted in adults. All articles were initially reviewed by two authors (YF and ALM) to determine inclusion in the review. In the case of disagreements, the third author (SMD) resolved the discrepancies.

2.3. Data Extraction

The data extracted included the authors, year of the publication, study location, experimental design, sample size, intervention, study duration, and relevance to brain and cognitive development, or the gut-brain axis.

3. Results

3.1. Study Selection

The PRISMA flow diagram [43] is shown in Figure 1. A total of 3474 articles were identified through the PubMed database. During screening by title and abstract, 3417 studies were outside the scope of our review and therefore excluded. In total, 57 studies underwent full-text review. An additional 31 articles were removed for not being relevant to MOS (n = 7), not relevant to early life (n = 5), and not related to cognition (n = 19). As a result, 26 publications met the inclusion criteria, reporting the associations between milk oligosaccharide exposure during the early developmental period and the brain or cognitive development of the offspring.

3.2. Study Characteristics

The characteristics of the 26 selected studies are presented in Tables 1 and 2. Most (69%) studies were intervention studies in animal models (n = 18) (Table 1), and the rest were observational studies involving human subjects (n = 8) (Table 2). The most common study interventions were milk oligosaccharide supplementation (n = 15) to either pig (n = 9) or rodent models (n = 6). There was a wide variety of methods used for the assessment of cognition and brain development. Magnetic resonance imaging (MRI), magnetic resonance spectroscopy (MRS), and Hippocampal gene expressions were the most common methods for investigating differences in brain structures between control and treatment groups.

Memory and learning in animal models are often accessed through observation of behaviors following a stimulus. The most common behavioral tests for cognitive function in the present review were novel object recognition (NOR), T-maze, and Y-maze. NOR refers to the evaluation of differences in the exploration time of the animal for novel and familiar objects [44,45]. The NOR task contains three phases: habituation, familiarization, and test phase. In habituation, the animals can freely explore an open-field arena without objects. For familiarization, a single animal will be introduced to two identical sample objects in the open field. Lastly, during the test phase, the animals will be returned to the open-field arena, where they encounter a sample project identical to the previous one and a novel one [44].

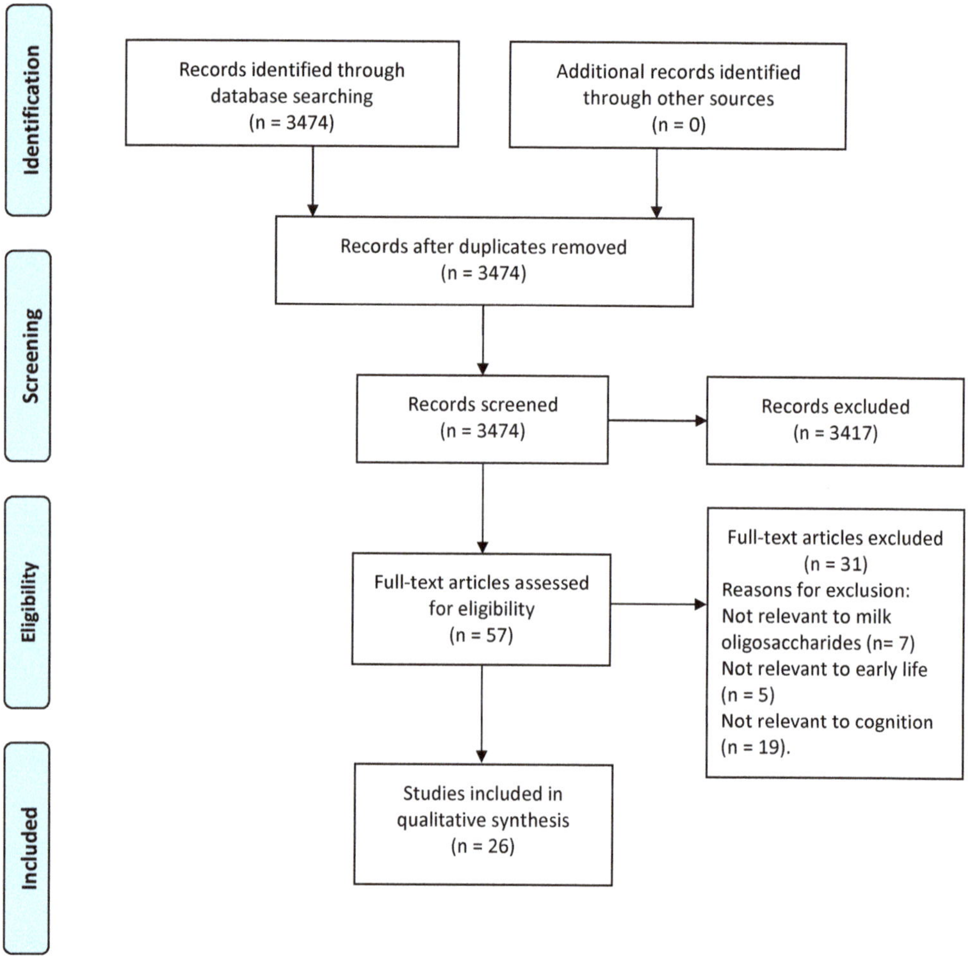

Figure 1. PRISMA flow diagram for the study selection process.

Because there is no reward involved in NOR, animals explore novel objects based on their natural preferences [44]. The increased time spent exploring novel objects reflects greater cognitive skills from the animal subjects [46], and it has been suggested that the dorsal hippocampus plays a vital role in NOR memory formation [47].

T-maze and Y-maze Spontaneous Alternative tests are two similar assessment tools for spatial working and reference memory, the only difference being the shape of the apparatus (Y versus T-shaped apparatus) [48]. Both mazes are based on the natural tendency of animals for preference to explore a novel arm compared to a familiar arm [49]. T-maze and Y-maze assess habit learning and short-term habituation in a novel environment [49,50].

Table 1. Characteristics of intervention studies in preclinical animal models.

Ref.	First Author and Year	Country	Subjects	Sample Size (*n*)	Study Duration	Intervention or Exposure
[51]	Tarr, 2015	US	Mice; male C57/BL6	54	Upon arrival for 20 days	Diets: • CON: AIN-93G semi-purified laboratory mouse diet • 6′-SL: CON + 5% 6′-SL • 3′-SL: CON + 5% 3′-SL Groups: • Stress (with social disruption stressor) • Non-stress
[52]	Jacobi, 2016	US	Pigs	54	21 days	Diets: • CON: formula adjusted for nutrient requirements of neonatal pigs • CON +2 g 3′-SL/L • CON +4 g 3′-SL/L • CON +2 g 6′-SL/L • CON +4 g 6′-SL/L • CON +2 g PDX/L + 2 g GOS/L
[53]	Oliveros, 2016	Spain	Rat pups; Lister Hooded & Sprague-Dawley	60 (Lister Hooded) & 60 (Sprague-Dawley)	PND 3 until weaning	Diets: • Control: BF + 1 g/kg body weight of water • 2′-FL: BF + 1 g/kg body weight of 2′-FL per day
[54]	Mudd, 2017	US	Pigs; vaginally delivered male	38	PND 2 until PND 32 or 33	Diets: • Control (CON): formula for nutritional needs of growing pigs • LOW: CON + bovine-derived modified why enriched with SL(SAL-10) (130 mg SL/L) • MOD: CON + SAL-10 (380 mg SL/L) • HIGH: CON + SAL-10 (760 mg SL/L)
[55]	Oliveros, 2018	Spain	Rats; Sprague-Dawley	30	PND 3 until weaning (PND 22)	Diets: • CON: BF + water • Neu5AC: BF + free Neu5AC to SA level in rat milk • 6′-SL: BF + free 6′-SL to mimic natural SA in rat milk
[56]	Fleming, 2018	US	Pigs; naturally farrowed male	36	PND 2 until PND 22	Diets: • CON: formula for nutritional needs of growing pigs • Sialyllactose: CON + SAL-10 (380 mg SL/L)
[57]	Obelitz-Ryom, 2019	Denmark	Piglets; male & female	40 (preterm), 14 (term, C-section), 12 (term, vaginal)	PND 0 until PND19	Diets: • PRE-CON: Raw bovine milk + 6 g/L lactose • PRE-SAL: Raw bovine milk + 8.5 g/L SAL-10 (380 mg SL/L) • TERM-CON: Raw bovine milk + 6 g/L lactose • TERM-NAT: Naturally BF

Table 1. *Cont.*

Ref.	First Author and Year	Country	Subjects	Sample Size (*n*)	Study Duration	Intervention or Exposure
[58]	Wang, 2019	Australia	Piglets; domestic *Sus scrofa*	46	PND 3 until PND 38	Diets: • CON: sow milk replacer • SL: Control + 3′-SL (7.6 g/kg) and 6′-SL (1.9 g/kg) • SL/SLN: Control + 3′-SL (7.04 g/kg), 6′-SL (1.74 g/kg), and 6′-sialyllactosamine (0.72 g/kg)
[59]	Lee, 2020	US	Mice; C57/BL6 male	36	Six weeks of age until 12 weeks	Diets: • LF: 10% kcal as fat diet • HF: 45% kcal as fat diet • HF 1% 2′-FL: HF + 98.4% purity 2′-FL 1% (*w/v*) • HF 2% 2′-FL: HF + 98.4% purity 2′-FL 2% (*w/v*) • HF 5% 2′-FL: HF + 98.4% purity 2′-FL 5% (*w/v*) • HF 10% 2′-FL: HF + 98.4% purity 2′-FL 10% (*w/v*)
[60]	Fleming, 2020	US	Pigs; male	36	PND 2 until PND 33	Diets: • CON: milk replacer • OF: CON + 5 g/L Oligofructose (OF) + 0 g/L 2′-FL • OF+2′-FL: CON + 5 g/L OF + 1 g/L 2′-FL
[61]	Fleming, 2020	US	Pigs; male	48	PND 2 until PND 33	Diets: • CON: sow milk replacer • BMOS [1]: CON + 12.4 g/L BMOS • HMO: CON + 1.0 g/L of 2′-FL + 0.5 g/L of LNnT • BMOS + HMO: CON + 12.4 g/L of BMOS + 1.0 g/L of 2′-FL + 0.5 g/L of LNnT
[62]	Tuplin, 2021	Canada	Rats; Sprague-Dawley both sex	40	PND 1 for Eight weeks	Diets: • CON: AIN-93G nutritionally complete diet • 3′-SL: CON + 0.625% wt/wt 3′-SL • 2′-FL: CON + 0.625% wt/wt 2′-FL • 3′-SL+2′-FL: CON + 0.625% wt/wt 3′-SL + 0.625% wt/wt 2′-FL
[63]	Pisa, 2021	Italy	Mice; male	28	PND 0 until 23 weeks	Genotypes: • WT: wild type • KO: knock-out for the gene synthesizing 3′-SL Diets: • CTRL: WT offspring with 3′-SL in milk • MILK: WT offspring with reduced 3′-SL in milk • GENE: KO offspring with 3′-SL in milk • GENE + MILK: KO offspring with reduced 3′-SL in milk

Table 1. *Cont.*

Ref.	First Author and Year	Country	Subjects	Sample Size (*n*)	Study Duration	Intervention or Exposure
[64]	Hauser, 2021	Italy	Mice; male	146	PND 0 until 25 weeks	Genotypes: • WT: wild type • KO: knock-out for the gene synthesizing 6′-SL Diets: • CTRL: WT offspring with 6′-SL in milk • MILK: WT offspring without 6′-SL in milk • GENE: KO offspring with 6′-SL in milk • GENE + MILK: KO offspring without 6′-SL in milk
[65]	Clouard, 2021	Denmark	Göttingen minipigs; female	64	Two weeks until 45 weeks	Diets: • Sow-reared: fed porcine milk until weaning. • Formula-fed: formula diets until weaning: • CON: Milk replacer with no additional oligosaccharides • FN: CON + 4 g/L mixture of fucosylated (2′-FL + di-FL) and neutral (LNT + LNnT) oligosaccharides • SL: CON + 0.68 g/L sialylated oligosaccharides (3′-SL + 6′-SL) • FN + SL: CON + 4 g/L FN + SL • After weaning to a high-energy, pelleted, obesogenic diet.
[66]	Lee, 2021	US	Mice; C57BL/6J male	32	Six weeks until 14 weeks	Diets: • LF/CON: 10% kcal as fat diet • HF/CON: 45% kcal as fat diet • LF/2′-FL: LF/CON + 10% 2′-FL (*w/w*) • HF/2′-FL: HF/CON + 10% 2′-FL (*w/w*)
[67]	Sutkus, 2022	US	Pigs; male	52	PND 2 until PND 34 or 35	Diets: • CON: Milk replacer supplemented with 0.532% lactose • FL: Con + 0.532% 2′-FL • BI: Con + 109 CFU/pig/d Bi-26 • FLBI: FL + BI

Table 1. *Cont.*

Ref.	First Author and Year	Country	Subjects	Sample Size (*n*)	Study Duration	Intervention or Exposure
[68]	Pisa, 2023	Italy	Mice; both sex	46 (Expt 1) 48 (Expt 2)	PND 0 until 25 weeks	Genotype: • WT: wild type • dKO: double-knock-out for the genes synthesizing 3′-SL and 6′-SL Diets—Experiment 1: • CTRL: WT offspring with WT BF • MILK: WT offspring with dKO BF • GENE: dKO offspring with WT BF • GENE + MILK: KO offspring with dKO BF Diets—Experiment 2: • CTRL-H_2O: WT offspring with WT BF + water • MILK-H_2O: WT offspring with dKO BF + water • CTRL-SL: WT offspring with WT BF + 3′SL and 6′SL • MILK-SL: WT offspring with dKO BF + 3′SL and 6′SL

[1] BMOS: Milk oligosaccharides derived from bovine whey, composed of primarily GOS + trace amount of 3′-SL and 6′-SL. Abbreviations: CON, control; PND, postnatal day; BF, breastfeeding; SA, sialic acid; LNT, Lacto-N-tetraose; LNnT, Lacto-N-neotetraose.

Table 2. Characteristics of human infant observational studies.

Ref.	First Author and Year	Country	Subjects	Sample Size	Study Duration	Exposure
[69]	Berger, 2020	US	Hispanic mother-term infant dyads (males and females)	50	• Milk collection at 1- and 6-months postpartum • Cognition assessment at 24 months of age	19 HMO concentrations
[70]	Cho, 2021	US	Mother-term infant dyads (males and females)	99	• Milk collection at study visit (infant at 2–25 months-old) • Cognition assessment at study visit	Eight HMO concentrations
[71]	Oliveros, 2021	Spain	Normal weight, overweight, obese, and GDM mother-term infant dyads (males and females)	82	• Milk collection at 1-month postpartum • Cognition assessment at 6 and 18 months-of-age	Two HMO concentrations

Table 2. *Cont.*

Ref.	First Author and Year	Country	Subjects	Sample Size	Study Duration	Exposure
[72]	Jorgensen, 2021	Malawi	Mother-term infant dyads (males and females)	659	• Milk collection at 6-months postpartum • Cognition assessment at 12 and 18 months-of-age	51 HMO relative abundances
[73]	Ferreira, 2021	Brazil	Mother-term infant dyads (males and females)	73	• Milk collection at 1-month postpartum • Cognition assessment at 1, 6, and 12 months-of-age	19 HMO concentrations
[74]	Rozé, 2022	France	Mother-preterm infants dyads (males and females)	137	• Milk collection for seven weeks from birth • Cognition assessment at two years of age	24 HMO and total sialic acid concentrations for mean impute values over samples from 7 weeks
[75]	Berger, 2022	US	Mother-term infant dyads (males and females)	20	• Milk collection at one month postpartum • MRI scanning at one month postpartum for infants	19 HMO concentrations
[76]	Willemsen, 2023	The Netherlands	Mother-term infant dyads (males and females)	63	• Milk collection at 2, 6 and 12 weeks postpartum • Cognition assessment at three years of age	24 HMO concentrations

Abbreviations: HMO, human milk oligosaccharides; GDM, gestational diabetes mellitus; MRI: magnetic resonance imaging.

3.3. *Sialyllactose and Cognition*

3.3.1. Term and Preterm Piglet Models

Six studies conducted intervention trials in piglets, analyzing the relationships between the milk oligosaccharide or SL intake on brain and/or cognitive developmental outcomes (Table 3). HMOS have been associated with increased SA delivery to the brain during development [27,77]. Among the sialylated HMOS, SL supplementation was most commonly investigated [31]. The most abundant SL are 6′-SL and 3′-SL [32], which are constitutional isomers sialylated by either α-(2,3) linkage(3′-SL) or α-(2,6) linkage(6′-SL); these two structures were reported to have similar biological functions [78].

Table 3. Sialyllactose and cognitive outcomes in preterm and term pigs.

Gestation	Diet	Analyses	Outcome	Ref.
Preterm piglets; 90% gestation (day 106) & Term piglets; C-section & Term piglets; Vaginally delivered	• PRE-CON: Raw BM + 6g/L lactose • PRE-SAL: Raw BM + 8.5 g/L SAL-10 (380 mg SL/L) • TERM-CON: Raw BM + 6 g/L lactose • TERM-NAT: Naturally BF	• Motor acquisition • Home cage activity • Open filed assessment • Spatial T-maze • Right cerebral hemisphere MRI • Hippocampal gangliosides SA quantification • qPCR hippocampal gene expression • In vitro computer-assisted fluorescence microscopy with H_2O_2 challenge for neuronal survival analysis	• PRE-SAL group had a higher ($p < 0.05$) percentage of pigs reaching the learning criteria of T-maze compared to PRE-CON pigs. • PRE-CON group spent a longer time ($p < 0.01$) on decision-making compared to TERM-CON pigs. • Hippocampal SA did not differ ($p > 0.05$) between PRE-CON and PRE-SAL pigs. • Hippocampal genes associated with myelination ($p < 0.05$) and SA metabolism ($p < 0.05$) were upregulated in PRE-SAL groups compared to PRE-CON pigs. • In vitro SAL and lactose treatment reduced cell death and promoted neuronal survival compared to control neurons ($p < 0.05$).	[57]
Term pigs; PND2	• CON: formula for nutritional needs of growing pigs • SAL: CON + SAL-10 (380 mg SL/L)	• NOR for object recognition memory • Accelerometers for home-cage activity analysis	• No difference in recognition memory was found between SAL and CON (all $p \geq 0.11$). • No difference in diurnal activity between SAL and CON (all $p \geq 0.56$)	[56]
Term pigs; PND2	• CON: formula for nutritional needs of growing pigs • LOW: CON + bovine-derived modified why enriched with SL(SAL-10) (130 mg SL/L) • MOD: CON + SAL-10 (380 mg SL/L) • HIGH: CON + SAL-10 (760 mg SL/L)	• Right hemisphere SA quantification (hippocampus, cerebellum, and prefrontal cortex) • Whole brain structural MRI • Whole brain MRS for brain metabolite quantification • DTI for white matter maturation and axonal tract integrity • Fractional anisotropy (FA) • Axial diffusivity (AD) • Mean diffusivity (MD) • Radial diffusivity (RD)	• No differences in total and free SA between treatments ($p > 0.05$). • Bound SA in the prefrontal cortex was higher in CON and HIGH groups compared to LOW and MOD groups ($p = 0.05$). • Free SA-to-bound SA in the hippocampus was higher in the MOD and LOW groups compared to the CON and HIGH groups ($p = 0.04$). • Corpus callosum MD ($p < 0.01$) and AD ($p < 0.01$) were higher in the MOD group compared to other groups.	[54]
Term pigs; PND3	• CON: SMR • SL: CON + 3′-SL (7.6 g/kg) and 6′-SL (1.9 g/kg) • SL/SLN: CON + 3′-SL (7.04 g/kg), 6′-SL (1.74 g/kg), and 6′-sialyllactosamine (0.72 g/kg)	• 3T MRS for brain neurotransmitter and metabolites concentrations (Whole brain, cerebrum, and cerebellum)	• SL/SLN increased ($p < 0.05$) absolute and relative amounts of myo-inositol (mlns) and glutamate + glutamine (Glx) • Positive correlations between 3′-SL and SLN intake and brain metabolite Glu ($p = 0.017$), mlns ($p = 0.013$) and Glx ($p = 0.032$) levels in SL and SL/SLN groups	[58]

Table 3. *Cont.*

Gestation	Diet	Analyses	Outcome	Ref.
Term Göttingen minipigs; 2 weeks old	• CON: Milk replacer with no additional oligosaccharides • FN: CON + 4 g/L mixture of fucosylated (2′-FL+di-FL) and neutral (LNT + LNnT) oligosaccharides • SL: CON + 0.68 g/L sialylated (3′-SL + 6′-SL) oligosaccharides • FN + SL: CON+ 4 g/L FN + SL • After weaning: high-energy, pelleted, obesogenic diet for all groups	• Behavioral procedure tasks • Spatial hole board • Open field • Novel object exposure • Runway • Single-feed test for appetite measurement • Home pen behavior observation	• SL group improved reference memory ($p \leq 0.010$) between 16 to 29 weeks compared to CON. • FN, SL, and FN+SL had longer trial durations ($p < 0.05$) compared to CON, between 16 to 29 weeks and 39–45 weeks. • FN group spent the most time displaying ingestive behaviors between 0 to 11 weeks ($p < 0.05$)	[65]
Term pigs; PND1	• CON: formula adjusted for nutrient requirements of neonatal pigs • CON + 2 g 3′-SL/L • CON + 4 g 3′-SL/L • CON + 2 g 6′-SL/L • CON + 4 g 6′-SL/L • CON + 2 g PDX/L + 2 g GOS/L	• Left hemisphere SA analysis (cerebral cortex, cerebellum, corpus callosum, and hippocampus) • Microbiota quantification	• 2 g 3′-SL and 6′-SL/L increased ($p \leq 0.05$) total SA concentration in the corpus callosum by 15% compared to CON • 4 g 3′-SL increased ($p \leq 0.05$) total and ganglioside SA concentration in the cerebellum by 10% compared to CON • Quadratic effect of dose for 3′-SL and 6′-SL in total and ganglioside-bound SA ($p \leq 0.05$) • Significant differences between proximal ($p = 0.001$) and distal colon ($p = 0.009$) microbiota of piglets fed the 4 g 6′-SL/L and CON • Significant differences between proximal ($p = 0.006$) and distal colon ($p = 0.032$) microbiota of piglets fed the 2 g PDX/L + 2 g GOS/L and CON	[52]

Abbreviations: BM, bovine milk; BMO, bovine milk oligosaccharide; BF, breastfeeding; DTI, diffusion tensor imaging; FN, fucosylated and neutral oligosaccharides; GOS, galactooligosaccharides; MRI, magnetic resonance imaging; MRS, magnetic resonance spectroscopy; PDX, polydextrose; SL, sialyllatose; SA, sialic acid; SMR, sow milk replacer.

Piglets are widely used as a preclinical model for human gut-brain-axis studies [79] due to their similarities with human gastrointestinal physiology [80] and brain development [81]. Only one study utilized preterm piglets to study the influence of dietary SL on cognition, finding that preterm piglets supplemented with SL were more likely to succeed in the learning criteria than the control group [57]. Although supplementation with SL did not directly affect the SA levels in the hippocampus of the preterm piglets, SL supplementation resulted in the up-regulation of the myelination-responsible genes, myelin-associated glycoprotein, myelin basic protein, and genes related to SA metabolism. However, the selected genes involved in memory formation and learning processes were not modified by SL enrichment [57].

Due to the lack of pure forms of synthesized SL, some previous studies have administered a bovine milk extract enriched in 3′-SL and 6′-SL (SAL) (43,45). For instance, in male term piglets, SAL was supplemented in varying amounts: control (55 mg SL/L), low (159 mg SL/L), moderate (429 mg SL/L), or high (779 mg SL/L) from postnatal day 2 through 32 or 33 [54]. The moderate SAL concentration group was selected to represent a concentration similar to human milk [54]. Higher levels of bound SA were found in the prefrontal cortex of the control and high groups compared to the low and moderate groups. Additionally, the moderate group showed a higher ratio of free-to-bound SA in the hippocampus than the control and high-concentration groups. As for brain structures, white matter maturation and the level of axonal tract integrity were measured with diffusion tensor imaging. Increased measures of corpus callosum mean diffusivity (MD), axial diffusivity (AD), and radial diffusivity (RD) were observed in the group with moderate SL supplementation compared to other levels of SAL supplementations and control [54]. Tract-based spatial statistics (TBSS) analysis revealed that the moderate SL group showed higher RD measures in the white matter of the left corpus callosum compared to the low SL group. This study suggests that the effects of SL supplementation are dose-dependent and specific to brain regions, including the corpus callosum, prefrontal cortex, and hippocampus [54].

Piglets receiving the SAL concentration comparable to human milk concentrations exhibited better effects on brain structural development. Similarly, Jacobi et al. compared the different SL isomer supplementation on full-term pigs from day 1 to 21 days. The left hemispheres of the pigs were divided into four regions, and their sialic acid concentrations were measured. The total incorporation of ganglioside-bound SA in the corpus callosum was higher for pigs supplemented with 3′-SL and 6′-SL than the control diet group. Ganglioside-bound SA was also increased in the cerebellum for supplementation with 3′-SL [52]. The corpus callosum is the largest white matter structure in the brain, containing diverse intra- and interhemispheric myelinated axonal projections [52,82]. The impact of dietary SL on the amount of ganglioside-bound SA in the corpus callosum suggests SL may play a role in supporting axonal myelination.

To investigate the effects of sialylated HMO on brain development, another piglet study explored the effects of supplementation of pure 3′-SL and 6′-SL or combined supplementation of pure forms of 3′-SL, 6′-SL, and 6′-sialyl-lactosamine (SLN) compared to a control group. At postnatal day 38, absolute concentrations of 33 brain metabolites were measured, and results showed that sialylated HMO supplementation significantly increased several important brain metabolites and neurotransmitters compared to the control group [58]. For example, with the combination of SL and SLN, the absolute and relative levels of glutamate were significantly increased ($p < 0.05$) compared to control. Thus, this study provides evidence that orally administered sialylated HMOS up-regulated brain levels of glutamate (Glu), which is one of the major excitatory neurotransmitters in the brain that has been suggested to support brain development such as influencing neurite sprouting, synaptogenesis and dendrite pruning [58].

Several studies investigated behavioral outcomes in piglets administered HMOS as measures of cognitive development. Fleming et al. reported that supplementation of SL to term male pigs (n = 38) did not affect exploratory behaviors, including time spent investigating objects, the number of object visits, or the mean time spent per object visit [56]. Clouard et al. [65] was the only study to compare the effects of sialylated, neutral, and fucosylated HMOS on cognitive outcomes. Dietary treatment of female Göttingen minipigs with HMOS between 2 and 11 weeks of age resulted in significant improvement in behavioral tasks as indicated by spending longer time in the trials compared to the control group. Also, reference memory was increased with SL supplementation compared to control [65]. However, the significant beneficial effects of dietary HMOS were time-dependent, where working and reference memory scores were found to be greater with SL treatment between 16–29 weeks of age (after HMOS treatment had ended) but not at 39–45 weeks. This period (between 16–29 weeks) is the time between weaning and sexual maturity, sometimes referred to as the adolescence age. The time-dependent effects observed in the study raise intriguing questions about the underlying mechanisms of HMOS and their interaction with neural circuits during critical periods of development.

The findings also imply that the benefits of HMOS supplementation might have the most pronounced effects during the adolescent period.

3.3.2. Rodent Models

Four studies used young mice to investigate the effects of sialylated milk oligosaccharide exposure in early life on cognitive outcomes (Table 4). Oliveros et al. used Sprague-Dawley rats (n = 47) to assess the impact of sialic acid and sialylated oligosaccharides supplementation from birth to postnatal day three on learning and memory outcomes. In the NOR test that evaluates the time rats explored a novel object compared to a familiar object, rats that received sialic acid supplementation in the form of both SA and 6′-SL spent more time exploring the novel object, demonstrating better cognitive abilities [55]. Long-term potentiation (LTP) for signal transmission between neurons, Y maze test and IntelliCage® Protocol test (an automated testing system for spontaneous and learning behavior of rodents) performance at one year were significantly improved with both Neu5Ac and 6′-SL supplementations during lactation [55].

Table 4. Sialyllactose and cognitive outcomes in rodent models.

Gestation	Diet	Analysis	Outcome	Ref.
Mice; PND 0	Genotyping • WT: wild type • KO: knock-out for the gene synthesizing 3′-SL Diets • CTRL: WT offspring with 3′-SL in milk • MILK: WT offspring with reduced 3′-SL in milk • GENE: KO offspring with 3′-SL in milk • GENE + MILK: KO offspring with reduced 3′-SL in milk	• NOR • T-maze Spontaneous Alternation Test • Elevated 0-maze for anxiety-relate behavior. • Pre-pulse inhibition • Barnes maze • Attentional set-shifting task • Sucrose preference • General locomotion • Glucose tolerance test • Electrophysiology Experiments	• MILK (p = 0.025), GENE (p < 0.05), and GENE+MILK (p < 0.05) mice had decreased spatial memory compared to CTRL mice • MILK mice had reduced (p < 0.05) attention and higher response to glucose injection compared to other groups • MILK mice had reduced (p = 0.03) number of spontaneous alternations compared to CTRL • MILK mice had reduced (p < 0.05) recognition memory compared to CTRL and GENE + MILK • LTP was lower in GENE + MILK (p < 0.05) and CTRL (p < 0.05) mice compared to GENE • LTP was lower (p < 0.05) in GENE + MILK mice compared to MILK	[63]
Mice; 6–8 weeks old	• CON: AIN-93G semi-purified laboratory mouse diet • 6′-SL: CON + 5% 6′-SL • 3′-SL: CON + 5% 3′-SL	• Social disruption stressor (SDR)-induced anxiety-like behavior assessment. • Open field and Light/Dark preference test • ELISA for serum corticosterone • Microbiota sequencing • Brain cell proliferation and immature neuronal assessment	• CON mice had higher (p < 0.05) microbiota Shannon Diversity Index compared to 6′-SL mice • 6′-SL and 3′-SL mice had altered microbial beta-diversity compared to CON mice (p < 0.01) • 6′-SL and 3′-SL mice resulted in significant taxonomic shifts at phylum and genus levels (p < 0.05) • SDR changed microbial beta-diversity in CON mice (p < 0.05) • SDR did not induce shifts in microbial beta-diversity in 6′-SL (p = 0.138) and 3′-SL (p = 0.077) mice • 6′-SL and 3′-SL mice spend less time in dark zone compared to CON mice under SDR (p < 0.05) • 6′-SL mice significantly decreased proliferation within the hippocampus compared to CON regardless of SDR (all p < 0.05) • 6′-SL and 3′-SL mice rescued reduction of immature neurons induced by SDR compared to CON (all p < 0.05)	[51]

Table 4. *Cont.*

Gestation	Diet	Analysis	Outcome	Ref.
Mice; PND 0	Genotyping • WT: wild type • KO: knock-out for the gene synthesizing 6′-SL Diets • CTRL: WT offspring with 6′-SL in milk • MILK: WT offspring without 6′-SL in milk • GENE: KO offspring with 6′-SL in milk • GENE + MILK: KO offspring without 6′-SL in milk	• Maternal behavior assessment • Fox scale for Neurodevelopmental milestones • NOR • T-maze test • PPI • Barnes maze • General locomotion • Attentional set-shifting task for executive functions • Electrophysiology experiments for LTP assessment • Gene expression analyses • Metabolomics • Microbiota analyses • Brain Neu5Ac quantification	• MILK and GENE + MILK mice increased ($p = 0.015$) general locomotion in adulthood • Only CTRL mice showed a preference for novel objects in the NOR test. • MILK mice had impaired spatial memory retention compared to CTRL mice ($p = 0.02$) • MILK mice required more trials for the CD phase compared to CTRL ($p = 0.0218$) and GENE ($p = 0.0041$) • GENE + MILK mice required more trials for the CD phase compared to GENE ($p = 0.023$) • MILK mice required more trials for the IDS phase compared to CTRL ($p = 0.003$) and GENE ($p = 0.017$) • MILK mice required more trials for the EDS phase compared to CTRL ($p = 0.008$), GENE ($p = 0.0005$), and GENE+MILK ($p = 0.006$). • CTRL and GENE mice showed PPI, but MILK and GENE + MILK mice failed to exhibit PPI • MILK mice had increased LTP compared to CTRL mice ($p = 0.04$) • At eye-opening, MILK mice had a downregulation of 53 genes involved in neuronal circuits formation and patterning compared to CTRL	[64]
Rats; PND 3	• CON: BF + water • Neu5AC: BF + free Neu5AC to mimic natural Sia level in rat milk • 6′-SL: BF + free 6′-SL to mimic natural Sia level in rat milk	• HPLC for SA content determination • Western blotting • In vivo LTP measurement • Classical behavioral tests • NOR • Y maze with blocked arm • IntelliCage® Protocol for spontaneous and learning behavior	• 6′-SL rats showed more PSA-NCAM in the frontal cortex at weaning compared to Neu5AC ($p = 0.012$) and CON ($p = 0.042$) • 6′-SL rats had improved LTP in male rats at one year compared to CTRL ($p \leq 0.05$) • 6′-SL ($p = 0.0352$) and Neu5Ac ($p = 0.0304$) rats displayed longer exploration time in NOR at one year • Higher percentage of 6′-SL ($p < 0.0001$) and Neu5AC ($p = 0.0004$) rats chose novel arm in the Y maze compared to CON • A higher percentage of 6′-SL ($p = 0.0279$) rats chose novel arm in the Y maze compared to Neu5AC rats • Higher percentage of 6′-SL ($p = 0.0483$) and Neu5AC ($p = 0.0237$) rats had better performance in IntelliCage® test	[55]

Table 4. *Cont.*

Gestation	Diet	Analysis	Outcome	Ref.
Mice; PND 0	Genotyping • WT: wild type • dKO: double-knock-out for milk reduced in 3′-SL and without 6′-SL Diets—Experiment 1 • CTRL: WT offspring with WT BF • MILK: WT offspring with dKO BF • GENE: dKO offspring with WT BF • GENE + MILK: KO offspring with dKO BF Diets—Experiment 2 • CTRL-H2O: WT offspring with WT BF+water • MILK-H2O: WT offspring with dKO BF + water • CTRL-SL: WT offspring with WT BF + 3′SL–6′SL solution • MILK-SL: WT offspring with dKO BF + 3′SL–6′SL solution	• NOR • T-maze • Bernes maze • PPI • Attentional set-shifting task • Glucose tolerance test	Experiment 1: • MILK and GENE + MILK groups showed reduced spontaneous alternation in T-maze compared to CTRL and GENE milk ($p = 0.005$) • All groups except for the MILK group showed significant preference ($p = 0.015$) • All groups showed reduced long-term spatial memory in the Bernes maze compared to CTRL ($p = 0.01$) • CTRL and GENE groups showed intact PPI, while MILK and GENE + MILK groups failed to • MILK subjects need more trials in the SD and CD phases of the attentional set-shifting task compared to CTRL ($p < 0.05$) Experiment 2: • No differences were observed for all behavioral tests between treatment groups.	[68]

Abbreviations: WT, wildtype; KO, knockout; dKO, double-knockout; CON, control; PND, postnatal day; SDR, social disruption stressor; PPI, Prepulse inhibition; ELISA, Interleukin-6 Enzyme-Linked Immunosorbant Assay; SL, sialyllatose; SA, sialic acid; SMR, sow milk replacer; CD, compound discrimination; CDR, compound discrimination reversal; IDS, intra-dimensional shift; EDS, extra-dimensional shift; BF, breastfeeding; SD, simple discrimination; CD, compound discrimination.

Tarr et al. [51] explored the effects of HMO supplementation on the gut microbiota community to investigate the impact of HMO on the gut-brain axis. To assess the potential role of HMOS supplementation in reducing anxiety behaviors, a social disruption stressor was given to the experimental animals for all groups. Supplementations of 5% 3′-SL and 6′-SL supported the maintenance of both normal behaviors and the number of immature neurons in the dentate gyrus under stress compared to the control group. Since it has been proven that immature neurons are important in anxiety-like behaviors and learning, the maintenance of the number of immature neurons by SL may explain the maintenance of normal behavior under stress. Additionally, the microbial community was not significantly affected by stressor exposure when 3′-SL and 6′-SL were supplied in the diet compared to the control group. These results suggest that MOS may support normal behavior under stress conditions by modulating gut microbiota and gut-brain signaling [51]. These findings contribute to the growing understanding of the complex interactions between the gut and the brain and highlight the potential role of HMOS in promoting mental well-being.

Instead of supplementing SL, three studies from the same laboratory used knock-out preclinical mice models to test the effects of sialylated MOS deficiencies [63,64,68]. The first study, Pisa et al. produced knockout (KO) dams that lack the gene that encodes α2,3-sialyltransferase for synthesizing 3′-SL in the mouse mammary gland, achieving around an 80% reduction in 3′-SL content in the milk provided to the pups [63]. Hauser et al., on the other hand, genetically engineered mice to lack the gene for synthesizing 6′-SL in the mammary gland, resulting in milk theoretically devoid of 6′-SL, but the levels in milk were not directly measured [64]. By cross-fostering wildtype (WT) pups to KO dams, the effect of consuming milk with reduced 3′-SL or 6′-SL diets during lactation was investigated in adulthood. The cognitive outcomes of the KO offspring reared in KO or WT dams were also evaluated to differentiate the effects of genetic deficiencies versus HMO reduction in milk [63]. Four groups were compared for behavioral outcomes: CTRL, WT offspring receiving WT milk; MILK, WT offspring receiving SL deficient milk; GENE, KO offspring receiving WT milk; and GENE + MILK, KO offspring receiving SL deficit milk [63]. WT pups that received milk with decreased 3′-SL showed a significant reduction in spatial memory, attention, NOR recognition memory, and altered hippocampal long-term potentiation compared to WT pups that received WT milk. In addition, the KO pups (both receiving WT milk and 3′-SL poor milk) exhibited impairment in spatial memory and general locomotion compared to CTRL mice. These results suggest that 3′-SL exposure in early life has long-term implications for cognitive functions [63].

Secondly, in the 6′-SL KO mouse model developed by Hauser et al. [64], the effects of 6′-SL deficiency were observed. After eye-opening, 53 genes involved in the formation and patterning of neuronal circuits were downregulated in WT and KO pups consuming 6′-SL deficient milk. Further, these mice had impaired recognition, sensorimotor gating, and LTP in adulthood, suggesting that the absence of SL during lactation may result in poorer cognitive function throughout life [64].

The third gene knock-out study from the same research group engineered double knock-out mice with deletion of genes synthesizing both 3′-SL and 6′-SL to investigate further the effects of reduced SL exposure on cognitive capabilities later in life [68]. As a secondary aim, they evaluated whether exogenous supplementation of 3′-SL and 6′-SL (compared to H_2O) would counteract the influences caused by the deficiencies in a second experiment. As expected, the concurrent deficiencies of 3′-SL and 6′-SL during lactation resulted in impairments in memory and attention functions, consistent with the previous two studies [63,64]. However, interestingly, in the second experiment, the researchers failed to reproduce the same phenotypic impairments in the WT pups receiving SL-poor milk (MILK group) and H_2O supplementation, as observed previously in the MILK group in their first experiment. Therefore, they were not able to conclude whether or not exogenous supplementation of MOS to mice that are receiving SL deficit milk would compensate for the observed neurocognitive deficits [68]. The researchers proposed that the failure to replicate these phenotypic impairments in the MILK group may have potentially resulted from the supplementation procedure introducing confounding in behavioral performances, warranting future studies.

Together, these studies in knock-out mice demonstrate the importance of exposure to milk-borne 3′-SL and 6′-SL during lactation for long-term cognitive and executive functioning in multiple domains, including spatial memory, recognition memory, attention, and synaptic plasticity.

3.4. *Fucosyllactose and Cognition*

3.4.1. Piglet Models

As noted above, 2′-FL is a predominant HMOS produced by secretor gene-positive mothers. 2′-FL contains fucose, a component of glycoconjugates in the brain [83], supporting a potential role for dietary 2′-FL in cognitive development. Three intervention trials explored the effects of 2′-FL supplementation on cognitive outcomes using piglet models (Table 5).

Table 5. Fucosylated milk oligosaccharides and cognitive outcomes in piglets.

Gestation	Diet	Test	Outcome	Ref.
Term pigs; PND 2	• CON: SMR supplemented with 0.532% lactose • FL: CON + 0.532% 2′-FL • BI: CON + 10^9 CFU/pig/d Bi-26 • FLBI: FL + BI	• NOR • Structural MRI • DTI	• FL resulted in a larger ($p = 0.046$) relative volume in the pons region • *B. infantis* Bi-26 resulted in smaller ($p < 0.05$) absolute volume in the corpus callosum, left and right internal capsules, left and right putamen-globus pallidus, left caudate, left cortex, lateral ventricles, and medulla; and smaller ($p < 0.03$) relative volume of the left and right putamen-globus pallidus. • No effects of FL and Bi-26 on novel recognition memory • FL group had a greater ($p < 0.05$) number of familiar object visits in NOR than in CON. • BI and FLBI groups spent less ($p = 0.002$) time investigating familiar object	[67]
Term pigs; PND 2	• CON: SMR • OF: Control + 5 g/L Oligofructose (OF) + 0 g/L 2′-FL • OF + 2′-FL: Control + 5 g/L OF + 1 g/L 2′-FL	• NOR • Structural MRI • DTI • MRS • Hippocampal gene expression	• CON failed to show recognition memory after a 1 or 48 h delay. • OF showed recognition memory only after 1 h delay ($p < 0.001$) • OF + 2′-FL showed recognition memory only after 48 h delay ($p = 0.001$) • OF showed higher ($p = 0.022$) novel object visit frequency than CON after 1 h delay • OF + 2′-FL had increased ($p = 0.038$) sample object exploration time through trial compared to CON • OF and OF + 2′-FL had increased ($p = 0.019$) olfactory bulbs relative volume compared to CON • OF showed lower hippocampal mRNA expression of DRD3, GABBR1, HDAC5/8, NCAM1, and CHRM2 (all $p < 0.045$) compared to CON • OF + 2′-FL had higher hippocampal mRNA expression of DRD3, GABBR1, HDAC5, and NCAM1 (all $p < 0.045$) compared to CON	[60]
Term pigs, PND 2	• CON: SMR • BMOS: CON + 12.4 g/L BMOS • HMO: CON + 1.0 g/L of 2′-FL + 0.5 g/L of LNnT • BMOS + HMO: CON + 12.4 g/L of BMOS + 1.0 g/L of 2′-FL + 0.5 g/L of LNnT	• NOR • Structural MRI • DTI • MRS • Hippocampal gene expression	• HMO showed recognition memory after a 1-h delay ($p = 0.038$) • BMOS + HMO showed recognition memory after 48-h delay ($p = 0.045$) • CON and BMOS + HMO showed similar absolute and relative volumes of caudate, lateral ventricles and pons as HMO and BMOS • HMO and BMOS+HMO had larger relative cortices and corpus callosum compared to BMOS (all $p < 0.05$) • HMO and BMOS downregulated many genes in the hippocampus, whereas BMOS + HMO upregulated many of the same genes	[61]

Abbreviations: CON, control; SMR, sow milk replacer; NOR, novel object recognition; MRI, magnetic resonance imaging; DTI, diffusion tensor imaging; MRS, magnetic resonance spectroscopy; PDX, polydextrose; SL, sialyllatose; SA, sialic acid; SMR, sow milk replacer; DRD3, dopamine receptor D3; GABBR1, GABA type B receptor subunit 1; HDAC5/8, histone deacetylases 5 and 8; NCAM1, neural cell adhesion molecule 1; CHRM2, cholinergic receptor muscarinic 2.

All three studies used male pigs fed a commercial sow milk replacer as the control diet and the control diet, plus exogenous oligosaccharides for the experimental diets. Sutkus et al. compared the effects of a control diet to 2′-FL- and prebiotic *B. infantis* Bi-26-supplemented diets on the gut-brain axis [67], while Fleming et al. conducted one study that assessed the impact of dietary oligofructose (OF) in combination with 2′-FL on brain development [60], and another study that assessed the impact of HMOS (2′-FL + LNnT), BMOS, and their combination on behavioral outcomes and brain structures [61]. Dietary OF is a non-HMO oligosaccharide of vegetable origin, which has been reported to impact brain-derived neurotrophic factor expression. HMO and non-HMO oligosaccharide benefits for cognitive development were evaluated individually and in combination (OF + 2′-FL). BMOS, on the other hand, are bovine milk-derived oligosaccharides that are less complex in structures but are structurally identical to those found in HMOS, such as 3′-SL and 6′-SL [84]. Supplementation of BMOS to infant formula has been reported as safe and may rescue deficits in weight, height, and head circumference measurements observed in formula-fed infants compared to breastfed infants [84].

Both Sutkus et al. [67] and the two studies by Fleming et al. [60,61] utilized the NOR test to investigate the recognition and working memory of the pigs. These studies found that 2′-FL, OF, and BMOS influenced recognition memory, as shown by increased object visits. However, the type of OS supplementation yielded varying results on recognition memory. Specifically, OF alone increased recognition memory after a 1 h delay, while OF+2′-FL increased recognition memory after a 48 h delay [60]. On the other hand, BMO supplementations (BMOS alone and BMOS+HMO) showed a lesser increase in distance moved per minute during the habituation phase in the NOR task compared to pigs fed no BMOS. HMOS supplementation of 2′-FL and LNnT increased recognition memory after the 1 h delay, but only HMOS in combination with BMOS was associated with increased recognition memory after the 48-h delay. As for the control group, no recognition memory was displayed either after a 1 h or 48 h delay [61]. These results suggest that the combination of HMOS and other oligosaccharide supplementation may result in longer recognition memory retention.

These studies also explored the effects of MOS supplementation on brain structures, which were investigated using structural MRI. Sutkus et al. [67] observed an increase in relative volume in the pons region of the 2′-FL-supplemented pigs compared to the control. Fleming et al. [60], however, did not find significant alterations in the brain structures, but trending effects ($0.05 < p < 0.10$) on absolute volumes of several brain regions, including olfactory bulbs and thalamus, were found between diets. When looking at HMOS and BMOS and their effects on brain structures, the results suggested that all diet groups with HMOS supplementation displayed larger relative and absolute volumes of cortices and corpus callosum [61].

3.4.2. Rodent Models

Four studies orally administered 2′-FL during lactation to investigate relationships with cognitive development in rodent models. Unlike the studies conducted in piglet models, the studies conducted in rodent models did not perform brain imaging but did conduct behavioral assessments (Table 6).

Table 6. Fucosylated milk oligosaccharides and cognitive outcomes in rodents.

Gestation	Diet	Analysis	Outcome	Ref.
Rats; PND 3	• CON: BF + 1 g/kg body weight of water • 2′-FL group: BF + 1 g/kg body weight of 2′-FL per day	• In vivo LTP at six weeks in the hippocampus for Sprague-Dawley rats • In vivo LTP at 1 year for Lister Hooded rats • NOR • Y maze • MWM	• 2′-FL evoked larger LTP compared to CON ($p < 0.05$) at six weeks and one year • 2′-FL spent longer time exploring the novel object than the familiar object ($p = 0.03$) • 2′-FL spent longer time exploring objects compared to CON at 1 year ($p = 0.0475$) • 2′-FL showed lower latency to the novel arm in the Y maze compared to CON at one year ($p = 0.0331$) • 2′-FL had a higher percentage of rats that visited the novel arm as the first choice in the Y maze compared to CON at one year ($p = 0.0138$)	[53]
Rats; PND21	• CON: AIN-93G nutritionally complete diet • 3′-SL: Control + 0.625% wt/wt 3′-SL • 2′-FL: Control + 0.625% wt/wt 2′-FL • 3′-SL+2′-FL: Control + 0.625% wt/wt 3′-SL + 0.625% wt/wt 2′-FL	• RNA extraction and cDNA • qPCR • Protein extraction and quantification for NAc and VAT tissue • Western blot procedure	• 3′-SL + 2′-FL females had decreased VAT DAT expression ($p = 0.032$) compared to CON females • 3′-SL + 2′-FL females had increased NAc leptin expression ($p < 0.05$) compared to CON females • Male CON rats had lower DAT expression ($p = 0.039$) had higher GhrelinR ($p < 0.05$) and leptin ($p < 0.05$) expression than females • Male rats had lower NAc leptin expression ($p = 0.047$) than females	[62]
Mice; 6-week-old	• LF: 10% kcal as fat research diet • HF: 45% kcal as fat research diet • HF 1% 2′-FL: HF + 98.4% purity 2′-FL 1% (*w/v*) • HF 2% 2′-FL: HF + 98.4% purity 2′-FL 2% (*w/v*) • HF 5% 2′-FL: HF + 98.4% purity 2′-FL 5% (*w/v*) • HF 10% 2′-FL: HF + 98.4% purity 2′-FL 10% (*w/v*)	• CCK sensitivity assessment • OGTT • RNA extraction and quantitative RT-PCR • Immunofluorescence • Histology • Hepatic lipid accumulation assessment • Blood analysis for LPS-bind protein • Microbiota DNA sequencing • Metabolomic analysis	• 10% 2′-FL results in less weight gain ($p < 0.001$) with the HF diet compared to the HF • 10% 2′-FL decreased food intake ($p < 0.05$) compared to HF • 10% 2′-FL suppressed ($p < 0.01$) the increase in fat mass resulting from HF • 10% 2′-FL restored the CCK-induced inhibition of food intake for HF mice ($p < 0.05$) • 10% 2′-FL resulted in compositional changes in the microbiota ($p < 0.05$) and metabolites ($p < 0.05$) compared to LF and HF mice • 10% 2′-FL attenuates the HF-induced inflammation ($p < 0.05$) compared to HF • 10% 2′-FL decreased ($p < 0.05$) the upregulation of PPARγ gene expression induced by HF	[59]

Table 6. *Cont.*

Gestation	Diet	Analysis	Outcome	Ref.
Mice; 6-week-old	• LF/CON: 10% kcal as fat diet • HF/CON: 45% kcal as fat diet • LF/2′-FL: LF/CON + 10% 2′-FL (*w/w*) • HF/2′-FL: HF/CON + 10% 2′-FL (*w/w*)	• Y-maze • Open field test for general locomotion • NOR • OGTT • Barrier function assessment • RNA extraction and quantitative RT-PCR • Immunohistochemistry • Histology • Hepatic lipid accumulation • Microbiota DNA sequencing • 16S metagenomic analysis • Metabolomic analysis	• HF/2′-FL decreased energy intake ($p < 0.05$ at weeks 4–8) and fat mass ($p < 0.05$ at weeks 2,4,6,8) compared to HF • HF/2′-FL decreased ($p = 0.001$) the upregulation of PPARγ gene expression induced by HF • HF/2′-FL downregulated ($p < 0.001$) the SREBP-1c gene expression compared to LF/2′-FL • 2′-FL decreased the size of adipocytes in visceral adipose tissues compared to control for both LF ($p < 0.01$) and HF ($p < 0.05$) group • 2′-FL decreased intestinal transcellular permeability ($p < 0.01$) in HF group • 2′-FL decreased intestinal para- ($p < 0.05$) and transcellular ($p < 0.05$) permeability in the LF group • 2′-FL increased IL-22 gene expression that regulates epithelial homeostasis in the ileum for both LF ($p < 0.05$) and HF ($p < 0.05$) group • HF/2′-FL restored vagally-mediated gut-brain signaling integrity compared to the HF group ($p < 0.05$) • No detectable effects were found on any cognitive outcome. • 2′-FL had different gut microbiota beta diversity compared to LF and HF groups (both $p = 0.001$) • 2′-FL significantly shifted microbiota composition and cecal metabolites	[66]

Abbreviations: NOR; Novel Object Recognition; MWM, Morris Water Maze; DA, dopamine; DAT, dopamine transporter; RNA, messenger RNA; NAc, nucleus accumbens; TH, tyrosine hydroxylase; VTA, ventral tegmental area; OGTT, oral glucose tolerate test; PPARγ, peroxisome proliferator-activated receptor gamma.

Oliveros et al. supplemented 2′-FL to rats during lactation, finding that 2′-FL supplementation resulted in significantly increased performance in NOR, Y maze, and long-term potentiation in their offspring at one year old [53], suggesting the long-lasting effect of 2′-FL exposure in early life, which is consistent with previous supplementation effects of 3′-SL and 6′-SL in rodents. One study tested the effects of combined SL and FL supplementation on the mesolimbic dopamine system in rats. The results showed that the HMOS supplementation exerted sex-dependent effects; 3′-SL + 2′-FL fortification decreased dopamine transporter expression in the ventral tegmental area and increased leptin expression in the nucleus accumbens in females only [62]. This study not only highlighted the impact of HMOS supplementation on the dopamine system but suggested for the first time that variations in response to the HMOS supplementation may be sex-dependent [62].

To investigate the beneficial effects of 2′-FL on the gut-brain axis and cognition in obesity, Lee et al. [59] conducted a study on high-fat diet-induced obese mice. They found that 10% 2′-FL supplementation resulted in compositional changes to the gut microbiota and improved gut-brain signaling [59]. Lower 2′-FL doses (1, 2, or 5%) did not significantly affect microbiota composition or attenuate inflammation induced by a high-fat diet, suggesting a dose-dependent effect of these HMOS.

Another laboratory study investigated the effects of 2′-FL supplementation with both low-fat (control) and high-fat diets on the gut-brain axis [66]. The 10% 2′-FL supplementations reduced intestinal para and transcellular permeability and restored the vagally-mediated gut-brain signaling in mice fed the high-fat diet compared to the low-fat diet. Thus, this study revealed potential new roles for 2′-FL in controlling gut-barrier function and gut-brain signaling during metabolic stress in high-fat-fed mice [66].

3.5. Human Studies on HMOS and Cognition

The current literature on the effects of HMOS on cognitive outcomes in human infants is limited compared to data from preclinical models and includes only observational trials. After the selection process, only eight studies involving human subjects were retained in the review (Table 7). The studies applied various cognitive measures and observed mixed associations between HMOS concentrations and cognitive outcomes.

Table 7. HMOS and cognitive outcomes in human observational studies.

Maternal Condition	HMO Assessment	Covariates Adjusted	Tests	Outcome	Ref.
At least partially BF at the study visit	• Complete expression of HM collected by pump from the right breast. • HMOS quantified with LC with fluorescence detection	• Infant age at milk collection • Milk collection site and batch • Multiple comparisons corrected with Holm-Bonferroni method	• S (MSEL) • Early learning composite (ELC) score	• Positive association ($p = 0.002$) between 3′-SL level and ELC scores of early learning in A-tetra positive group • Positive association between 3′-SL level and receptive ($p = 0.015$) and expressive ($p = 0.048$) language scores in A-tetra positive group • Interaction effect ($p = 0.03$) between 3′-SL level and age for receptive language scores A-tetra positive group	[70]
Hispanic mothers with pre-pregnancy normal or overweight Exclusively BF for six months	• Complete expression of HM collected after 1.5 h fasting by pump from one breast. • HMOS quantified with HPLC-MS and internal standards	• Maternal secretor status • Maternal age at delivery • Education level • Infant sex • Infant age • Infant birth weight • Not corrected for multiple comparisons	Bayley Scales of Infant Development (Bayley III)	• Maternal pre-pregnancy BMI negative predicted ($p = 0.03$) infant cognitive development score • 2′-FL at one month ($p \leq 0.01$), LNH ($p \leq 0.02$) and FLNH ($p \leq 0.02$) at six months were associated with higher infant cognitive development score • DSLNT at one month ($p = 0.02$) and LSTb at six months ($p < 0.01$) were negatively associated with infant cognitive development scores	[69]
Study groups: Healthy normal weight Overweight Obese GDM No information is available on BF	• HM collected before and after each feed throughout one day • HMOS quantified with UHPLC-MS/MS and 2′-FL/6′-SL external standards	• GWG • Maternal IQ • Maternal education • Study groups • Prepregnancy BMI • Not corrected for multiple comparisons	Bayley III	• Positive association ($p = 0.041$) between 6′-SL and composite cognitive scores in infants at 18 months when adjusted for GWG, maternal IQ and education, and study groups • Positive association between 6′-SL and composite cognitive scores ($p = 0.019$) and motor scores ($p = 0.043$) in infants at 18 months when adjusted for prepregnancy BMI and study groups • Positive association between 2′-FL and motor scores ($p = 0.041$) in infants at six months when adjusted for prepregnancy BMI and study groups	[71]

Table 7. *Cont.*

Maternal Condition	HMO Assessment	Covariates Adjusted	Tests	Outcome	Ref.
Exclusively BF for seven weeks	• Complete expression of HM by manual breast pump from one breast • HMOS and SA quantified with LC and fluorescence detection	• Maternal age • Pregravid BMI • Self-perceived income • Educational level • Tobacco use • Number of previously breastfed children • Course of pregnancy and delivery process • Multiple comparisons corrected with Benjamini-Hochberg procedure	Ages and Stages Questionnaire (ASQ)	• Positive association (p = 0.009) between LNFP-III content and total ASQ scores at two years old for infants born to secretor mothers	[74]
Healthy women 67.0% Exclusively BF at one month	• HM collected manually by hand • HMOS quantified by HPLC with fluorescence detection and internal standards	• Gestational age at birth • GWG • Prepregnancy BMI • Maternal age • Parity • Mode of BF at one month • Multiple comparisons corrected with Benjamini-Hochberg procedure	Brazilian Ages and Stages Questionnaire (ASQ-BR)	Negative associations between: • LNT and risk of inadequate development for personal-social skills (HR = 0.06) and $\geq$2 developmental domains (HR = 0.06) • LNT and risk of inadequate development for personal-social skills (HR = 0.09) and $\geq$2 developmental domains (HR = 0.05) in secretor mothers only	[73]
Women from the iLiNS project No information is available on BF	• HM was collected manually for a single full breast. • HMOS absolute abundance by nano-LC-chip/time-of-flight MS with standards or relative abundance where standards are not available.	• Maternal age • Maternal height • Maternal BMI • Parity • Education • Food security • HIV status • Hemoglobin • Household assets • Residential location • Infant sex • Season of milk sample collection • Family Care Indicator Score (only for developmental outcomes at 18 mos) • Child's mood, activity level, and willingness to interact with the tester (only for motor development/executive function and working memory model) • Multiple comparisons corrected with Benjamini–Hochberg method	• Motor development (Kilifi Development Inventory • Language development (MacArthur–Bates Communicative Development Inventory) • Socioemotional development (Profile of Social and Emotional Development) • Working memory and executive function (A-not-B task)	• Positive association between HMO 5311a and motor skills (p = 0.003) • Negative association between HMO 5130a and language at 18 months (p = 0.002) • Positive association between total fucosylated (p = 0.007) and total sialyated (p = 0.033) HMOS relative abundances and language at 18 months in infants of secretor mothers • Negative association (p = 0.003) between 6′-SL and walking at 12 months in infants of secretor mothers • Positive association (p = 0.049) between LNnT and walking at 12 months in infants of secretor mothers • Positive associations between F-LSTc (p = 0.004) and DFLNnO II (p = 0.044) and motor skills at 18 months in infants of secretor mothers • Positive associations between DFLNHa (p = 0.02) working memory and executive function at 18 months in infants of secretor mothers • Positive association (p = 0.007) between LSTb relative abundances and working memory and executive function at 18 months in infants of nonsecretor mothers	[72]

Table 7. *Cont.*

Maternal Condition	HMO Assessment	Covariates Adjusted	Tests	Outcome	Ref.
Healthy mothers in the Netherlands 71.4% Exclusively BF for 12 weeks	• HM collected manually or with a breast pump • HMOS quantified by UPLC-MS and HPAEC-PAD	• Gestational age at birth • Maternal education level • Parent(s) executive functioning • Sample-to-sample variations • Estimated daily milk intake • Proportion of human milk feeding • Multiple comparisons corrected with Bonferroni adjustments	• The Behavior Rating Inventory of Executive Function-Preschool Version (BRIEF-P) • Ratings of Everyday Executive Functioning (REEF)	Analyses with exclusively breastfed infants: • Higher 2′-FL ($p = 0.02$) and grouped fucosylated HMOS ($p = 0.03$) were associated with higher executive functioning at three years old (REEF) Analyses including partially breastfed infants: • Higher levels of grouped sialylated HMOS ($p = 0.05$) were associated with worse executive functioning (BRIEF-P)	[76]
Healthy mothers with full-term singleton birth Exclusively BF at one month	• HM collected with a breast pump for a single full breast • HMOS isolated with high-throughput SPE and quantified with MS	• Prepreganancy BMI • Postmenstrual age at the time of MRI scan • Infant birthweight • Infant sex • Multiple comparisons corrected with Benjamini–Yekutieli procedure	• MRI • DTI • ASL	At one month postpartum: Negative associations between: • 2′-FL and FA values in the cortex ($p = 0.001$) • 2′-FL and rCBF in the cortical gray matter of the frontal, temporal, parietal, and occipital lobes (all $p < 0.01$) • 3-FL and MD values in left IC ($p = 0.007$) and posterior white matter ($p < 0.001$) • 3′-SL and MD values in the posterior white matter ($p = 0.007$) Positive associations between: • 2′-FL and MD values in the posterior cortical gray matter, posterior white matter, and subcortical gray matter nuclei (all $p < 0.01$) • 3-FL and FA values in the white matter throughout the frontal, temporal, parietal, and occipital lobes, and left IC and right aCR (all $p < 0.05$) • 3-FL and rCBF in the most part of the cortex, the white matter of the frontal, temporal, parietal, and occipital lobes, and subcortical gray matter nuclei (all $p < 0.05$) • 3′-SL and FA values in the white matter throughout the brain ($p < 0.05$) • 3′-SL and rCBF in the white matter bilaterally (all $p < 0.01$) and in the cortical gray matter of the frontal lobe ($p < 0.001$) 6′SL was not significantly associated with any MRI measures	[75]

Abbreviations: BF, breastfeeding; GDM, gestational diabetes mellitus; GWG, Gestational weight gain; SA, sialic acid; HR, hazard ratio; iLiNS, International Lipid-Based Nutrient Supplements; PGC-UPLC-MS, porous graphitized carbon-ultra high-performance liquid chromatography–mass spectrometry; HPAEC-PAD, high-performance anion exchange chromatography with pulsed amperometric detection; SPE, solid phase extraction; MS, mass-spectrometry; MRI, Magnetic Resonance Imaging; DTI, diffusion tensor imaging; ASL, arterial spin labeling; FA, Fractional anisotropy; MD, mean diffusivity; AD, axial diffusivity; RD, radial diffusivity; rCBF, Regional cerebral blood flow; IC, internal capsule; aCR, anterior corona radiata.

Berger et al. [69] investigated the relationship between 19 HMOS concentrations in human milk and cognitive development in Hispanic infants ($n = 50$) living in Los Angeles, California. This observational study collected human milk samples at 1- and 6-months postpartum and measured cognitive development using the Bayley Scales of Infant Development, third edition (Bayley-III) at 24 months-of-age. The Bayley III was administered by trained personnel to measure the functions of cognitive, language, and motor skills. In the study, only the age-standardized scores for cognitive development were utilized as the dependent variable. The concentration of 2′-FL in milk at one month postpartum was associated with higher infant cognitive development scores at 24 months of age, whereas milk disialyllacto-N-tetraose (DSLNT) concentration at one month was associated with lower cognitive scores at 24 months of age. 2′-FL concentration from milk collected at six months postpartum was no longer related to 24-month cognitive scores. However, several other HMOS concentrations, lactose-N-hexaose (LNH) and fucosyllacto-N-hexaose (FLNH) were related to greater, while LSTb related to lower cognitive development scores at 24 months [69]. This study corroborates findings for the beneficial effects of 2′-FL exposure during lactation for cognitive development in preclinical studies. It implies the potential relevance of other fucosylated and sialylated HMOS for cognitive development. Additionally, associations between HMOS levels of 1- and 6-months were found with child cognitive outcomes at 24 months of age, suggesting sustained effects of early-life HMOS exposure on child development.

Another study by Jorgensen et al. [72] conducted in Malawian mother-infant pairs ($n = 659$) also collected milk samples at six months postpartum, observing mixed relationships between HMOS structures and later child development, including motor and language skills. These findings were mostly secretor status dependent. For example, in infants born to secretor mothers only, the relative abundances of total fucosylated and total sialylated HMOS were positively associated with infant language ability at 18 months. Infants of secretor mothers with milk samples containing a relative abundance of fucosylated HMOS above the median also showed greater vocabulary at 12 months old than those below the median. On the other hand, positive associations between the relative abundance of sialyllacto-*N*-tetraose b (LSTb) and working memory and executive function were only observed in non-secretors [72].

While Berger et al. reported LNH concentrations were positively related to greater cognitive development scores at 24 months [69], Jorgensen et al. instead found a negative association between LNH relative abundance and language at 18 months, but only in infants born by secretor mothers [72]. The lack of consistency in the findings regarding the association between MOS and child development highlights the complexity of the relationship. These inconsistencies may arise from various factors, including maternal secretor status, differences in sample populations, methodologies, outcome measurements, and potential confounding variables. It is important to consider that child development is a multifaceted process influenced by a wide range of genetic, environmental, and nutritional factors, not solely dependent on milk oligosaccharides.

Another observational study of children 2-25 months old ($n = 99$) quantified eight HMOS in milk collected at each study visit [70]. Positive associations between 3′-SL concentrations were observed with receptive and expressive language functions, supporting a higher composite score of early learning criteria, as measured by Mullen Scales of Early Learning. However, the positive association was only observed in mothers with alpha-tetrasaccharide (A-tetra +) in milk, which has been suggested to only be present in mothers with blood type A [70]. This finding is consistent with the study of Malawian children mentioned previously, which found that infants of secretor mothers with higher 6-month total relative abundances of sialylated HMOS had higher language skills at 18 months [72]. Thus, these data indicated the beneficial effects of sialylated HMOS on infant language development. Further, relationships between sialylated HMOS and language may be confounded by maternal genetic background, warranting further investigations.

Two studies [73,74] measured neurodevelopmental outcomes with the Ages and Stages Questionnaire (ASQ), which measures five domains of development: communication, gross motor skills, fine motor skills, problem-solving, and personal-social skills [85]. Ferreira et al. studied full-term infants and utilized a version of the ASQ tailored for the Brazilian children population [73]. They reported that infants of mothers with lower median HMOS concentrations had a higher risk of various developmental inadequacies at one month of age. For example, a lower 3-FL concentration was associated with the risk of inadequate communication skill development; a lower FLNH concentration was related to inadequate fine motor skills. However, after adjusting for multiple comparisons, only an inverse relationship between LNT concentration and risk for personal-social skill inadequacies remains significant in total samples and in secretor mothers only [73]. The second was an exploratory study in preterm infants that assessed associations between HMOS in milk collected from birth to 7 weeks and infant neurocognitive outcomes measured at two years of age. This is the only study investigating the beneficial effects of HMOS on cognitive development in preterm infants. Aside from receiving their mother's milk with standardized fortification, the preterm infants were on parental nutrition, and donor milk was used on rare occasions to ensure adequate nutrition. Only Lacto-N-fucopentaose III (LNFP III) concentration and total ASQ scores were positively related in infants of secretor mothers, which was not reported by other studies before [74]. This study extends the relevance of HMOS for cognition and its possible dependence on maternal genetic factors, such as the secretor genes, to preterm infants.

While there are numerous outcomes of infant cognitive development, assessing executive function in children has become increasingly prevalent [86] due to its critical roles in academic achievement [87], self-regulation and the development of social and cognitive competencies [88]. The core domains of executive functioning include working memory, attention control, cognitive flexibility, and inhibitory control [89]. Several studies in this review explored the relationships between HMOS and executive functioning. Consistent with findings from preclinical studies, a recent study in the Netherlands reported concentrations of 2′-FL and total fucosylated HMOS in the first 12 weeks being related to better parent-reported executive functioning at three years of age in exclusively breastfed infants [76]. This study contributed further evidence of 2′-FL acting as a crucial component for cognitive outcomes. Of note, this study also reported that higher levels of sialylated HMOS were associated with worse executive functioning, but only in partially breastfed infants [76]. To account for formula intake in partially breastfed infants, Willemsen et al. corrected the HMO concentrations by the human milk intake. For example, if the infant received 30% formula, the HMO concentrations will be multiplied by 0.7 [76]. However, among the other studies that included mixed-fed infants [70,73,76], the amount of formula intake was not adjusted in the analysis. Also, two studies [71,72] did not provide information on the mode of feeding. This limitation potentially introduces confounding effects and hinders the accurate interpretation of the observed associations between HMOs and cognitive outcomes.

One study from Spain recruited lactating women with overweight, obesity, or gestational diabetes in pregnancy to investigate potential confounding factors related to maternal health status [71]. Maternal weight status and gestational diabetes did not impact the HMOS levels in milk. However, concentrations of 6′-SL at one month postpartum were positively associated with infant cognitive and motor scale scores at 18 months of age; additionally, 2′-FL was positively correlated with motor scale scores at six months old. Collectively, 6′-SL and 2′-FL levels are linked to better language and motor skills in infants, consistent with findings in preclinical animal models discussed previously [71].

All the human studies discussed above used standardized behavioral assessment questionnaires to evaluate the cognitive development of infants later in life. Although the surveys are standardized, the results were mostly obtained through parent reports, which may not be sensitive enough to detect subtle neurodevelopment variations in infants [74]. However, one study included in the review explored the effects of HMOS exposure on infant brain tissue organization using MRI scanning, and the study was done in the same cohort of infants from Los Angeles [69]. Berger et al. [75] reported that fucosylated and sialylated HMOS were differentially associated with the microstructure of numerous brain tissues [75]. Specifically, the 2′-FL concentration at one month postpartum is associated with greater MD values in the posterior cortical gray matter, posterior white matter, and subcortical gray matter nuclei; 2′-FL exposure was also inversely associated with regional cerebral blood flow (rCBF) and fractional anisotropy (FA) throughout much of the cortical mantle. 3-FL and 3′-SL exposure exhibited differential effects, where 3-FL and 3′-SL concentrations were negatively associated with MD values and positively associated with FA values and rCBF in the white matter throughout the brain [75].

4. Discussion

The purpose of this narrative review was to summarize current evidence for the impact of MOS consumption in early life on the neurocognitive and brain developmental outcomes in both preclinical models and human subjects. Most studies assessed the effects of milk oligosaccharide supplementation in piglet or rodent models. However, observational analyses conducted in mother-infant pairs assessed associations between human milk HMOS content and cognitive outcomes, providing additional evidence that supports the findings from animal model interventions.

More than 200 individual HMOS structures are reported in human milk [16], but only a few HMOS have been tested in clinical studies. Among the 26 studies in the current review, the preclinical model studies have only investigated the influence of SL or FL supplementation or SL gene knockout on brain and cognitive development. On the other hand, analyses conducted in human subjects focused on the associations between the absolute concentrations or relative abundances of the most abundant HMOS and infant cognition. Beyond SL and FL that were investigated in preclinical models, significant associations have also been observed between various infant learning and memory outcomes and the less abundant HMOS, including LNH [69] and LNFP III [74]. Some HMOS, such as DSLNT and LSTb, was reported to have a negative effect on infant cognitive development [69]. This suggests that individual HMOS with different structures might have differential effects on infant brain development. Given the scarcity of research on less abundant HMOS, further investigation is warranted, especially through well-designed preclinical trials or well-controlled observational studies.

4.1. *Sialylated MOS and Cognition*

Human milk provides infants with about 20% more SA compared to formula [90]. Various studies have shown that the SA component of HMOS is crucial for facilitating infant brain development [77,91]. SA is significantly more abundant in neural cell membranes than other types of membranes, suggesting that SA plays a distinct role in the structure of neural cells [92]. The function of the brain in learning and memory appears to be related to the high recognition abilities of the glycoproteins in the brain [29], and there is evidence indicating that the SA content of brain glycoproteins is involved in memory formation [93,94]. Given that around 70–83% of SA in human milk is bound to HMOS, sialylated HMOS can potentially serve as the source of SA for neurologic development [95]. Animal studies revealed that 3′-SL and 6′-SL supplementation during lactation increased cognitive performance [51,52,54,55,57,58,65], suggesting that sialylated HMOS play an essential role in cognitive development by improving recognition and working memory.

Piglet studies provide evidence for the provision of SA by sialylated HMOS: formula 3′-SL or 6′-SL supplementation increased bound SA concentration in piglet prefrontal cortex, corpus callosum, and cerebellum [52,54] and upregulated expression of genes related to SA metabolism [57].

To investigate the individual effect of SL on brain development, genetically modified rodent models were also developed to generate milk deficient in 3′-SL or 6′-SL or both [63,64,68]. Mouse pups who received SL-deficient milk during lactation demonstrated impairments in spatial and recognition memory, suggesting that early life exposure to SL was critical for optimal memory formation.

Aside from SA within HMO, dietary SA found in other milk components may have a beneficial effect on cognitive development as well. One study utilized three-day-old male piglets to investigate the effect of dietary SA on brain growth, learning, and memory, finding that a protein-bound SA, casein glycomacropeptide, enhanced learning performance and increasing the expression of two genes, *ST8SIA4* and *GNE*, related to learning [96]. Likewise, another study suggested that supplementation of isolated dietary SA led to increased cortical ganglioside SA content in developing rats, suggesting that the beneficial effects of sialic acid on cognitive function may be due to its alteration of brain composition to support early brain development [97]. However, there is a lack of evidence on whether SL promotes its cognitive effects through its SA content or indirectly, such as modulating the gut-brain axis. Interestingly, 6′-SL supplementation resulted in a greater positive effect on enhancing learning than free SA supplementation [55]. The underlying mechanisms driving this differential effect remain to be replicated and fully elucidated.

4.2. Fucosylated MOS and Cognition

Fucosylated HMOS, especially 2′-FL, are usually the most abundant HMOS in secretor mothers [98]. Many studies included in this review supported the role of 2′-FL and fucosylated HMOS in learning and memory formation processes [53,59–62,66,67]. This may be explained by the neuroprotective effects of 2′-FL in animal models [99,100], although the exact mechanism for this effect is unclear. LTP is often considered the cellular analog of learning and memory [101] and is widely used to assess synaptic transmission in neurons [102]. An increase in LTP indicates improved synaptic transmission and suggests that neurons are more capable of adapting to new information and retaining it [103]. While multiple brain regions are involved in learning and memory, the hippocampus is particularly critical for memory formation [104]. Most animal studies included in the current review assessed the effects of milk oligosaccharide supplementation on memory through measurement of hippocampal LTP by implanting stimulating and recording electrodes in the hippocampus [55], consistently demonstrating that 3′-SL and 2′-FL may be involved in the maintenance of LTP for rodents in early life [55,63,64]. Oral administration of L-fucose [105] and 2′-FL significantly improved hippocampal LTP memory skills and impacted synaptic plasticity in rodents [106,107]. However, D-fucose or 3-FL infusion [35] did not generate the same improvements as 2′-FL or L-fucose on hippocampal LTP and other measures of memory performance. This may suggest that the benefits of the fucose moiety versus FL for cognition are structurally dependent.

Nonetheless, a recent mouse study examined the role of 2′-FL and fucose on cognition with stable isotope (^{13}C) labeling, finding that benefits from 2′-FL intake were not explained by fucose absorption, as fucose did not cross the blood-brain barrier [40]. Thus, the specific role of 2′-FL on cognition outcomes should be further studied. Also, it is worth noting that the direct link between LTP and cognitive performance is not well-established [108]. Although some studies have shown improved LTP in animals following HMOS supplementation, this association has not yet been confirmed in human subjects.

4.3. HMOS and Infant Cognition

The effects of HMOS on brain and cognitive development in human infants are sparsely explored, and the participants of these studies are relatively limited to certain geographic locations. Among the eight human observational studies included in the current review, two found positive associations for 2′-FL concentrations [69,76], while two found positive associations for SL (3′-SL and 6′-SL) with cognitive development measured via infant behavioral assessment questionaries [70,71]. One study reported a unique association between LNFP III concentration and cognitive scores in infants born to secretor mothers [74], while another found negative associations between several less abundant HMO levels (DSLNT and LSTb) and cognitive outcomes [69]. The inconsistency observed in these observational studies may be due to several reasons. First, methods of assessing cognitive development and motor skills varied, with most assessments being parent-reported surveys. The use of questionnaires or surveys to assess cognitive development in infants and children may not provide a complete picture of the phenomenon under investigation. This could be due to the complexity of cognitive development processes that involve a multitude of factors [109], including genetics and environment [110], and cognitive outcomes can be largely influenced by parent-child relationships and the home environment for children before the start of school [111]. Besides, only two studies [72,76] looked at the effect of HMO groups, namely total fucosylated and/or total sialylated HMOS concentrations, on cognitive outcomes. Most studies mainly focused on associations between single HMO concentrations and cognitive measures, leaving a significant knowledge gap in understanding their combined influence or synergistic effects on neurocognitive development. Therefore, bioinformatics tools are needed for HMO diversity and cluster analyses.

While most human infant studies measured HMO concentrations, Jorgensen et al. [72] reported associations between HMOS and infant cognitive outcomes based on the relative abundances of each HMO structure. Although relative abundance measurements offer insight into the proportions of different HMOS in breast milk, they have inherent limitations that must be acknowledged. One significant concern with relying solely on relative abundance is that it does not provide a direct assessment of the absolute concentration of each HMO. In cases where one specific HMO is relatively high in abundance, it may indicate a corresponding decrease in the relative abundance of other HMOS.

Remarkably, only one [76] study estimated the breastmilk intake by infants, which limits the precision of calculating the absolute amount of HMO intake. This becomes especially pertinent when considering the inclusion of formula feeding in the infants' diet. For infants who are not exclusively breastfed, the amount of HMO consumed will be even less accurate since both human milk and formula intake are rarely collected. To address this limitation, future research should consider implementing a more precise methodology, such as weighing before and after each breastfeeding session or the use of doubly labeled water to determine milk intake. For combination-fed infants, researchers need to carefully report how they account for formula feeding to ensure the results are accurately interpreted. For example, as mentioned previously, the approach used by Willemsen et al. [76] could be implemented.

4.4. Potential Mechanisms of MO Functions in Cognition

Only one of the eight observational studies utilized a brain MRI scanning procedure to investigate the associations between HMOS exposure and infant brain microstructures [75]. Significant relationships between HMO concentrations and brain structures were identified, suggesting a role for HMO in brain maturation processes. For example, 2′-FL concentrations at one month were associated with reduced FA and increased MD in the cortical mantle [75]. A previous study suggested that the decline of FA, coupled with an increase in MD, indicates increased dendritic arborization and synapse formation in the cortical region of the brain [112,113]. Since dendritic arborization and synaptogenesis form the structural basis of learning and memory [75,114,115], maintaining their integrity is important for preventing cognitive dysfunction. Thus, the positive association between 2′-FL and cognitive function may be achieved through enhancing dendritic arborization and synaptic formation. In addition, Berger et al. [75] also reported that 3-FL and 3′-SL concentrations at one month postpartum are associated with increased FA and decreased MD in white matter across most brain areas. Studies suggested that the increased FA in white matter is associated with myelination and axon tract development, which are important for cognitive development [75]. The changes in brain microstructures provide invaluable insight into the potential mechanism of HMO to support the structural maturation of the brain.

Interestingly, a piglet study in which a combination of 3′-SL and 6′-SL was supplemented to formula at concentrations typically found in mature human milk (61-120 days of lactation) significantly increased corpus callosum white matter MD and AD [54]. However, similar effects were not reported by other animal model studies, and the findings are not consistent with the results from the infant observational study [75]. Since an elevation in MD in the white matter may be related to decreased synaptic density, further investigations are needed [116]. Future studies in humans should continue employing more robust markers of cognitive development, such as brain imaging, neuroelectric measurement, and researcher-administrated cognitive tasks, preferably in a longitudinal setting.

Another confounding factor in human studies of HMO relationships with cognitive outcomes may stem from other factors that influence cognitive and brain development, including genetics, maternal health conditions, and environmental factors [117]. For example, it has been reported that the association between breastfeeding and infant cognition was modified by maternal genetic variants of the fatty acid desaturase (FADS) gene, which is involved in polyunsaturated fatty acid metabolism [118], where children of mothers with lower FADS1 and higher FADS2 activities showed a significant advantage in cognition at 14 months [118]. Other human studies also demonstrate the interaction effects of FADS2 polymorphism on the breastfeeding IQ relationship [119,120], although the directionality was inconsistent. Among the studies included in the current review, two studies [72,74] reported associations between several HMOS concentrations and cognitive outcome measures only in secretor mothers and their infants. However, the detailed genetic information was not obtained for the mothers. Another study reported differential effects of HMOS on cognitive outcomes by A-tetra blood groups [70]. Thus, maternal genetics could potentially impact the functions of HMOS on infant cognitive development. It would be practical to investigate infant genetics and interactions with HMO exposure in early life.

Other maternal characteristics, such as pre-pregnancy BMI [121], gestational diabetes [122], as well as mode of delivery [123], have been demonstrated to influence HMOS concentrations in human milk. Thus, it is likely that associations between HMOS and infant cognition can be affected by other maternal factors. Few studies included these factors as covariates in their analyses. However, one study included mothers who developed gestational diabetes and mothers with overweight and obese weight status in the study design [71] but reported no effects of these conditions on the relationships between HMOS and infant cognition when considering pre-pregnancy BMI and diabetic status as covariates [71]. Future clinical trials on HMO and cognition should explore maternal and child genetics, maternal health status, mode of delivery, and other environmental factors as potential confounders.

Additionally, most of the studies were conducted on full-term animal models or human infants, with the exception of one study of preterm pig models [57] and an exploratory analysis on preterm infants [74]. The results suggested that SAL supplementation to preterm pigs ameliorated deficiencies observed in making correct choices in spatial T-maze navigation, such that they performed similarly to term pigs [57]. Even though the supplementation was bovine milk oligosaccharide-enriched whey with SL, the 3′-SL and 6′-SL content still played an essential role in supporting cognitive functions in preterm pigs. The study on preterm infants did not compare differences between term and preterm infants in their responses to HMOS in human milk. However, they observed greater LNFP III concentrations in human milk related to better ASQ scores in preterm infants, corresponding to five domains (communication, gross motor, fine motor, problem-solving and personal-social skills) [74]. Thus, it is important to further examine this relationship, particularly through controlled clinical trials in preterm infants, as they may be at higher risk for developmental delays and cognitive impairments [124]. Aside from potential cognitive benefits, preterm infants reap numerous benefits from human milk consumption [125], and HMOS are thought to play important roles; infants fed human milk demonstrated a reduced incidence of viral and nosocomial infections compared to formula-fed preterm infants [126].

Although the mechanisms by which MOS promote cognitive function are not yet fully understood, several studies suggested that the beneficial effects of MOS occur via modulation of gut microbiota. It has been proposed that differences in microbial colonization patterns and microbiome composition between breastfed and formula-fed infants are largely driven by HMOS [127]. Likewise, it has been reported that bifidobacterial colonization was delayed for infants consuming HM from non-secretor mothers, who lack the enzyme for making 2′-FL compared to secretor mothers [128]. Thus, variations in HMOS composition likely contribute to the differences in *Bifidobacterium* colonization early in life [127], an interaction that may represent a mechanism by which HMOS promote cognitive development. Savignac et al. discovered that supplementation with = *B. longum* 1714 = produced a positive effect on cognition in male mice [129].

Further, in human infants, Carlson et al. conducted a cluster analysis and identified associations between microbiome and cognitive measurements [130]. In addition, upon the investigation of the metabolite fate of ^{13}C-labelled 3′-SL (^{13}C-3′-SL) and ^{13}C-N-acetylneuraminic acid (^{13}C-Neu5Ac) in mice, Galuska et al. [131] claimed that ^{13}C-Neu5Ac is taken by the gut epithelial cells and not incorporated in the brain. They proposed that gut microbiota is involved in the metabolism of 3′-SL and sialic acid. Together, these findings support the brain–gut–microbiome axis. However, most current studies on the effects of prebiotics on the gut-brain axis are descriptive and limited to investigating indirect influences of prebiotics on brain physiology and behavior. However, there is still a lack of comprehensive understanding of the mechanisms [132].

Wang et al. [133] investigated the modulation effect of BMOS and HMOS on the gut microbiota composition in the same pig models from Fleming et al. [61], and they found that BMOS supplementation altered the relative abundance of bacterial taxa in both ascending colon and feces. Specifically, *Bacteroides* abundance was increased by BMOS and BMOS+HMO supplementations, and HMO alone increased the proportion of several taxa, such as *Blautia*. Taken together with the behavioral outcomes, where the pigs with BMOS+HMO supplementation showed long-term recognition memory and increased volumes in the cortices and corpus callosum, suggested that BMOS and HMO could play a role in microbiota composition and cognition. To elucidate the mechanism between gut-brain signaling in the context of HMOS, mediation analyses of the existing data were performed by Fleming et al. [134]. The mediation analysis revealed mediators between gut microbiota, cognitive functions, and brain structures in young pigs, including hippocampal genes related to myelination and neurotransmitters. They pointed out that mediating variables between the gut and brain varied with oligosaccharide intake but in a similar pattern [134]. Therefore, the relationship between HMO consumption, gut microbiome, and cognitive needs additional investigation [134].

Another area for further research is the potential long-term effects of early-life HMOS exposure on cognitive development in children, as long-term benefits of breastfeeding on cognitive development have been demonstrated [135–138]. Most studies in our review focused on early-life cognitive development, but the potential effects of HMOS may extend beyond infancy and early childhood. In several animal model studies, the beneficial effects of HMOS supplementation are detected through adulthood [53,55,63]. Current data available for cognitive development assessment of human infants ranges from 1 month- to 3 years of age.

In our review, some studies did not account for multiple comparisons [69,71], raising concerns about the risk of Type 1 errors [42]. With numerous HMOS tested and multiple cognitive measures explored, the probability of obtaining false-positive results increases. To address this issue, researchers should apply appropriate statistical corrections to ensure the reliability of findings. Transparent reporting and replication of significant results across independent studies will strengthen the validity of associations between HMOS and cognitive outcomes.

While the collective results from preclinical models are promising, another significant concern for animal studies is the risk of publication bias, where the studies with positive results are more likely to be published [139]. This bias can lead to an overrepresentation of positive outcomes in the literature, potentially skewing the overall perception of the effects of HMOS on neurodevelopment. Thus, clinical studies on mother-infant pairs are needed in combination to fully understand the role of HMOS in cognitive development in humans. Current evidence suggests the benefits of several individual HMOS components and total sialylated or fucosylated HMOS for improving cognitive development and brain maturation. Routine supplementation of HMO in the formula may benefit infants that cannot be breastfed [140], although more controlled clinical trials are necessary before this can be widely applied.

5. Conclusions

The results from this review demonstrate a consistent link between early life HMOS consumption and cognitive developmental outcomes, including motor skills, language development, working and reference memory, and IQ. Although most of the relationships were correlations and non-causal, 2′-FL, 3-FL, 3′-SL, and 6′-SL were consistently shown to provide a supportive role in brain and cognitive outcomes. These results underscore the potential importance of these specific HMOS in promoting optimal cognitive development in early life. This review highlights the need for clinical studies investigating the mechanism by which MOS promote learning and memory formation in infants. For example, longitudinal studies with neuroimaging components may be informative in shedding light on the neural basis of HMO-related effects on cognitive development.

Author Contributions: Conceptualization, Y.F. and S.M.D.; methodology, Y.F., A.L.M. and S.M.D.; formal analysis, Y.F. and S.M.D.; writing—original draft preparation, Y.F.; writing—review and editing, Y.F., A.L.M. and S.M.D.; supervision, S.M.D.; funding acquisition, S.M.D. All authors have read and agreed to the published version of the manuscript.

Funding: This research was funded by the National Dairy Council, the National Institutes of Health (R01 DK107561), the Gerber Foundation, and USDA Hatch funding. Y.F. was supported by the Jeanette Chu and Winston Y. Lo Endowed Fellowship from the Department of Food Science and Human Nutrition at the University of Illinois Urbana-Champaign. A.L.M. was supported a USDA National Needs fellowship (2017-09548) to the Division of Nutritional Sciences at the University of Illinois Urbana-Champaign.

Institutional Review Board Statement: Not applicable.

Informed Consent Statement: Not applicable.

Data Availability Statement: Not applicable.

Conflicts of Interest: The authors declare no conflict of interest.

References

1. Bhatnagar, S.; Taneja, S. Zinc and cognitive development. *Br. J. Nutr.* **2001**, *85*, S139–S145. [CrossRef] [PubMed]
2. Johnson, M.H. Functional brain development in humans. *Nat. Rev. Neurosci.* **2001**, *2*, 475–483. [CrossRef] [PubMed]
3. Clark, C.A.; Pritchard, V.E.; Woodward, L.J. Preschool executive functioning abilities predict early mathematics achievement. *Dev. Psychol.* **2010**, *46*, 1176. [CrossRef]
4. Nyaradi, A.; Li, J.; Hickling, S.; Foster, J.; Oddy, W.H. The role of nutrition in children's neurocognitive development, from pregnancy through childhood. *Front. Hum. Neurosci.* **2013**, *7*, 97. [CrossRef]
5. Martorell, R. Undernutrition during pregnancy and early childhood and its consequences for cognitive and behavioral development. In *Early Child Development: Investing in Our Children's Future*; Young, M.E., Ed.; Elsevier: Amsterdam, The Netherlands; New York, NY, USA, 1997; pp. 39–83.
6. Engle, P.L.; Fernández, P.D. INCAP studies of malnutrition and cognitive behavior. *Food Nutr. Bull.* **2010**, *31*, 83–94. [CrossRef] [PubMed]
7. Andreas, N.J.; Kampmann, B.; Le-Doare, K.M. Human breast milk: A review on its composition and bioactivity. *Early Hum. Dev.* **2015**, *91*, 629–635. [CrossRef]
8. Breastfeeding, S.O.; Eidelman, A.I.; Schanler, R.J.; Johnston, M.; Landers, S.; Noble, L.; Szucs, K.; Viehmann, L. Breastfeeding and the use of human milk. *Pediatrics* **2012**, *129*, e827–e841. [CrossRef]
9. Young, B. Breastfeeding and human milk: Short and long-term health benefits to the recipient infant. In *Early Nutrition and Long-Term Health*; Woodhead Publishing: Sawston, UK, 2017; pp. 25–53.
10. Martin, C.R.; Ling, P.-R.; Blackburn, G.L. Review of infant feeding: Key features of breast milk and infant formula. *Nutrients* **2016**, *8*, 279. [CrossRef]

11. Horta, B.; Loret de Mola, C.; Victora, C. Breastfeeding and intelligence: A systematic review and meta-analysis. *Acta Paediatr.* **2015**, *104*, 14–19. [CrossRef]
12. Bernard, J.Y.; De Agostini, M.; Forhan, A.; Alfaiate, T.; Bonet, M.; Champion, V.; Kaminski, M.; de Lauzon-Guillain, B.; Charles, M.-A.; Heude, B. Breastfeeding duration and cognitive development at 2 and 3 years of age in the EDEN mother–child Cohort. *J. Pediatr.* **2013**, *163*, 36–42.e31. [CrossRef]
13. Angelsen, N.; Vik, T.; Jacobsen, G.; Bakketeig, L. Breast feeding and cognitive development at age 1 and 5 years. *Arch. Dis. Child.* **2001**, *85*, 183–188. [CrossRef] [PubMed]
14. Lucas, A.; Morley, R.; Cole, T.J. Randomised trial of early diet in preterm babies and later intelligence quotient. *BMJ* **1998**, *317*, 1481–1487. [CrossRef] [PubMed]
15. Chiurazzi, M.; Cozzolino, M.; Reinelt, T.; Nguyen, T.D.; Elke Chie, S.; Natalucci, G.; Miletta, M.C. Human milk and brain development in infants. *Reprod. Med.* **2021**, *2*, 107–117. [CrossRef]
16. Zheng, J.; Xu, H.; Fang, J.; Zhang, X. Enzymatic and chemoenzymatic synthesis of human milk oligosaccharides and derivatives. *Carbohydr. Polym.* **2022**, *291*, 119564. [CrossRef]
17. Tao, N.; DePeters, E.; Freeman, S.; German, J.; Grimm, R.; Lebrilla, C.B. Bovine milk glycome. *J. Dairy Sci.* **2008**, *91*, 3768–3778. [CrossRef]
18. Urashima, T.; Taufik, E.; Fukuda, K.; Asakuma, S. Recent advances in studies on milk oligosaccharides of cows and other domestic farm animals. *Biosci. Biotechnol. Biochem.* **2013**, *77*, 455–466. [CrossRef]
19. Zivkovic, A.M.; Barile, D. Bovine milk as a source of functional oligosaccharides for improving human health. *Adv. Nutr.* **2011**, *2*, 284–289. [CrossRef]
20. Vandenplas, Y.; Berger, B.; Carnielli, V.P.; Ksiazyk, J.; Lagström, H.; Sanchez Luna, M.; Migacheva, N.; Mosselmans, J.-M.; Picaud, J.-C.; Possner, M. Human milk oligosaccharides: 2′-fucosyllactose (2′-FL) and lacto-N-neotetraose (LNnT) in infant formula. *Nutrients* **2018**, *10*, 1161. [CrossRef] [PubMed]
21. Parschat, K.; Melsaether, C.; Jäpelt, K.R.; Jennewein, S. Clinical evaluation of 16-week supplementation with 5HMO-mix in healthy-term human infants to determine tolerability, safety, and effect on growth. *Nutrients* **2021**, *13*, 2871. [CrossRef]
22. Lasekan, J.; Choe, Y.; Dvoretskiy, S.; Devitt, A.; Zhang, S.; Mackey, A.; Wulf, K.; Buck, R.; Steele, C.; Johnson, M. Growth and gastrointestinal tolerance in healthy term infants fed milk-based infant formula supplemented with five human milk oligosaccharides (HMOs): A randomized multicenter trial. *Nutrients* **2022**, *14*, 2625. [CrossRef]
23. Cheng, Y.-J.; Yeung, C.-Y. Recent advance in infant nutrition: Human milk oligosaccharides. *Pediatr. Neonatol.* **2021**, *62*, 347–353. [CrossRef]
24. Carabotti, M.; Scirocco, A.; Maselli, M.A.; Severi, C. The gut-brain axis: Interactions between enteric microbiota, central and enteric nervous systems. *Ann. Gastroenterol.* **2015**, *28*, 203.
25. LeMay-Nedjelski, L.; Yonemitsu, C.; Asbury, M.R.; Butcher, J.; Ley, S.H.; Hanley, A.J.; Kiss, A.; Unger, S.; Copeland, J.K.; Wang, P.W. Oligosaccharides and microbiota in human milk are interrelated at 3 months postpartum in a cohort of women with a high prevalence of gestational impaired glucose tolerance. *J. Nutr.* **2021**, *151*, 3431–3441. [CrossRef]
26. Singh, R.P.; Niharika, J.; Kondepudi, K.K.; Bishnoi, M.; Tingirikari, J.M.R. Recent understanding of human milk oligosaccharides in establishing infant gut microbiome and roles in immune system. *Food Res. Int.* **2022**, *151*, 110884. [CrossRef] [PubMed]
27. Wang, B. Sialic acid is an essential nutrient for brain development and cognition. *Annu. Rev. Nutr.* **2009**, *29*, 177–222. [CrossRef]
28. Schnaar, R.L.; Gerardy-Schahn, R.; Hildebrandt, H. Sialic acids in the brain: Gangliosides and polysialic acid in nervous system development, stability, disease, and regeneration. *Physiol. Rev.* **2014**, *94*, 461–518. [CrossRef] [PubMed]
29. Wang, B.; Brand-Miller, J. The role and potential of sialic acid in human nutrition. *Eur. J. Clin. Nutr.* **2003**, *57*, 1351–1369. [CrossRef] [PubMed]
30. Wang, B.; Brand-Miller, J.; McVeagh, P.; Petocz, P. Concentration and distribution of sialic acid in human milk and infant formulas. *Am. J. Clin. Nutr.* **2001**, *74*, 510–515. [CrossRef]
31. Martín-Sosa, S.; Martín, M.-J.; García-Pardo, L.-A.; Hueso, P. Sialyloligosaccharides in human and bovine milk and in infant formulas: Variations with the progression of lactation. *J. Dairy Sci.* **2003**, *86*, 52–59. [CrossRef]
32. Monaco, M.H.; Wang, M.; Pan, X.; Li, Q.; Richards, J.D.; Chichlowski, M.; Berg, B.M.; Dilger, R.N.; Donovan, S.M. Evaluation of sialyllactose supplementation of a prebiotic-containing formula on growth, intestinal development, and bacterial colonization in the neonatal piglet. *Curr. Dev. Nutr.* **2018**, *2*, nzy067. [CrossRef]
33. Zhu, Y.; Wan, L.; Li, W.; Ni, D.; Zhang, W.; Yan, X.; Mu, W. Recent advances on 2′-fucosyllactose: Physiological properties, applications, and production approaches. *Crit. Rev. Food Sci. Nutr.* **2022**, *62*, 2083–2092. [CrossRef] [PubMed]
34. Mountford, C.; Quadrelli, S.; Lin, A.; Ramadan, S. Six fucose-α (1–2) sugars and α-fucose assigned in the human brain using in vivo two-dimensional MRS. *NMR Biomed.* **2015**, *28*, 291–296. [CrossRef] [PubMed]
35. Matthies, H.; Staak, S.; Krug, M. Fucose and fucosyllactose enhance in-vitro hippocampal long-term potentiation. *Brain Res.* **1996**, *725*, 276–280. [CrossRef]
36. Tosh, N.; Quadrelli, S.; Galloway, G.; Mountford, C. Two new fucose-α (1–2)-glycans assigned in the healthy human brain taking the number to seven. *Sci. Rep.* **2019**, *9*, 18806. [CrossRef] [PubMed]
37. Wetzel, W.; Popov, N.; Lössner, B.; Schulzeck, S.; Honza, R.; Matthies, H. Effect of L-fucose on brain protein metabolism and retention of a learned behavior in rats. *Pharmacol. Biochem. Behav.* **1980**, *13*, 765–771. [CrossRef]

38. Kelly, R.J.; Rouquier, S.; Giorgi, D.; Lennon, G.G.; Lowe, J.B. Sequence and expression of a candidate for the human secretor blood group A (1, 2) fucosyltransferase gene (Fut2): Homozygosity for an enzyme-inactivating nonsense mutation commonly correlates with the non-secretor phenotype. *J. Biol. Chem.* **1995**, *270*, 4640–4649. [CrossRef]
39. Kuntz, S.; Kunz, C.; Borsch, C.; Vazquez, E.; Buck, R.; Reutzel, M.; Eckert, G.P.; Rudloff, S. Metabolic fate and distribution of 2-fucosyllactose: Direct influence on gut microbial activity but not on brain. *Mol. Nutr. Food Res.* **2019**, *63*, 1900035. [CrossRef]
40. Rudloff, S.; Kuntz, S.; Borsch, C.; Vazquez, E.; Buck, R.; Reutzel, M.; Eckert, G.P.; Kunz, C. Fucose as a cleavage product of 2′Fucosyllactose does not cross the blood-brain barrier in mice. *Mol. Nutr. Food Res.* **2021**, *65*, 2100045. [CrossRef]
41. Docq, S.; Spoelder, M.; Wang, W.; Homberg, J.R. The protective and long-lasting effects of human milk oligosaccharides on cognition in mammals. *Nutrients* **2020**, *12*, 3572. [CrossRef]
42. Berger, P.K.; Ong, M.L.; Bode, L.; Belfort, M.B. Human Milk Oligosaccharides and Infant Neurodevelopment: A Narrative Review. *Nutrients* **2023**, *15*, 719. [CrossRef]
43. Moher, D.; Liberati, A.; Tetzlaff, J.; Altman, D.G.; Prisma Group. Preferred reporting items for systematic reviews and meta-analyses: The PRISMA statement. *Ann. Intern. Med.* **2009**, *151*, 264–269. [CrossRef]
44. Antunes, M.; Biala, G. The novel object recognition memory: Neurobiology, test procedure, and its modifications. *Cogn. Process.* **2012**, *13*, 93–110. [CrossRef] [PubMed]
45. Lueptow, L.M. Novel object recognition test for the investigation of learning and memory in mice. *J. Vis. Exp.* **2017**, e55718.
46. Silvers, J.M.; Harrod, S.B.; Mactutus, C.F.; Booze, R.M. Automation of the novel object recognition task for use in adolescent rats. *J. Neurosci. Methods* **2007**, *166*, 99–103. [CrossRef] [PubMed]
47. Goulart, B.; De Lima, M.; De Farias, C.; Reolon, G.; Almeida, V.; Quevedo, J.; Kapczinski, F.; Schröder, N.; Roesler, R. Ketamine impairs recognition memory consolidation and prevents learning-induced increase in hippocampal brain-derived neurotrophic factor levels. *Neuroscience* **2010**, *167*, 969–973. [CrossRef]
48. Kraeuter, A.-K.; Guest, P.C.; Sarnyai, Z. The Y-maze for assessment of spatial working and reference memory in mice. *Methods Mol. Biol.* **2019**, *1916*, 105–111. [CrossRef]
49. d'Isa, R.; Comi, G.; Leocani, L. Apparatus design and behavioural testing protocol for the evaluation of spatial working memory in mice through the spontaneous alternation T-maze. *Sci. Rep.* **2021**, *11*, 21177. [CrossRef] [PubMed]
50. Wenk, G.L. Assessment of spatial memory using the T maze. *Curr. Protoc. Neurosci.* **1998**, *4*, 8.5 B. 1–8.5 A. 7. [CrossRef]
51. Tarr, A.J.; Galley, J.D.; Fisher, S.E.; Chichlowski, M.; Berg, B.M.; Bailey, M.T. The prebiotics 3′ Sialyllactose and 6′ Sialyllactose diminish stressor-induced anxiety-like behavior and colonic microbiota alterations: Evidence for effects on the gut–brain axis. *Brain Behav. Immun.* **2015**, *50*, 166–177. [CrossRef] [PubMed]
52. Jacobi, S.K.; Yatsunenko, T.; Li, D.; Dasgupta, S.; Yu, R.K.; Berg, B.M.; Chichlowski, M.; Odle, J. Dietary isomers of sialyllactose increase ganglioside sialic acid concentrations in the corpus callosum and cerebellum and modulate the colonic microbiota of formula-fed piglets. *J. Nutr.* **2016**, *146*, 200–208. [CrossRef]
53. Oliveros, E.; Ramirez, M.; Vazquez, E.; Barranco, A.; Gruart, A.; Delgado-Garcia, J.M.; Buck, R.; Rueda, R.; Martin, M.J. Oral supplementation of 2′-fucosyllactose during lactation improves memory and learning in rats. *J. Nutr. Biochem.* **2016**, *31*, 20–27. [CrossRef]
54. Mudd, A.T.; Fleming, S.A.; Labhart, B.; Chichlowski, M.; Berg, B.M.; Donovan, S.M.; Dilger, R.N. Dietary sialyllactose influences sialic acid concentrations in the prefrontal cortex and magnetic resonance imaging measures in corpus callosum of young pigs. *Nutrients* **2017**, *9*, 1297. [CrossRef] [PubMed]
55. Oliveros, E.; Vázquez, E.; Barranco, A.; Ramírez, M.; Gruart, A.; Delgado-García, J.M.; Buck, R.; Rueda, R.; Martín, M.J. Sialic acid and sialylated oligosaccharide supplementation during lactation improves learning and memory in rats. *Nutrients* **2018**, *10*, 1519. [CrossRef] [PubMed]
56. Fleming, S.A.; Chichlowski, M.; Berg, B.M.; Donovan, S.M.; Dilger, R.N. Dietary sialyllactose does not influence measures of recognition memory or diurnal activity in the young pig. *Nutrients* **2018**, *10*, 395. [CrossRef] [PubMed]
57. Obelitz-Ryom, K.; Bering, S.B.; Overgaard, S.H.; Eskildsen, S.F.; Ringgaard, S.; Olesen, J.L.; Skovgaard, K.; Pankratova, S.; Wang, B.; Brunse, A. Bovine milk oligosaccharides with sialyllactose improves cognition in preterm pigs. *Nutrients* **2019**, *11*, 1335. [CrossRef]
58. Wang, H.X.; Chen, Y.; Haque, Z.; de Veer, M.; Egan, G.; Wang, B. Sialylated milk oligosaccharides alter neurotransmitters and brain metabolites in piglets: An In vivo magnetic resonance spectroscopic (MRS) study. *Nutr. Neurosci.* **2021**, *24*, 885–895. [CrossRef]
59. Lee, S.; Goodson, M.; Vang, W.; Kalanetra, K.; Barile, D.; Raybould, H. 2′-fucosyllactose supplementation improves gut-brain signaling and diet-induced obese phenotype and changes the gut microbiota in high fat-fed mice. *Nutrients* **2020**, *12*, 1003. [CrossRef]
60. Fleming, S.A.; Mudd, A.T.; Hauser, J.; Yan, J.; Metairon, S.; Steiner, P.; Donovan, S.M.; Dilger, R.N. Dietary oligofructose alone or in combination with 2′-fucosyllactose differentially improves recognition memory and hippocampal mrna expression. *Nutrients* **2020**, *12*, 2131. [CrossRef]
61. Fleming, S.A.; Mudd, A.T.; Hauser, J.; Yan, J.; Metairon, S.; Steiner, P.; Donovan, S.M.; Dilger, R.N. Human and bovine milk oligosaccharides elicit improved recognition memory concurrent with alterations in regional brain volumes and hippocampal mRNA expression. *Front. Neurosci.* **2020**, *14*, 770. [CrossRef]
62. Tuplin, E.W.N.; Chleilat, F.; Alukic, E.; Reimer, R.A. The Effects of Human Milk Oligosaccharide Supplementation During Critical Periods of Development on the Mesolimbic Dopamine System. *Neuroscience* **2021**, *459*, 166–178. [CrossRef]

63. Pisa, E.; Martire, A.; Chiodi, V.; Traversa, A.; Caputo, V.; Hauser, J.; Macrì, S. Exposure to 3′ Sialyllactose-Poor Milk during Lactation Impairs Cognitive Capabilities in Adulthood. *Nutrients* **2021**, *13*, 4191. [CrossRef] [PubMed]
64. Hauser, J.; Pisa, E.; Arias Vásquez, A.; Tomasi, F.; Traversa, A.; Chiodi, V.; Martin, F.-P.; Sprenger, N.; Lukjancenko, O.; Zollinger, A. Sialylated human milk oligosaccharides program cognitive development through a non-genomic transmission mode. *Mol. Psychiatry* **2021**, *26*, 2854–2871. [CrossRef] [PubMed]
65. Clouard, C.; Reimert, I.; Fleming, S.A.; Koopmans, S.-J.; Schuurman, T.; Hauser, J. Dietary sialylated oligosaccharides in early-life may promote cognitive flexibility during development in context of obesogenic dietary intake. *Nutr. Neurosci.* **2021**, *25*, 2461–2478. [CrossRef] [PubMed]
66. Lee, S.; Goodson, M.L.; Vang, W.; Rutkowsky, J.; Kalanetra, K.; Bhattacharya, M.; Barile, D.; Raybould, H.E. Human milk oligosaccharide 2′-fucosyllactose supplementation improves gut barrier function and signaling in the vagal afferent pathway in mice. *Food Funct.* **2021**, *12*, 8507–8521. [CrossRef] [PubMed]
67. Sutkus, L.T.; Joung, S.; Hirvonen, J.; Jensen, H.M.; Ouwehand, A.C.; Mukherjea, R.; Donovan, S.M.; Dilger, R.N. Influence of 2′-Fucosyllactose and Bifidobacterium longum Subspecies infantis Supplementation on Cognitive and Structural Brain Development in Young Pigs. *Front. Neurosci.* **2022**, *16*, 860368. [CrossRef]
68. Pisa, E.; Traversa, A.; Caputo, V.; Ottomana, A.M.; Hauser, J.; Macrì, S. Long-term consequences of reduced availability and compensatory supplementation of sialylated HMOs on cognitive capabilities. *Front. Cell. Neurosci.* **2023**, *17*, 1091890. [CrossRef]
69. Berger, P.K.; Plows, J.F.; Jones, R.B.; Alderete, T.L.; Yonemitsu, C.; Poulsen, M.; Ryoo, J.H.; Peterson, B.S.; Bode, L.; Goran, M.I. Human milk oligosaccharide 2′-fucosyllactose links feedings at 1 month to cognitive development at 24 months in infants of normal and overweight mothers. *PLoS ONE* **2020**, *15*, e0228323. [CrossRef]
70. Cho, S.; Zhu, Z.; Li, T.; Baluyot, K.; Howell, B.R.; Hazlett, H.C.; Elison, J.T.; Hauser, J.; Sprenger, N.; Wu, D. Human milk 3′-Sialyllactose is positively associated with language development during infancy. *Am. J. Clin. Nutr.* **2021**, *114*, 588–597. [CrossRef]
71. Oliveros, E.; Martín, M.; Torres-Espínola, F.; Segura-Moreno, M.; Ramírez, M.; Santos, A.; Buck, R.; Rueda, R.; Escudero, M.; Catena, A. Human milk levels of 2-fucosyllactose and 6-sialyllactose are positively associated with infant neurodevelopment and are not impacted by maternal BMI or diabetic status. *J. Nutr. Food Sci.* **2021**, *4*, 100024.
72. Jorgensen, J.M.; Young, R.; Ashorn, P.; Ashorn, U.; Chaima, D.; Davis, J.C.; Goonatilleke, E.; Kumwenda, C.; Lebrilla, C.B.; Maleta, K. Associations of human milk oligosaccharides and bioactive proteins with infant growth and development among Malawian mother-infant dyads. *Am. J. Clin. Nutr.* **2021**, *113*, 209–220. [CrossRef]
73. Ferreira, A.L.L.; Alves-Santos, N.H.; Freitas-Costa, N.C.; Santos, P.P.; Batalha, M.A.; Figueiredo, A.C.; Yonemitsu, C.; Manivong, N.; Furst, A.; Bode, L. Associations Between Human Milk Oligosaccharides at 1 Month and Infant Development Throughout the First Year of Life in a Brazilian Cohort. *J. Nutr.* **2021**, *151*, 3543–3554. [CrossRef] [PubMed]
74. Rozé, J.-C.; Hartweg, M.; Simon, L.; Billard, H.; Chen, Y.; Austin, S.; Boscher, C.; Moyon, T.; Darmaun, D.; Rodenas, C.L.G. Human milk oligosaccharides in breast milk and 2-year outcome in preterm infants: An exploratory analysis. *Clin. Nutr.* **2022**, *41*, 1896–1905. [CrossRef]
75. Berger, P.K.; Bansal, R.; Sawardekar, S.; Yonemitsu, C.; Furst, A.; Hampson, H.E.; Schmidt, K.A.; Alderete, T.L.; Bode, L.; Goran, M.I. Associations of human milk oligosaccharides with infant brain tissue organization and regional blood flow at 1 month of age. *Nutrients* **2022**, *14*, 3820. [CrossRef]
76. Willemsen, Y.; Beijers, R.; Gu, F.; Vasquez, A.A.; Schols, H.A.; de Weerth, C. Fucosylated human milk oligosaccharides during the first 12 postnatal weeks are associated with better executive functions in toddlers. *Nutrients* **2023**, *15*, 1463. [CrossRef] [PubMed]
77. McVeagh, P.; Miller, J.B. Human milk oligosaccharides: Only the breast. *J. Paediatr. Child Health* **1997**, *33*, 281–286. [CrossRef]
78. EFSA Panel on Nutrition, N.F.; Allergens, F.; Turck, D.; Bohn, T.; Castenmiller, J.; De Henauw, S.; Hirsch-Ernst, K.I.; Maciuk, A.; Mangelsdorf, I.; McArdle, H.J.; et al. Safety of 6′-sialyllactose (6′-SL) sodium salt produced by derivative strains of Escherichia coli BL21 (DE3) as a novel food pursuant to Regulation (EU) 2015/2283. *EFSA J.* **2022**, *20*, e07645.
79. Gieling, E.T.; Schuurman, T.; Nordquist, R.E.; van der Staay, F.J. The pig as a model animal for studying cognition and neurobehavioral disorders. *Mol. Funct. Model. Neuropsychiatry* **2011**, *7*, 359–383.
80. Odle, J.; Lin, X.; Jacobi, S.K.; Kim, S.W.; Stahl, C.H. The suckling piglet as an agrimedical model for the study of pediatric nutrition and metabolism. *Annu. Rev. Anim. Biosci.* **2014**, *2*, 419–444. [CrossRef]
81. Mudd, A.T.; Dilger, R.N. Early-life nutrition and neurodevelopment: Use of the piglet as a translational model. *Adv. Nutr.* **2017**, *8*, 92–104. [CrossRef] [PubMed]
82. van der Knaap, L.J.; van der Ham, I.J. How does the corpus callosum mediate interhemispheric transfer? A review. *Behav. Brain Res.* **2011**, *223*, 211–221. [CrossRef]
83. Palmano, K.; Rowan, A.; Guillermo, R.; Guan, J.; Mc Jarrow, P. The role of gangliosides in neurodevelopment. *Nutrients* **2015**, *7*, 3891–3913. [CrossRef]
84. Meli, F.; Puccio, G.; Cajozzo, C.; Ricottone, G.L.; Pecquet, S.; Sprenger, N.; Steenhout, P. Growth and safety evaluation of infant formulae containing oligosaccharides derived from bovine milk: A randomized, double-blind, noninferiority trial. *BMC Pediatr.* **2014**, *14*, 306. [CrossRef]
85. Singh, A.; Yeh, C.J.; Blanchard, S.B. Ages and stages questionnaire: A global screening scale. *Boletín Médico Del Hosp. Infant. De México* **2017**, *74*, 5–12.

86. Müller, U.; Kerns, K. The development of executive function. In *Handbook of Child Psychology and Developmental Science*; Lerner, R.R.M., Ed.; John Wiley & Sons, Inc.: Hoboken, NJ, USA, 2015; pp. 1–53.
87. Blair, C.; Razza, R.P. Relating effortful control, executive function, and false belief understanding to emerging math and literacy ability in kindergarten. *Child Dev.* **2007**, *78*, 647–663. [CrossRef] [PubMed]
88. San Diego, R.J.; Franke, N.; Harding, J.E.; Wouldes, T.A. Cross-cultural validity and reliability of the BRIEF-P at age 2 and 4.5 years in children born at risk of neonatal hypoglycemia. *Child Neuropsychol.* **2023**, *29*, 340–356. [CrossRef]
89. Nejati, V.; Salehinejad, M.A.; Nitsche, M.A.; Najian, A.; Javadi, A.-H. Transcranial direct current stimulation improves executive dysfunctions in ADHD: Implications for inhibitory control, interference control, working memory, and cognitive flexibility. *J. Atten. Disord.* **2020**, *24*, 1928–1943. [CrossRef] [PubMed]
90. Heine, W.; Wutzke, K.; Radke, M. Sialic acid in breast milk and infant formula food. *Mon. Kinderheilkd.* **1993**, *141*, 946–950.
91. Zhang, X.; Liu, Y.; Liu, L.; Li, J.; Du, G.; Chen, J. Microbial production of sialic acid and sialylated human milk oligosaccharides: Advances and perspectives. *Biotechnol. Adv.* **2019**, *37*, 787–800. [CrossRef] [PubMed]
92. Schauer, R. *Sialic Acids: Chemistry, Metabolism, and Function*; Springer Science & Business Media: Berlin, Germany, 2012; Volume 10.
93. Bogoch, S. Recognins and their chemoreciprocals. In *Behavioral Neurochemistry*; Spectrum-Wiley Press: New York, NY, USA, 1977; p. 270.
94. Schmidt, R. Glycoproteins Involved in Long Lasting Plasticity in the Teleost Brain. 1989. Available online: https://jlupub.ub.uni-giessen.de/bitstream/handle/jlupub/16860/SchmidtRupert-Glycoproteinsin.pdf?sequence=1&isAllowed=y (accessed on 4 April 2023).
95. Lis-Kuberka, J.; Orczyk-Pawiłowicz, M. Sialylated oligosaccharides and glycoconjugates of human milk. The impact on infant and newborn protection, development and well-being. *Nutrients* **2019**, *11*, 306. [CrossRef]
96. Wang, B.; Yu, B.; Karim, M.; Hu, H.; Sun, Y.; McGreevy, P.; Petocz, P.; Held, S.; Brand-Miller, J. Dietary sialic acid supplementation improves learning and memory in piglets. *Am. J. Clin. Nutr.* **2007**, *85*, 561–569. [CrossRef]
97. Scholtz, S.A.; Gottipati, B.S.; Gajewski, B.J.; Carlson, S.E. Dietary sialic acid and cholesterol influence cortical composition in developing rats. *J. Nutr.* **2013**, *143*, 132–135. [CrossRef] [PubMed]
98. Castanys-Muñoz, E.; Martin, M.J.; Prieto, P.A. 2′-Fucosyllactose: An abundant, genetically determined soluble glycan present in human milk. *Nutr. Rev.* **2013**, *71*, 773–789. [CrossRef] [PubMed]
99. Hung, T.-W.; Wu, K.-J.; Wang, Y.-S.; Bae, E.-K.; Song, Y.; Yoon, J.; Yu, S.-J. Human milk oligosaccharide 2′-fucosyllactose induces neuroprotection from intracerebral hemorrhage stroke. *Int. J. Mol. Sci.* **2021**, *22*, 9881. [CrossRef]
100. Wu, K.-J.; Chen, Y.-H.; Bae, E.-K.; Song, Y.; Min, W.; Yu, S.-J. Human milk oligosaccharide 2′-fucosyllactose reduces neurodegeneration in stroke brain. *Transl. Stroke Res.* **2020**, *11*, 1001–1011. [CrossRef]
101. Hayashi, Y. Molecular mechanism of hippocampal long-term potentiation–Towards multiscale understanding of learning and memory. *Neurosci. Res.* **2022**, *175*, 3–15. [CrossRef] [PubMed]
102. Teyler, T.J.; DiScenna, P. Long-term potentiation. *Annu. Rev. Neurosci.* **1987**, *10*, 131–161. [CrossRef]
103. Bliss, T.V.; Collingridge, G.L. A synaptic model of memory: Long-term potentiation in the hippocampus. *Nature* **1993**, *361*, 31–39. [CrossRef]
104. Lynch, M.A. Long-term potentiation and memory. *Physiol. Rev.* **2004**, *84*, 87–136. [CrossRef]
105. Krug, M.; Wagner, M.; Staak, S.; Smalla, K.-H. Fucose and fucose-containing sugar epitopes enhance hippocampal long-term potentiation in the freely moving rat. *Brain Res.* **1994**, *643*, 130–135. [CrossRef]
106. Vazquez, E.; Barranco, A.; Ramirez, M.; Gruart, A.; Delgado-Garcia, J.M.; Jimenez, M.L.; Buck, R.; Rueda, R. Dietary 2′-fucosyllactose enhances operant conditioning and long-term potentiation via gut-brain communication through the vagus nerve in rodents. *PLoS ONE* **2016**, *11*, e0166070. [CrossRef]
107. Vázquez, E.; Barranco, A.; Ramírez, M.; Gruart, A.; Delgado-García, J.M.; Martínez-Lara, E.; Blanco, S.; Martín, M.J.; Castanys, E.; Buck, R. Effects of a human milk oligosaccharide, 2′-fucosyllactose, on hippocampal long-term potentiation and learning capabilities in rodents. *J. Nutr. Biochem.* **2015**, *26*, 455–465. [CrossRef]
108. Cooke, S.F.; Bliss, T.V. Plasticity in the human central nervous system. *Brain* **2006**, *129*, 1659–1673. [CrossRef] [PubMed]
109. Bruner, J.S. The course of cognitive growth. *Am. Psychol.* **1964**, *19*, 1. [CrossRef]
110. Rutter, M. Family and school influences on cognitive development. *J. Child Psychol. Psychiatry* **1985**, *26*, 683–704. [CrossRef] [PubMed]
111. McMath, A.L.; Aguilar-Lopez, M.; Cannavale, C.N.; Khan, N.A.; Donovan, S.M. A systematic review on the impact of gastrointestinal microbiota composition and function on cognition in healthy infants and children. *Front. Neurosci.* **2023**, *17*, 1171970. [CrossRef]
112. Hüppi, P.S.; Maier, S.E.; Peled, S.; Zientara, G.P.; Barnes, P.D.; Jolesz, F.A.; Volpe, J.J. Microstructural development of human newborn cerebral white matter assessed in vivo by diffusion tensor magnetic resonance imaging. *Pediatr. Res.* **1998**, *44*, 584–590. [CrossRef]
113. Dean, J.M.; McClendon, E.; Hansen, K.; Azimi-Zonooz, A.; Chen, K.; Riddle, A.; Gong, X.; Sharifnia, E.; Hagen, M.; Ahmad, T. Prenatal cerebral ischemia disrupts MRI-defined cortical microstructure through disturbances in neuronal arborization. *Sci. Transl. Med.* **2013**, *5*, 168ra167. [CrossRef]

114. Zhong, J.; Li, J.; Ni, C.; Zuo, Z. Amantadine alleviates postoperative cognitive dysfunction possibly by preserving neurotrophic factor expression and dendritic arborization in the hippocampus of old rodents. *Front. Aging Neurosci.* **2020**, *12*, 605330. [CrossRef] [PubMed]
115. Knutson, D.; Mitzey, A.; Talton, L.; Clagett-Dame, M. Mice null for NEDD9 (HEF1) display extensive hippocampal dendritic spine loss and cognitive impairment. *Brain Res.* **2016**, *1632*, 141–155. [CrossRef]
116. Filippi, C.G.; Watts, R.; Duy, L.A.; Cauley, K.A. Diffusion-tensor imaging derived metrics of the corpus callosum in children with neurofibromatosis type I. *Am. J. Roentgenol.* **2013**, *200*, 44–49. [CrossRef]
117. Stiles, J.; Brown, T.T.; Haist, F.; Jernigan, T.L. Brain and cognitive development. In *Handbook of Child Psychology and Developmental Science*; John Wiley and Sons: Hoboken, NJ, USA, 2015; pp. 1–54.
118. Morales, E.; Bustamante, M.; Gonzalez, J.R.; Guxens, M.; Torrent, M.; Mendez, M.; Garcia-Esteban, R.; Julvez, J.; Forns, J.; Vrijheid, M. Genetic variants of the FADS gene cluster and ELOVL gene family, colostrums LC-PUFA levels, breastfeeding, and child cognition. *PLoS ONE* **2011**, *6*, e17181. [CrossRef]
119. Caspi, A.; Williams, B.; Kim-Cohen, J.; Craig, I.W.; Milne, B.J.; Poulton, R.; Schalkwyk, L.C.; Taylor, A.; Werts, H.; Moffitt, T.E. Moderation of breastfeeding effects on the IQ by genetic variation in fatty acid metabolism. *Proc. Natl. Acad. Sci. USA* **2007**, *104*, 18860–18865. [CrossRef] [PubMed]
120. Steer, C.D.; Davey Smith, G.; Emmett, P.M.; Hibbeln, J.R.; Golding, J. FADS2 polymorphisms modify the effect of breastfeeding on child IQ. *PLoS ONE* **2010**, *5*, e11570. [CrossRef] [PubMed]
121. McGuire, M.K.; Meehan, C.L.; McGuire, M.A.; Williams, J.E.; Foster, J.; Sellen, D.W.; Kamau-Mbuthia, E.W.; Kamundia, E.W.; Mbugua, S.; Moore, S.E. What's normal? Oligosaccharide concentrations and profiles in milk produced by healthy women vary geographically. *Am. J. Clin. Nutr.* **2017**, *105*, 1086–1100. [CrossRef]
122. Dou, Y.; Luo, Y.; Xing, Y.; Liu, H.; Chen, B.; Zhu, L.; Ma, D.; Zhu, J. Human Milk Oligosaccharides Variation in Gestational Diabetes Mellitus Mothers. *Nutrients* **2023**, *15*, 1441. [CrossRef]
123. Samuel, T.M.; Binia, A.; de Castro, C.A.; Thakkar, S.K.; Billeaud, C.; Agosti, M.; Al-Jashi, I.; Costeira, M.J.; Marchini, G.; Martínez-Costa, C. Impact of maternal characteristics on human milk oligosaccharide composition over the first 4 months of lactation in a cohort of healthy European mothers. *Sci. Rep.* **2019**, *9*, 11767. [CrossRef]
124. Maxwell, J.R.; Yellowhair, T.R.; Oppong, A.Y.; Camacho, J.E.; Lowe, J.R.; Jantzie, L.L.; Ohls, R.K. Cognitive development in preterm infants: Multifaceted deficits reflect vulnerability of rigorous neurodevelopmental pathways. *Minerva Pediatr.* **2017**, *69*, 298–313. [CrossRef] [PubMed]
125. Moro, G.E.; Arslanoglu, S.; Bertino, E.; Corvaglia, L.; Montirosso, R.; Picaud, J.-C.; Polberger, S.; Schanler, R.J.; Steel, C.; van Goudoever, J. XII. Human milk in feeding premature infants: Consensus statement. *J. Pediatr. Gastroenterol. Nutr.* **2015**, *61*, S16–S19. [CrossRef] [PubMed]
126. Moukarzel, S.; Bode, L. Human milk oligosaccharides and the preterm infant: A journey in sickness and in health. *Clin. Perinatol.* **2017**, *44*, 193–207. [CrossRef]
127. Davis, E.C.; Wang, M.; Donovan, S.M. The role of early life nutrition in the establishment of gastrointestinal microbial composition and function. *Gut Microbes* **2017**, *8*, 143–171. [CrossRef]
128. Lewis, Z.T.; Totten, S.M.; Smilowitz, J.T.; Popovic, M.; Parker, E.; Lemay, D.G.; Van Tassell, M.L.; Miller, M.J.; Jin, Y.-S.; German, J.B. Maternal fucosyltransferase 2 status affects the gut bifidobacterial communities of breastfed infants. *Microbiome* **2015**, *3*, 13. [CrossRef]
129. Savignac, H.; Tramullas, M.; Kiely, B.; Dinan, T.; Cryan, J. Bifidobacteria modulate cognitive processes in an anxious mouse strain. *Behav. Brain Res.* **2015**, *287*, 59–72. [CrossRef] [PubMed]
130. Carlson, A.L.; Xia, K.; Azcarate-Peril, M.A.; Goldman, B.D.; Ahn, M.; Styner, M.A.; Thompson, A.L.; Geng, X.; Gilmore, J.H.; Knickmeyer, R.C. Infant gut microbiome associated with cognitive development. *Biol. Psychiatry* **2018**, *83*, 148–159. [CrossRef] [PubMed]
131. Galuska, C.E.; Rudloff, S.; Kuntz, S.; Borsch, C.; Reutzel, M.; Eckert, G.; Galuska, S.P.; Kunz, C. Metabolic fate and organ distribution of 13C-3′-sialyllactose and 13C-N-acetylneuraminic acid in wild-type mice–No evidence for direct incorporation into the brain. *J. Funct. Foods* **2020**, *75*, 104268. [CrossRef]
132. Cryan, J.F.; O'Riordan, K.J.; Cowan, C.S.; Sandhu, K.V.; Bastiaanssen, T.F.; Boehme, M.; Codagnone, M.G.; Cussotto, S.; Fulling, C.; Golubeva, A.V. The microbiota-gut-brain axis. *Physiol. Rev.* **2019**, *99*, 1877–2013. [CrossRef]
133. Wang, M.; Monaco, M.H.; Hauser, J.; Yan, J.; Dilger, R.N.; Donovan, S.M. Bovine milk oligosaccharides and human milk oligosaccharides modulate the gut microbiota composition and volatile fatty acid concentrations in a preclinical neonatal model. *Microorganisms* **2021**, *9*, 884. [CrossRef]
134. Fleming, S.A.; Hauser, J.; Yan, J.; Donovan, S.M.; Wang, M.; Dilger, R.N. A mediation analysis to identify links between gut bacteria and memory in context of human milk oligosaccharides. *Microorganisms* **2021**, *9*, 846. [CrossRef]
135. Keim, S.A.; Sullivan, J.A.; Sheppard, K.; Smith, K.; Ingol, T.; Boone, K.M.; Malloy-McCoy, A.; Oza-Frank, R. Feeding infants at the breast or feeding expressed human milk: Long-term cognitive, executive function, and eating behavior outcomes at age 6 years. *J. Pediatr.* **2021**, *233*, 66–73.e61. [CrossRef]
136. Richards, M.; Hardy, R.; Wadsworth, M.E. Long-term effects of breast-feeding in a national birth cohort: Educational attainment and midlife cognitive function. *Public Health Nutr.* **2002**, *5*, 631–635. [CrossRef]

137. Oddy, W.H.; Kendall, G.E.; Li, J.; Jacoby, P.; Robinson, M.; De Klerk, N.H.; Silburn, S.R.; Zubrick, S.R.; Landau, L.I.; Stanley, F.J. The long-term effects of breastfeeding on child and adolescent mental health: A pregnancy cohort study followed for 14 years. *J. Pediatr.* **2010**, *156*, 568–574. [CrossRef]
138. Lenehan, S.M.; Boylan, G.B.; Livingstone, V.; Fogarty, L.; Twomey, D.M.; Nikolovski, J.; Irvine, A.D.; Kiely, M.; Kenny, L.C.; Hourihane, J.O. The impact of short-term predominate breastfeeding on cognitive outcome at 5 years. *Acta Paediatr.* **2020**, *109*, 982–988. [CrossRef] [PubMed]
139. Nair, A.S. Publication bias-Importance of studies with negative results! *Indian J. Anaesth.* **2019**, *63*, 505. [CrossRef] [PubMed]
140. Chouraqui, J.-P. Does the contribution of human milk oligosaccharides to the beneficial effects of breast milk allow us to hope for an improvement in infant formulas? *Crit. Rev. Food Sci. Nutr.* **2021**, *61*, 1503–1514. [CrossRef] [PubMed]

nutrients

MDPI

Review

Potential Epigenetic Effects of Human Milk on Infants' Neurodevelopment

Giannoula Gialeli [1], Ourania Panagopoulou [1], Georgios Liosis [2] and Tania Siahanidou [1,*]

1 First Department of Pediatrics, Medical School, National & Kapodistrian University of Athens, 11527 Athens, Greece; giannoula.g@gmail.com (G.G.); niakinder@yahoo.gr (O.P.)
2 Neonatal Intensive Care Unit, "Elena Venizelou" General and Maternal Hospital, 11521 Athens, Greece; gtliosis@yahoo.gr
* Correspondence: siahan@med.uoa.gr; Tel.: +30-21-3201-3517

Abstract: The advantages of human milk feeding, especially in preterm babies, are well recognized. Infants' feeding with breast milk lowers the likelihood of developing a diverse range of non-communicable diseases later in life and it is also associated with improved neurodevelopmental outcomes. Although the precise mechanisms through which human milk feeding is linked with infants' neurodevelopment are still unknown, potential epigenetic effects of breast milk through its bioactive components, including non-coding RNAs, stem cells and microbiome, could at least partly explain this association. Micro- and long-non-coding RNAs, enclosed in milk exosomes, as well as breast milk stem cells, survive digestion, reach the circulation and can cross the blood–brain barrier. Certain non-coding RNAs potentially regulate genes implicated in brain development and function, whereas nestin-positive stem cells can possibly differentiate into neural cells or/and act as epigenetic regulators in the brain. Furthermore, breast milk microbiota contributes to the establishment of infant's gut microbiome, which is implicated in brain development via epigenetic modifications and key molecules' regulation. This narrative review provides an updated analysis of the relationship between breast milk feeding and infants' neurodevelopment via epigenetics, pointing out how breast milk's bioactive components could have an impact on the neurodevelopment of both full-term and preterm babies.

Keywords: epigenetics; human milk; neurodevelopment; miRNAs; long non-coding RNAs; stem cells; microbiome

1. Introduction

Almost fifty years ago, the international scientific community believed that a person's health and the expression of non-communicable diseases was solely a matter of that individual's gene pool, which was not influenced by external factors. However, primitive genetic patterns could not explain the explosive increase in cancer and other non-communicable metabolic disorders [1]. Barker's hypothesis provided a revolutionary answer to this issue. Based on the observation that coronary heart disease, obesity and type 2 diabetes had a higher incidence in the poorest areas of England, Professor Barker was able to link low birth weight and poor prenatal conditions to adult disease [2]. The fetal origins of adult disease (FOAD) hypothesis of Professor Barker holds that the embryo's genome exhibits developmental plasticity [3]. Stressors, such as malnutrition, may remodel the embryos genome in order to prepare it for adverse extrauterine conditions, thus allowing a single genotype to produce multiple phenotypes depending on intrauterine conditions [4]. Over the following years, the FOAD was extended to "the Developmental Origins of Health and Disease" (DOHaD) hypothesis, which suggests that environmental exposures during early life, in both prenatal and postnatal period, can permanently influence health and the vulnerability to disease in later life by "programming" the phenotype without altering the genotype [5–8]. This programming process involves heritable changes in gene expression, which are mediated through epigenetic modifications such as DNA methylation, histone modification, and the activation or silencing of genes associated with non-coding RNAs [6,9,10]. These epigenetic mechanisms are suspected to play a crucial role in developmental programming [11]. Maternal stressors such as obesity or malnutrition, smoking and diabetes, among others, are known triggers for epigenetic modifications in the offspring [6,12].

The majority of human development occurs in the first 1000 days starting from conception. This time period of perinatal programming is considered critical in determining further development and health [13,14]. Postnatally, human breast milk is known to reduce the probability of expression of a wide variety of non-communicable diseases [15,16]. Breast milk may modify the epigenetic mechanisms of the infants and influence their health intergenerationally [17,18]. It is hypothesized that breast milk promotes epigenetic modifications via its bioactive components, including growth factors, microbiota, stem cells, micro-RNAs (miRNAs) and long-non-coding-RNAs [16,17,19,20]. Several studies have also shown that breast milk feeding, especially with mother's own milk, is associated with improved neurodevelopmental outcomes in both full-term and preterm infants [21–23], whereas longer duration of exclusive breastfeeding has been linked to higher intelligence quotients [24] and improved cognitive development [25,26]. A positive impact of breast milk feeding on structural brain development in preterm babies has been demonstrated using brain magnetic resonance imaging (MRI) [27].

The underlying mechanisms that explain the connections between the consumption of breast milk—particularly the mother's own milk—and the subsequent neurodevelopmental outcomes, especially in the vulnerable population of very-low-birth-weight (VLBW, <1500 g) infants, have not yet been clarified. The potential epigenetic effects of human milk could mediate the associations between breast milk feeding and brain development/neurodevelopment. Interestingly, Xu et al. have recently demonstrated that the percentage of the mother's own milk intake during the hospital stay of VLBW infants was linked to changes in DNA methylation (DNAm) patterns of genes related to neurodevelopment at 5.5 years of age. Certain DNAm variations were associated with differences in brain structure and intelligence quotient (IQ) [28].

In this article, we discuss the potential epigenetic role of miRNAs and long non-coding RNAs, stem cells and microbiome of human milk on infants' neurodevelopment.

2. Methods

For this narrative review, a literature search was conducted using the databases PubMed, Medline, ScienceDirect and Google Scholar (last accessed on 4 August 2023). Specific keywords such as breast milk, epigenetics, non-coding RNAs, miRNAs, long non-coding RNAs, stem cells, microbiome, brain development, neurodevelopment, infants, and preterm birth or prematurity were used. The inclusion criteria were as follows: all types of articles, articles published in PubMed, and studies using both humans and animals. Articles not written in the English language, or for which full text was not available, or were grey literature were excluded. From the articles retrieved in the first round of search, additional articles were identified via a manual search among the cited references (Table 1).

Table 1. Characteristics of the included studies.

Sources	Type of Articles	No. of Articles	Human Studies	Preclinical Studies (Mice, Pups, Rats, In Vitro, In Situ)
PubMEd Medline ScienceDirect GoogleScholar	Research articles	64	52	12
	Reviews	58		
	Total	122		

3. MiRNAs

A number of recent publications have demonstrated that human milk contains components recently described as extracellular vesicles (EVs) [29]. Extracellular vesicles is a term for all phospholipid bilayer-enclosed particles that are released by cells into their environment and include exosomes and microvesicles [29]. Exosomes carry bioactive substances like proteins, DNA, messenger RNA (mRNA) and miRNAs [29,30]. Breast milk exosomes, being resistant to digestion [31], are able to transport their cargo and miRNAs to peripheral tissues via the systemic circulation and facilitate the epigenetic programming of various tissues and organs [20]. For this reason, they are considered important signaling molecules (signalosomes) between mother and child [20,32]. Since exosomes are also able to cross the blood–brain barrier, it is possible that the positive impact of breast milk on neurodevelopment is associated with miRNAs' activity [33].

MiRNAs are small, single-stranded, non-coding RNA molecules containing 18 to 25 nucleotides. MiRNAs are also found in plants, animals and viruses, among others [34], and they are capable of controlling up to 60% of gene expression [35,36] by inhibiting mRNA translation into protein. These particles are, thus, involved in post-transcriptional gene regulation [37–39]. Breast milk has been categorized as one of the biological fluids that possesses a high concentration of miRNAs encapsulated in exosomes or as free molecules, with more than 1400 distinct miRNAs identified [36,40]. Not only is human milk highly enriched in miRNAs, but it has also the highest concentration of miRNAs compared to other body fluids, including plasma [20,40]. While previous research was focused on analyzing miRNAs in the skim fraction of breast milk, recent studies investigating the lipid and cell fractions of milk have revealed a larger quantity and diversity of miRNAs compared to the skim fraction [36]. A systematic review of 30 studies on non-coding RNAs of human breast milk showed that 10 miRNAs, including miR-148a-3p, miR-30a-5p, miR-30d-5p, miR-22-3p, miR-146b-5p, miR-200a-3p, miR-200c-3p, let-7a-5p, let-7b-5p and let-7f-5p, were the most abundant miRNAs in all breast milk fractions examined [19].

Several factors have been identified to affect the miRNAs' composition of breast milk. For example, there is evidence that the miRNAs' concentration in human milk is influenced by the stage of lactation. Hatmall et al. reported that the total concentration of miRNA in colostrum was significantly higher than that of mature milk [40]. Similarly, Xi et al. found that the concentrations of let-7a and miRNA-378 were higher, whereas the concentration of miRNA-30B was lower, in colostrum than in mature milk [41]. On the contrary, in another study, similar levels of let-7a, mi-R16, miR-21, miR-146b, miR-181a, miR-150, and miR-223 were found across various lactation stages [42]. Differences have also been observed in species and in the expression of several miRNAs between fore- and hind-milk [18]. Although the majority of known miRNAs were identified in both pre- and post-feed milk, a number of miRNAs were found to be specific to pre-feed (n = 159) or post-feed milk (n = 180); none of the pre-feed milk-specific miRNAs was found in any post-feed samples, and vice versa [43]. Interestingly, freezer storage at −80 °C did not affect the variations in miRNAs of breast milk, indicating their stability [18].

In addition, maternal conditions such as diabetes mellitus, overweight or obesity, diet or even psychosocial factors and stress can influence the human milk miRNAs. In a study conducted by Shat et al., the levels of miRNA-148a, miRNA-30b, miRNA-let-7a, and miRNA-let-7d were found to be lower in the milk of mothers with gestational diabetes mellitus [44]. Aberrant levels of several miRNAs have also been detected in breast milk of mothers with type 1 diabetes [45]. Furthermore, in a study from Kupso et al., the expression of the majority (374 out of the 419) of miRNAs analyzed in human milk extracellular vesicles was found to correlate negatively with maternal BMI [46]. Similarly, Shah et al. showed that the exosomal content of breast milk in selected miRNAs, such as miR-148a and miR-30b, was lower by 30% and 42%, respectively, in overweight/obese mothers in comparison with a normal-weight control group [47]. In another study, 19 miRNAs including miR-575, miR-630, miR-642a-3p, and miR-652-5p, which are associated both per se and by their target genes with neurological diseases and psychological disorders, were differentially expressed in breast milk exosomes of obese nursing mothers [48]. Concerning maternal diet, animals fed an obesogenic dietary pattern exhibited higher concentrations of miR-222 and lower levels of miR-200 and miR-26 compared to the control group [49]. In humans, the expression of novel miRNAs, specifically miR-67 and miR-27, was increased in milk fat globules of women following a high-fat diet compared to those following a high-carbohydrate diet with similar calorie and protein content [50]. Additionally, maternal lifetime stress and negative life events during pregnancy were associated with the detection and expression of certain miRNAs in breast milk, such as hsa-miR-96-5p and hsa-miR-155-5p, which may be related to stress, postnatal development, and cognitive function of the offspring [51].

Concerning the association between breast milk miRNAs and improved infants' neurodevelopment, there is evidence that several miRNAs of breast milk, such as let-7a, miR-15b miR-21, miR-29b, miR-30, miR-132, miR-138, miR-148, miR-210 and miR-574, among others, may play important roles in brain development and function [52]. For example, let-7 miRNAs are highly expressed in the developing mammalian brain and regulate neural cell proliferation and differentiation [53–55]. Furthermore, Walgrave et al. have demonstrated that introducing miR-132, an miRNA existing also in human milk [52], into the hippocampus of adult mice with Alzheimer's disease restores adult hippocampal neurogenesis and improves memory deficits associated with the disease [56]. These findings highlight the potential therapeutic value of targeting miR-132 in addressing neurodegeneration. Similarly, studies in animals and humans have shown that miR-148a, which is one of the most abundant miRNAs in human milk exosomes [19], is involved in many cellular pathways, regulates neural development and exerts neuroprotective effects [18,57]. Moreover, researchers have found that several miRNAs are linked to autism spectrum disorder and may be used as potential biomarkers both for the diagnosis and prognosis of this disorder [58]. The neuroprotective effect of selected exosomal miRNAs, such as miR-21, miR-29b, miR-30 and miR-138, which can also be present in human milk, was also discussed by Nasirishargh et al. in a review article [59]. The neuroprotective effects of these miRNAs are exerted by promoting neurogenesis, neurite remodeling and survival, and neuroplasticity [59]. Especially regarding neuroplasticity, many miRNAs are involved in synaptic plasticity [60], whereas several human milk exosomal miRNAs are implicated in the gene regulation of brain synapses and in synaptic vesicle trafficking [61]. It is worth mentioning that almost half of miRNAs with possible effects on synaptic development in mammals were found to be present in the top 288 miRNAs identified in human milk exosomes [62].

Although there are studies showing that the majority of miRNAs expressed in term milk are also present in preterm milk (derived from mothers with term and preterm birth, respectively) [63,64], differences in several miRNAs have been reported between preterm and term breast milk [63,65]. For example, Shiff et al. noted higher levels of miR-148 and lower levels of miRNA-320 in both the skim and lipid fractions of colostrum samples of preterm compared to term breast milk [65]. There is also evidence that the expression patterns of nine miRNAs (miR378a-3p, miR378c, miR-378g, miR-1260a, miR-1260b, miR-4783-5p, miR-4784, miR-5787, and miR-7975) in lipid and skim fraction of preterm breast milk exhibited variations compared to those in term breast milk. The targeted genes of these miRNAs were functionally associated with elemental metabolism and lipid biosynthesis [63]. In the same study, it was also demonstrated that a total of 113 miRNAs exhibited significant differences in expression between the lipid samples of term and preterm breast milk. Among those, 68 miRNAs showed downregulation in the preterm breast milk lipid fractions, while 45 miRNAs displayed upregulation [63]. Studies in animals also provided evidence that the exosomal content of human preterm breast milk has the potential to enable tissue healing in preterms with intestinal inflammation and protect against necrotizing enterocolitis [66]. Recent evidence has also shown significant differences between preterm and term human breast milk exosomes in several miRNAs associated with brain development and neurodevelopment including miR-3196, miR-1249-3p, miR-7847-3p, miR-1908-3p and miR-23b-3p, among others [61]. Further research in this area is needed.

Overall, these findings show that miRNAs, which are well-established epigenetic modulators, are abundant in human breast milk and they are influenced by several factors relevant to lactation per se, maternal health and disease and preterm birth. They can reach the brain by crossing the blood–brain barrier, whereas several of them possess neuroprotective effects and can regulate the expression of genes implicated in infants' brain development and function (Figure 1).

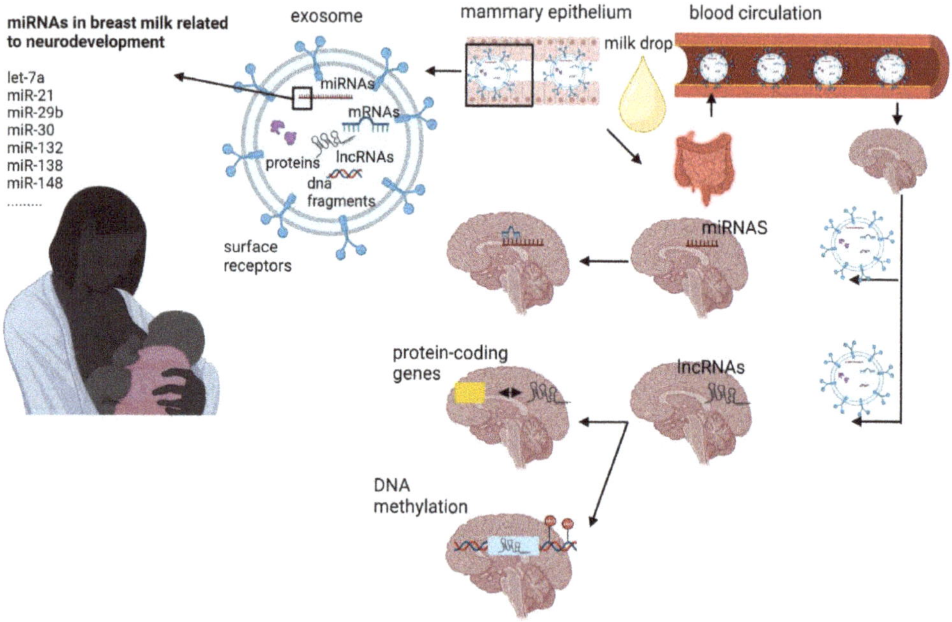

Figure 1. Potential mechanisms through which breast milk miRNAs and lncRNAs may be implicated in brain signaling cascade of breastfed infants. Mammary gland cells produce and release exosomes into the breast milk. Exosomes are taken up by the infant's intestinal cells and are capable to cross the blood–brain barrier. Once inside brain cells, exosomes release their cargo (including miRNAs and lncRNAs). MiRNAs target mRNA and this binding results in modulation of gene expression. LncRNAs can interact with near protein coding genes and this interaction may involve cis-regulation of nearby genes or trans-regulation of genes in distant regions. Illustration created with BioRender.com accessed on 16 August 2023.

4. Long Non-Coding RNAs

In addition to miRNAs, breast milk also contains other types of regulatory non-coding RNAs, such as long non-coding RNAs (lncRNAs). Long non-coding RNAs are RNA molecules that are typically composed of at least 200 nucleotides [67]. They are often formed through the splicing of two or more exons derived from genomic regions located near protein-coding genes [19].

LncRNAs have a crucial role in processes such as neurogenesis, synaptogenesis, and the development of the brain (Figure 1). The utilization of high-throughput technologies has revealed their specific expression in distinct cell types, subcellular compartments, and various brain regions [68,69]. Numerous lncRNAs exhibit expression patterns that vary with age [70] and actively contribute to the determination of neural cell fate [71]. Given their involvement in these essential processes, any abnormal expression of these transcripts has the potential to lead to neurodevelopmental or neuropsychiatric disorders, including, but not limited to, autism spectrum disorder and schizophrenia [71,72].

Karlsson et al. detected 55 lncRNAs (out of 87 screened) in human milk exosomes; of them, 5 lncRNAs (CRNDE, DANCR, GAS5, SRA1 and ZFAS1) were found to be present in more than 90% of milk samples. Many of the detected lncRNAs are known to have important epigenetic roles in immune function and metabolism and are potentially related to children's development and health [73].

Additionally, Mourtzi et al. [74] screened 88 lncRNAs in breast milk exosomes and showed that 13 lncRNAs were detected in more than 85% of milk samples, whereas 31 lncRNAs were detected in more than 50% of samples. In the same study, the expression of lncRNAs was compared between preterm and term breast milk. Differential expression analysis demonstrated at least two-fold differences in the expression of lncRNAs between the two groups, with levels of lncRNAs being higher in term breast milk as compared to the preterm one [74]. Interestingly, although the non-coding RNA activated at DNA damage (NORAD) was abundant in exosomes in both preterm and term breast milk, its expression was found to be significantly downregulated in the preterm milk exosomes. In previous studies, NORAD is a lncRNA involved in the DNA damage response and repair pathway and it is referred to as "the guardian of the human genome". NORAD has been proven to demonstrate a protective role in mitigating brain damage, cellular apoptosis, oxidative stress, and inflammation induced by cerebral ischemia/reperfusion injury [75]. Its protective mechanism involves the regulation of miR-30a-5p and subsequent upregulation of YWHAG expression [75]. It could be suggested that utilizing lncRNAs, especially NORAD, isolated from human milk may offer a potential way to safeguard premature infants and improve their neurodevelopmental outcomes.

Another lncRNA exhibiting specific expression patterns during brain development and progenitor cell differentiation is the Sox2OT (Sox2 overlapping transcript). It has been demonstrated that by suppressing the expression of Sox2OT in mice, sepsis-induced deficits in hippocampal neurogenesis and cognitive function were improved. This improvement was achieved through the downregulation of the transcription factor SOX2. Thus, inhibiting the signaling pathway involving Sox2OT and SOX2 may hold promise as a potential therapeutic approach for treating or preventing neurological damage associated with sepsis-induced encephalopathy [76]. However, it has not yet been studied whether Sox2OT or factors inhibiting this lncRNA is/are present in human breast milk.

From the above, it is evident that, compared to miRNAs, lncRNAs of breast milk have been much less studied to date and only from an immunological and metabolic point of view. NORAD, referred to as "the guardian of the human genome" and shown to have a neuroprotective epigenetic role, was found to be abundant in human breast milk; however, it was downregulated in preterm compared to term human milk. Further studies are needed to investigate human milk non-coding RNAs related to brain development and neurodevelopment in full-term and preterm babies.

5. Stem Cells

Stem cells possess a remarkable capacity for both self-renewal, sustaining their undifferentiated state, and differentiation into various cell types and tissues in specific conditions [77–79]. In contrast, adult cells traditionally maintain their lineage commitment, yet recent studies have revealed promising approaches to induce cellular plasticity, allowing them to potentially transform into diverse cell types. This breakthrough holds significant implications for cell-based therapies in the field of regenerative medicine [79].

The discovery of stem cells within human milk dates back to 2007 [80], highlighting their presence in this unique fluid. Breastfeeding has long been recognized for its protective effects against diseases that may arise later in life, although their precise mechanism remains elusive. The presence of stem cells in both preterm and term human breast milk [81] offers one potential explanation for these beneficial effects. Interestingly, in animal studies, breast milk stem cells survive digestion and enter into the circulation and the brain, where they can be differentiated into neuronal and glial cells [82].

Stem cells from human milk contain both genetic material and bioactive molecules, such as microRNAs, which can act as epigenetic regulators [83]. The beneficial effects of breast milk stem cells may also be mediated through the paracrine action of exosomes released by these cells [84,85]. Moreover, by using the marker nestin, Cregan et al. identified nestin-positive putative stem cells in human breast milk [80]. Nestin (acronym for neuroepithelial stem cell protein) is a marker for multipotent stem cells that can differentiate into neural cells [86]. Indeed, Hosseini et al. [87] showed that human breast milk derived stem cells can differentiate into neural lineages (oligodendrocytes, astrocytes, and neurons). This differentiation capacity of milk stem cells offers valuable insights into the beneficial effects of human milk on neurodevelopment. That discovery also indicates the potential use of these cells as a suitable and easy source for cell replacement therapies targeting brain diseases. Thus, breast milk stem cells, either through their differentiation into neural cells or/and by acting as epigenetic regulators in the brain (Figure 2), seem to have opened up new horizons in the explanation of the positive short- and long-term impact of human milk. However, further research is required to elucidate their exact mechanism(s) of action after breastfeeding and define the extent of their capabilities.

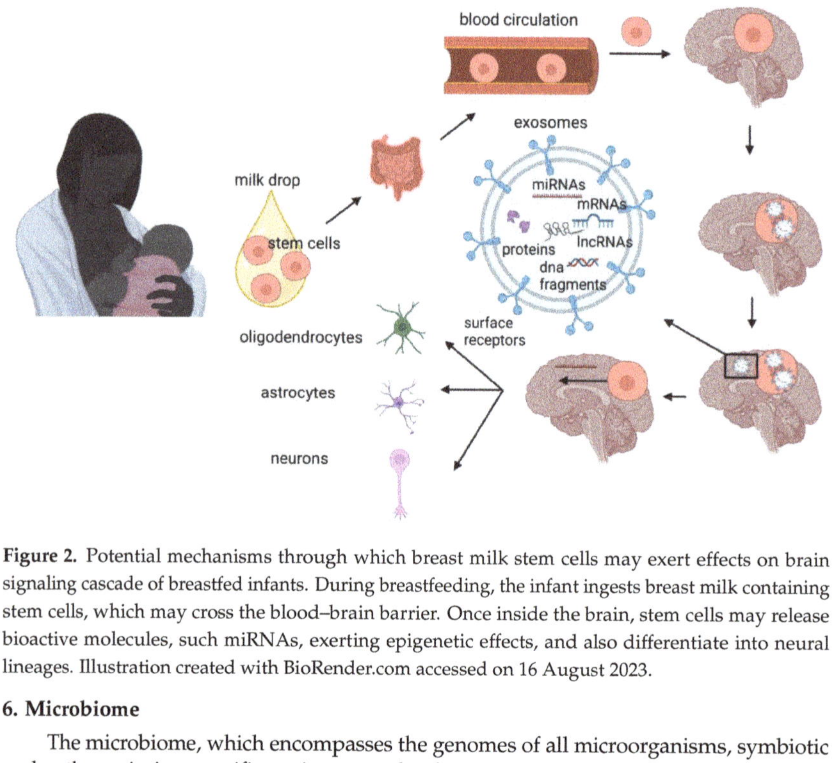

Figure 2. Potential mechanisms through which breast milk stem cells may exert effects on brain signaling cascade of breastfed infants. During breastfeeding, the infant ingests breast milk containing stem cells, which may cross the blood–brain barrier. Once inside the brain, stem cells may release bioactive molecules, such miRNAs, exerting epigenetic effects, and also differentiate into neural lineages. Illustration created with BioRender.com accessed on 16 August 2023.

6. Microbiome

The microbiome, which encompasses the genomes of all microorganisms, symbiotic and pathogenic, in a specific environment, has been extensively studied [88,89]. Previous assumptions regarding the existence of bacteria in human milk attributed their presence to contamination or mastitis [90,91]. However, during the early 2000s, research emerged revealing the existence of commensal bacteria in human milk and provided evidence that the DNA of these bacteria differed from that found on the surface of the breast skin, indicating that they were distinct entities [92–94]. By using next-generation sequencing techniques, it was found that half of the microorganism population was the same in all milk samples composing the core bacterial microbiota (bacteriome) [95]. The predominant phyla reported in human milk are Proteobacteria, Firmicutes, Actinobacteria, and Bacteroidetes. When examining the genus level, the most abundant taxa include Bifidobacterium, Lactobacillus, Streptococcus, Staphylococcus, Ralstonia, Bacteroides, Enterobacter, and Enterococcus, among others [96,97].

The composition of breast milk microbiota may be influenced by various factors. Among them, the impact of the stage of lactation on the composition of microbiota in breast milk has been investigated in several studies [98–102]. Findings have been inconsistent, with some studies reporting higher total bacterial loads in colostrum compared to mature milk [98,99], while others have observed an increase in bacterial loads throughout the lactation period [100,101]. On the contrary, certain studies did not detect significant alterations in bacterial numbers in breast milk samples collected within the first month after delivery, suggesting stability in microbial composition during this early period [102]. These varying results highlight the complexity and diversity of microbiota present in breast milk.

The complexity and diversity of breast milk microbiota have implications for understanding the influence of other factors on its composition. Probiotic administration during pregnancy did not influence the composition of the microbiota of breast milk, according to three separate studies involving participant sizes of 84, 125, and 20 women [97,103–105]. Similarly, the impact of smoking on the diversity and composition of the breast milk microbiota was examined in a study involving 393 participants, revealing no significant effects [96]. When considering milk expression methods, it was observed that using a breast pump rather than manual expression was associated with lower bacterial richness in breast milk; this could be attributed to the non-aseptic protocol used for milk collection [96].

Maternal factors, such as body mass index (BMI) and health conditions, like allergies and celiac disease, can also influence the composition of the human milk microbiota. For instance, women with higher BMI tend to exhibit a less diverse bacterial community in the breast milk microbiota, along with higher total bacterial loads and increased abundance of Lactobacillus in colostrum [106]. Nonetheless, it is important to note that in other studies, no significant impact of BMI on the composition of the breast milk microbiota was observed [96,107]. Moreover, it has been demonstrated that allergic mothers have significantly lower counts of Bifidobacteria in their breast milk compared to non-allergic mothers, as assessed using specific primers [108]. Similarly, women with celiac disease were found to have lower relative levels of Bifidobacterium and Bacteroides in their breast milk [109].

A recent cross-sectional study was carried out to examine the correlation between the milk microbiome and neurodevelopment, specifically focusing on head circumference-for-age z-scores (HCAZ) in breastfed infants [110]. Significant differences in the milk microbiota composition were found between infants with HCAZ ≥ -1 SD and HCAZ < -1 SD at both early ($\leq$46 days postpartum) and late stages of lactation (109–184 days postpartum). The HCAZ ≥ -1 SD group had a higher abundance of Streptococcus species associated with human milk, while the HCAZ < -1 SD group, particularly at the late stage of lactation, exhibited a higher abundance of differentially abundant taxa associated with environmentally and potentially opportunistic species. These findings suggest a potential association between the milk microbiome and brain growth in breastfed infants during lactation, necessitating, however, further investigation into the interplay between the human milk microbiome and infant neurodevelopment [110].

The microbiome of breast milk shares common characteristics with the gut microbiome. After the establishment of bacterial colonization in infants, the composition of intestinal microbes becomes distinct and individualized [111]. While there is variability among individuals, the majority of these microbes can be categorized into the following four main phyla: Firmicutes, Bacteroidetes, Actinobacteria, and Proteobacteria [111]. This pattern of phyla is also observed in the microbial composition of human milk [96,97]. A study conducted by Pannaraj et al. showed that the bacterial communities of maternal milk contributed to the establishment and development of the infant gut microbiome [112]. These results emphasize the significance of the microbiome of breast milk in shaping the intestinal microbiome, including colonization with beneficial bacteria. Similarly, in the study of Solis et al., certain strains of bifidobacteria, which displayed identical genetic profiles as determined via Random Amplified Polymorphic DNA analyses, were found both in the breast milk samples of mothers and in the fecal samples of their infants taken at several time points during the first 3 months after birth. This finding suggests that there is a vertical transfer of specific bifidobacterial strains from the mother's milk to the infant [99].

There is evidence that the gut microbiome during early life contributes to the establishment of epigenetic modifications and it is also associated with brain development and neurodevelopment [113–115]. The colonization of the infant's intestine after birth, influenced by maternal flora, delivery method, early skin-to-skin contact, and neonatal diet, results in specific epigenetic patterns that can influence the protective function of the gut mucosa against future insults [116]. Furthermore, the gut microorganisms secrete molecules which can reach the brain via the circulatory system after absorption and affect the brain's development (Figure 3), especially during sensitive periods (gut–brain axis) [117]. Interestingly, in a recent study in a humanized mouse model, the aberrant gut microbiome of preterm infants had negative effects on brain organization and maturation, and brain metabolism, as well as on behavior and memory [114]. The connection between the gut microbiome and brain function has led to investigations into its potential role in neurobehavioral disorders, such as autism spectrum disorder (ASD), anxiety and attention-deficit-hyperactivity disorder [118]. It has been reported that children with ASD have a dysbiotic microbiome with an abundance of Bacteroidetes in feces [119]. The presence of these bacteria in fecal samples could potentially explain the occurrence of gastrointestinal symptoms in certain individuals with ASD [120,121]. As neurodevelopmental impairments are often linked to the degree of prematurity, optimizing the microbial environment in early life becomes crucial for promoting healthy neurodevelopment in this vulnerable population [122]. Considering that the maternal breast milk microbiome colonizes the infant's gut and presents similar species to the gut microbiome of the infants, it can possibly be extrapolated that mother's breast milk microbiome also has epigenetic influences and it is associated with infants' brain function and neurodevelopment. The precise mechanisms through which the breast milk microbiome carries out such effects on infants' brains remain to be elucidated.

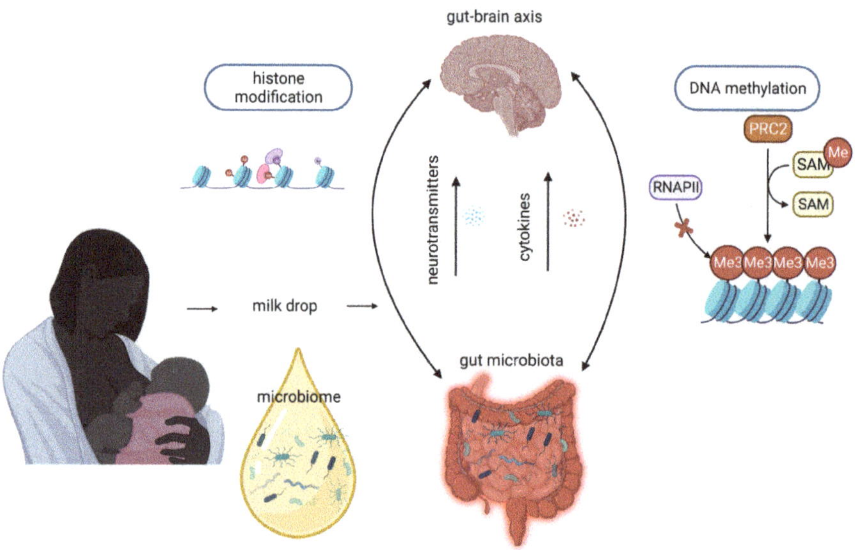

Figure 3. Potential mechanisms through which breast milk microbiota may exert effects on brain signaling cascades of breastfed infants. Breast milk microbiome colonizes the infant's gut and possibly shares similar epigenetic influences on the infant's brain. Illustration created with BioRender.com accessed on 16 August 2023.

7. Conclusions

This article discusses the impact of breast milk bioactive factors, such as microRNAs (miRNAs), long non-coding RNAs (lncRNAs), stem cells, and the microbiome, on the neurodevelopment of preterm-born children through epigenetic mechanisms.

MiRNAs, small RNA molecules that regulate gene expression, are abundant in human milk and can be transferred to peripheral tissues through exosomes, which are resistant to digestion and capable of crossing the blood–brain barrier. These miRNAs, including let-7a, miR-15b, miR-21, miR-29b, miR-30, miR-132, miR-138, miR-148, miR-210, and miR-574, among others, play crucial roles in neurodevelopment. Additionally, human milk contains lncRNAs, such as NORAD, which exhibit protective properties against brain damage, oxidative stress, and inflammation. Stem cells, including neural stem cells, have also been identified in breast milk, contributing to its beneficial effects on neurodevelopment. Furthermore, the breast milk microbiome, composed of bacteria that seed and colonize the infant's gut, likely shares with the gut microbiome similar effects on infant's epigenetics and neurodevelopment. The comprehensive insights shared in this review aim to provide clarity on the link between breastfeeding and the fundamental mechanisms driving the Developmental Origins of Health and Disease (DOHaD) concept. By discussing the potential contributions of bioactive elements in breast milk, such as miRNAs, lncRNAs, stem cells, and the microbiome, to neurodevelopment through epigenetic processes, this study provides a compelling link between early life experiences and enduring health consequences in both preterm- and term-born infants.

Author Contributions: Conceptualization, G.L. and T.S.; methodology, G.L. and G.G.; formal analysis, T.S.; investigation, G.G. and T.S.; resources, G.G. and O.P.; data curation, G.G. and O.P.; writing—original draft preparation, G.G. and O.P.; writing—review and editing, T.S.; visualization, G.L.; supervision, T.S. and G.L. All authors have read and agreed to the published version of the manuscript.

Funding: This research received no external funding.

Institutional Review Board Statement: Not applicable.

Informed Consent Statement: Not applicable.

Data Availability Statement: Not applicable.

Conflicts of Interest: The authors declare no conflict of interest.

References

1. GBD 2015 Obesity Collaborators; Afshin, A.; Forouzanfar, M.H.; Reitsma, M.B.; Sur, P.; Estep, K.; Lee, A.; Marczak, L.; Mokdad, A.H.; Moradi-Lakeh, M.; et al. Health Effects of Overweight and Obesity in 195 Countries over 25 Years. *N. Engl. J. Med.* **2017**, *377*, 13–27. [CrossRef] [PubMed]
2. Wilson, J. The Barker hypothesis. An analysis. *Aust. N. Z. J. Obstet. Gynaecol.* **1999**, *39*, 1–7. [CrossRef] [PubMed]
3. Calkins, K.; Devaskar, S.U. Fetal origins of adult disease. *Curr. Probl. Pediatr. Adolesc. Health Care* **2011**, *41*, 158–176. [CrossRef] [PubMed]
4. Barker, D.J.; Osmond, C.; Kajantie, E.; Eriksson, J.G. Growth and chronic disease: Findings in the Helsinki Birth Cohort. *Ann. Hum. Biol.* **2009**, *36*, 445–458. [CrossRef]
5. Barker, D.J. The developmental origins of adult disease. *J. Am. Coll. Nutr.* **2004**, *23*, 588S–595S. [CrossRef] [PubMed]
6. Goyal, D.; Limesand, S.W.; Goyal, R. Epigenetic responses and the developmental origins of health and disease. *J. Endocrinol.* **2019**, *242*, T105–T119. [CrossRef]
7. Holme, A.M.; Sitras, V. Developmental origin of health and disease—Evidence and time for action. *Acta Obstet. Gynecol. Scand.* **2020**, *99*, 961–962. [CrossRef]
8. Heindel, J.J.; Balbus, J.; Birnbaum, L.; Brune-Drisse, M.N.; Grandjean, P.; Gray, K.; Landrigan, P.J.; Sly, P.D.; Suk, W.A.; Cory Slechta, D.; et al. Developmental Origins of Health and Disease: Integrating Environmental Influences. *Endocrinology* **2015**, *156*, 3416–3421. [CrossRef]
9. Petronis, A. Epigenetics as a unifying principle in the aetiology of complex traits and diseases. *Nature* **2010**, *465*, 721–727. [CrossRef]
10. Deichmann, U. Epigenetics: The origins and evolution of a fashionable topic. *Dev. Biol.* **2016**, *416*, 249–254. [CrossRef]
11. Chen, M.; Zhang, L. Epigenetic mechanisms in developmental programming of adult disease. *Drug Discov. Today* **2011**, *16*, 1007–1018. [CrossRef] [PubMed]

12. Banik, A.; Kandilya, D.; Ramya, S.; Stünkel, W.; Chong, Y.S.; Dheen, S.T. Maternal Factors that Induce Epigenetic Changes Contribute to Neurological Disorders in Offspring. *Genes* **2017**, *8*, 150. [CrossRef] [PubMed]
13. Barker, D.J.P. Sir Richard Doll Lecture. Developmental origins of chronic disease. *Public Health* **2012**, *126*, 185–189. [CrossRef] [PubMed]
14. Plagemann, A. Maternal diabetes and perinatal programming. *Early Hum. Dev.* **2011**, *87*, 743–747. [CrossRef]
15. Horta, B.L.; de Lima, N.P. Breastfeeding and Type 2 Diabetes: Systematic Review and Meta-Analysis. *Curr. Diab. Rep.* **2019**, *19*, 1. [CrossRef]
16. Camacho-Morales, A.; Caba, M.; García-Juárez, M.; Caba-Flores, M.D.; Viveros-Contreras, R.; Martínez-Valenzuela, C. Breastfeeding Contributes to Physiological Immune Programming in the Newborn. *Front. Pediatr.* **2021**, *9*, 744104. [CrossRef]
17. Ozkan, H.; Tuzun, F.; Taheri, S.; Korhan, P.; Akokay, P.; Yılmaz, O.; Duman, N.; Özer, E.; Tufan, E.; Kumral, A.; et al. Epigenetic Programming Through Breast Milk and Its Impact on Milk-Siblings Mating. *Front. Genet.* **2020**, *11*, 569232. [CrossRef]
18. Chutipongtanate, S.; Morrow, A.L.; Newburg, D.S. Human Milk Extracellular Vesicles: A Biological System with Clinical Implications. *Cells* **2022**, *11*, 2345. [CrossRef]
19. Tingö, L.; Ahlberg, E.; Johansson, L.; Pedersen, S.A.; Chawla, K.; Sætrom, P.; Cione, E.; Simpson, M.R. Non-Coding RNAs in Human Breast Milk: A Systematic Review. *Front. Immunol.* **2021**, *12*, 725323. [CrossRef]
20. Melnik, B.C.; Stremmel, W.; Weiskirchen, R.; John, S.M.; Schmitz, G. Exosome-Derived MicroRNAs of Human Milk and Their Effects on Infant Health and Development. *Biomolecules* **2021**, *11*, 851. [CrossRef]
21. Koh, K. Maternal breastfeeding and children's cognitive development. *Soc. Sci. Med.* **2017**, *187*, 101–108. [CrossRef] [PubMed]
22. Wallenborn, J.T.; Levine, G.A.; Santos, A.C.D.; Grisi, S.; Brentani, A.; Fink, G. Breastfeeding, Physical Growth, and Cognitive Development. *Pediatrics* **2021**, *147*, e2020008029. [CrossRef]
23. Lewallen, L.P. Breastfeeding is important for cognitive development in term and preterm infants. *Evid. Based Nurs.* **2012**, *15*, 85–86. [CrossRef] [PubMed]
24. Horta, B.L.; de Mola, C.L.; Victora, C.G. Breastfeeding and intelligence: A systematic review and meta-analysis. *Acta Paediatr.* **2015**, *104*, 14–19. [CrossRef]
25. Kramer, M.S.; Aboud, F.; Mironova, E.; Vanilovich, I.; Platt, R.W.; Matush, L.; Igumnov, S.; Fombonne, E.; Bogdanovich, N.; Ducruet, T.; et al. Breastfeeding and child cognitive development: New evidence from a large randomized trial. *Arch. Gen. Psychiatry* **2008**, *65*, 578–584. [CrossRef] [PubMed]
26. Chetta, K.E.; Schulz, E.V.; Wagner, C.L. Outcomes improved with human milk intake in preterm and full-term infants. *Semin. Perinatol.* **2021**, *45*, 151384. [CrossRef] [PubMed]
27. Sullivan, G.; Vaher, K.; Blesa, M.; Galdi, P.; Stoye, D.Q.; Quigley, A.J.; Thrippleton, M.J.; Norrie, J.; Bastin, M.E.; Boardman, J.P. Breast Milk Exposure is Associated with Cortical Maturation in Preterm Infants. *Ann. Neurol.* **2022**, *93*, 591–603. [CrossRef] [PubMed]
28. Xu, J.; Shin, J.; McGee, M.; Unger, S.; Bando, N.; Sato, J.; Vandewouw, M.; Patel, Y.; Branson, H.M.; Paus, T.; et al. Intake of mother's milk by very-low-birth-weight infants and variation in DNA methylation of genes involved in neurodevelopment at 5.5 years of age. *Am. J. Clin. Nutr.* **2022**, *116*, 1038–1048. [CrossRef] [PubMed]
29. Hu, Y.; Thaler, J.; Nieuwland, R. Extracellular Vesicles in Human Milk. *Pharmaceuticals* **2021**, *14*, 1050. [CrossRef] [PubMed]
30. He, S.; Liu, G.; Zhu, X. Human breast milk-derived exosomes may help maintain intestinal epithelial barrier integrity. *Pediatr. Res.* **2021**, *90*, 366–372. [CrossRef]
31. Shandilya, S.; Rani, P.; Onteru, S.K.; Singh, D. Small Interfering RNA in Milk Exosomes Is Resistant to Digestion and Crosses the Intestinal Barrier In Vitro. *J. Agric. Food Chem.* **2017**, *65*, 9506–9513. [CrossRef] [PubMed]
32. Melnik, B.C.; John, S.M.; Schmitz, G. Milk is not just food but most likely a genetic transfection system activating mTORC1 signaling for postnatal growth. *Nutr. J.* **2013**, *12*, 103. [CrossRef] [PubMed]
33. Chen, C.C.; Liu, L.; Ma, F.; Wong, C.W.; Guo, X.E.; Chacko, J.V.; Farhoodi, H.P.; Zhang, S.X.; Zimak, J.; Ségaliny, A.; et al. Elucidation of Exosome Migration across the Blood–Brain Barrier Model In Vitro. *Cell. Mol. Bioeng.* **2016**, *9*, 509–529. [CrossRef] [PubMed]
34. Green, D.; Dalmay, T.; Chapman, T. Microguards and micromessengers of the genome. *Heredity* **2016**, *116*, 125–134. [CrossRef] [PubMed]
35. Ying, S.-Y.; Chang, D.C.; Lin, S.-L. The microRNA (miRNA): Overview of the RNA genes that modulate gene function. *Mol. Biotechnol.* **2008**, *38*, 257–268. [CrossRef] [PubMed]
36. Carrillo-Lozano, E.; Sebastián-Valles, F.; Knott-Torcal, C. Circulating microRNAs in Breast Milk and Their Potential Impact on the Infant. *Nutrients* **2020**, *12*, 3066. [CrossRef] [PubMed]
37. Bartel, D.P. Metazoan MicroRNAs. *Cell* **2018**, *173*, 20–51. [CrossRef]
38. Bartel, D.P. MicroRNAs: Genomics, biogenesis, mechanism, and function. *Cell* **2004**, *116*, 281–297. [CrossRef]
39. Wang, Z. MicroRNA: A matter of life or death. *World J. Biol. Chem.* **2010**, *1*, 41–54. [CrossRef]
40. Hatmal, M.M.; Al-Hatamleh, M.A.I.; Olaimat, A.N.; Alshaer, W.; Hasan, H.; Albakri, K.A.; Alkhafaji, E.; Issa, N.N.; Al-Holy, M.A.; Abderrahman, S.M.; et al. Immunomodulatory Properties of Human Breast Milk: MicroRNA Contents and Potential Epigenetic Effects. *Biomedicines* **2022**, *10*, 1219. [CrossRef]
41. Xi, Y.; Jiang, X.; Li, R.; Chen, M.; Song, W.; Li, X. The levels of human milk microRNAs and their association with maternal weight characteristics. *Eur. J. Clin. Nutr.* **2016**, *70*, 445–449. [CrossRef]

42. Alsaweed, M.; Lai, C.T.; Hartmann, P.E.; Geddes, D.T.; Kakulas, F. Human Milk Cells and Lipids Conserve Numerous Known and Novel miRNAs, Some of Which Are Differentially Expressed during Lactation. *PLoS ONE* **2016**, *11*, e0152610. [CrossRef] [PubMed]
43. Alsaweed, M.; Lai, C.T.; Hartmann, P.E.; Geddes, D.T.; Kakulas, F. Human Milk Cells Contain Numerous miRNAs that May Change with Milk Removal and Regulate Multiple Physiological Processes. *Int. J. Mol. Sci.* **2016**, *17*, 956. [CrossRef] [PubMed]
44. Shah, K.B.; Fields, D.A.; Pezant, N.P.; Kharoud, H.K.; Gulati, S.; Jacobs, K.; Gale, C.A.; Kharbanda, E.O.; Nagel, E.M.; Demerath, E.W.; et al. Gestational Diabetes Mellitus Is Associated with Altered Abundance of Exosomal MicroRNAs in Human Milk. *Clin. Ther.* **2022**, *44*, 172–185.e1. [CrossRef] [PubMed]
45. Mirza, A.H.; Kaur, S.; Nielsen, L.B.; Størling, J.; Yarani, R.; Roursgaard, M.; Mathiesen, E.R.; Damm, P.; Svare, J.; Mortensen, H.B.; et al. Breast Milk-Derived Extracellular Vesicles Enriched in Exosomes from Mothers With Type 1 Diabetes Contain Aberrant Levels of microRNAs. *Front. Immunol.* **2019**, *10*, 2543. [CrossRef] [PubMed]
46. Kupsco, A.; Prada, D.; Valvi, D.; Hu, L.; Petersen, M.S.; Coull, B.; Grandjean, P.; Weihe, P.; Baccarelli, A.A. Human milk extracellular vesicle miRNA expression and associations with maternal characteristics in a population-based cohort from the Faroe Islands. *Sci. Rep.* **2021**, *11*, 5840. [CrossRef]
47. Shah, K.B.; Chernausek, S.D.; Garman, L.D.; Pezant, N.P.; Plows, J.F.; Kharoud, H.K.; Demerath, E.W.; Fields, D.A. Human Milk Exosomal MicroRNA: Associations with Maternal Overweight/Obesity and Infant Body Composition at 1 Month of Life. *Nutrients* **2021**, *13*, 1091. [CrossRef]
48. Cho, Y.E.; Vorn, R.; Chimenti, M.; Crouch, K.; Shaoshuai, C.; Narayanaswamy, J.; Harken, A.; Schmidt, R.; Gill, J.; Lee, H. Extracellular vesicle miRNAs in breast milk of obese mothers. *Front. Nutr.* **2022**, *9*, 976886. [CrossRef]
49. Pomar, C.A.; Castro, H.; Picó, C.; Serra, F.; Palou, A.; Sánchez, J. Cafeteria Diet Consumption during Lactation in Rats, Rather than Obesity Per Se, alters miR-222, miR-200a, and miR-26a Levels in Milk. *Mol. Nutr. Food Res.* **2019**, *63*, e1800928. [CrossRef]
50. Munch, E.M.; Harris, R.A.; Mohammad, M.; Benham, A.L.; Pejerrey, S.M.; Showalter, L.; Hu, M.; Shope, C.D.; Maningat, P.D.; Gunaratne, P.H.; et al. Transcriptome profiling of microRNA by next-gen deep sequencing reveals known and novel miRNA species in the lipid fraction of human breast milk. *PLoS ONE* **2013**, *8*, e50564. [CrossRef]
51. Bozack, A.K.; Colicino, E.; Rodosthenous, R.; Bloomquist, T.R.; Baccarelli, A.A.; Wright, R.O.; Wright, R.J.; Lee, A.G. Associations between maternal lifetime stressors and negative events in pregnancy and breast milk-derived extracellular vesicle microRNAs in the programming of intergenerational stress mechanisms (PRISM) pregnancy cohort. *Epigenetics* **2021**, *16*, 389–404. [CrossRef] [PubMed]
52. Leroux, C.; Chervet, M.L.; German, J.B. Perspective: Milk microRNAs as Important Players in Infant Physiology and Development. *Adv. Nutr. Int. Rev. J.* **2021**, *12*, 1625–1635. [CrossRef]
53. Prieto-Colomina, A.; Fernández, V.; Chinnappa, K.; Borrell, V. MiRNAs in early brain development and pediatric cancer: At the intersection between healthy and diseased embryonic development. *Bioessays* **2021**, *43*, e2100073. [CrossRef]
54. Deng, Z.; Wei, Y.; Yao, Y.; Gao, S.; Wang, X. Let-7f promotes the differentiation of neural stem cells in rats. *Am. J. Transl. Res.* **2020**, *12*, 5752–5761. [PubMed]
55. Fairchild, C.L.A.; Cheema, S.K.; Wong, J.; Hino, K.; Simó, S.; La Torre, A. Let-7 regulates cell cycle dynamics in the developing cerebral cortex and retina. *Sci. Rep.* **2019**, *9*, 15336. [CrossRef] [PubMed]
56. Walgrave, H.; Balusu, S.; Snoeck, S.; Eynden, E.V.; Craessaerts, K.; Thrupp, N.; Wolfs, L.; Horré, K.; Fourne, Y.; Ronisz, A.; et al. Restoring miR-132 expression rescues adult hippocampal neurogenesis and memory deficits in Alz-heimer's disease. *Cell Stem Cell* **2021**, *28*, 1805–1821.e8. [CrossRef] [PubMed]
57. Zhang, H.; Liu, W.; Ge, H.; Li, K. Aberrant expression of miR-148a-3p in Alzheimer's disease and its protective role against amyloid-beta induced neurotoxicity. *Neurosci. Lett.* **2021**, *756*, 135953. [CrossRef]
58. Schepici, G.; Cavalli, E.; Bramanti, P.; Mazzon, E. Autism Spectrum Disorder and miRNA: An Overview of Experimental Models. *Brain Sci.* **2019**, *9*, 265. [CrossRef]
59. Nasirishargh, A.; Kumar, P.; Ramasubramanian, L.; Clark, K.; Hao, D.; Lazar, S.V.; Wang, A. Exosomal microRNAs from mesenchymal stem/stromal cells: Biology and applications in neuroprotection. *World J. Stem Cells* **2021**, *13*, 776–794. [CrossRef]
60. Aksoy-Aksel, A.; Zampa, F.; Schratt, G. MicroRNAs and synaptic plasticity—A mutual relationship. *Philos. Trans. R. Soc. B Biol. Sci.* **2014**, *369*, 20130515. [CrossRef]
61. Freiría-Martínez, L.; Iglesias-Martínez-Almeida, M.; Rodríguez-Jamardo, C.; Rivera-Baltanás, T.; Comís-Tuche, M.; Rodrígues-Amorím, D.; Fernández-Palleiro, P.; Blanco-Formoso, M.; Diz-Chaves, Y.; González-Freiria, N.; et al. Human Breast Milk microRNAs, Potential Players in the Regulation of Nervous System. *Nutrients* **2023**, *15*, 3284. [CrossRef] [PubMed]
62. Lonnerdal, B. Human Milk MicroRNAs/Exosomes: Composition and Biological Effects. *Nestle Nutr. Inst. Workshop Ser.* **2019**, *90*, 83–92. [PubMed]
63. Carney, M.C.; Tarasiuk, A.; DiAngelo, S.L.; Silveyra, P.; Podany, A.; Birch, L.L.; Paul, I.M.; Kelleher, S.; Hicks, S.D. Metabolism-related microRNAs in maternal breast milk are influenced by premature delivery. *Pediatr. Res.* **2017**, *82*, 226–236. [CrossRef]
64. Kahn, S.; Liao, Y.; Du, X.; Xu, W.; Li, J.; Lönnerdal, B. Exosomal MicroRNAs in Milk from Mothers Delivering Preterm Infants Survive in Vitro Digestion and Are Taken Up by Human Intestinal Cells. *Mol. Nutr. Food Res.* **2018**, *62*, e1701050. [CrossRef] [PubMed]
65. Shiff, Y.E.; Reif, S.; Marom, R.; Shiff, K.; Reifen, R.; Golan-Gerstl, R. MiRNA-320a is less expressed and miRNA-148a more expressed in preterm human milk compared to term human milk. *J. Funct. Foods* **2019**, *57*, 68–74. [CrossRef]

66. Wang, X.; Yan, X.; Zhang, L.; Cai, J.; Zhou, Y.; Liu, H.; Hu, Y.; Chen, W.; Xu, S.; Liu, P.; et al. Identification and Peptidomic Profiling of Exosomes in Preterm Human Milk: Insights into Necrotizing Enterocolitis Prevention. *Mol. Nutr. Food Res.* **2019**, *63*, e1801247. [CrossRef]
67. Aliperti, V.; Skonieczna, J.; Cerase, A. Long Non-Coding RNA (lncRNA) Roles in Cell Biology, Neurodevelopment and Neurological Disorders. *Non Coding RNA* **2021**, *7*, 36. [CrossRef]
68. Ng, S.Y.; Lin, L.; Soh, B.S.; Stanton, L.W. Long noncoding RNAs in development and disease of the central nervous system. *Trends Genet.* **2013**, *29*, 461–468. [CrossRef]
69. Shi, C.; Zhang, L.; Qin, C. Long non-coding RNAs in brain development, synaptic biology, and Alzheimer's disease. *Brain Res. Bull.* **2017**, *132*, 160–169. [CrossRef]
70. Lipovich, L.; Tarca, A.L.; Cai, J.; Jia, H.; Chugani, H.T.; Sterner, K.N.; Grossman, L.I.; Uddin, M.; Hof, P.R.; Sherwood, C.C.; et al. Developmental changes in the transcriptome of human cerebral cortex tissue: Long noncoding RNA transcripts. *Cereb. Cortex* **2014**, *24*, 1451–1459. [CrossRef]
71. Li, L.; Zhuang, Y.; Zhao, X.; Li, X. Long Non-coding RNA in Neuronal Development and Neurological Disorders. *Front. Genet.* **2018**, *9*, 744. [CrossRef] [PubMed]
72. Wilkinson, B.; Campbell, D.B. Contribution of long noncoding RNAs to autism spectrum disorder risk. *Int. Rev. Neurobiol.* **2013**, *113*, 35–59. [CrossRef] [PubMed]
73. Karlsson, O.; Rodosthenous, R.S.; Jara, C.; Brennan, K.J.; Wright, R.O.; Baccarelli, A.A.; Wright, R.J. Detection of long non-coding RNAs in human breastmilk extracellular vesicles: Implications for early child development. *Epigenetics* **2016**, *11*, 721–729. [CrossRef] [PubMed]
74. Mourtzi, N.; Siahanidou, T.; Tsifintaris, M.; Karamichali, E.; Tasiopoulou, A.; Sertedaki, A.; Pesmatzoglou, M.; Kapetanaki, A.; Liosis, G.; Baltatzis, G.; et al. lncRNA *NORAD* is consistently detected in breastmilk exosomes and its expression is downregulated in mothers of preterm infants. *Int. J. Mol. Med.* **2021**, *48*, 216. [CrossRef]
75. Zhou, X.; Wang, Z.; Xu, B.; Ji, N.; Meng, P.; Gu, L.; Li, Y. Long non-coding RNA NORAD protects against cerebral ischemia/reperfusion injury induced brain damage, cell apoptosis, oxidative stress and inflammation by regulating miR-30a-5p/YWHAG. *Bioengineered* **2021**, *12*, 9174–9188. [CrossRef]
76. Yin, J.; Shen, Y.; Si, Y.; Zhang, Y.; Du, J.; Hu, X.; Cai, M.; Bao, H.; Xing, Y. Knockdown of long non-coding RNA SOX_2OT downregulates SOX_2 to improve hippocampal neurogenesis and cognitive function in a mouse model of sepsis-associated encephalopathy. *J. Neuroinflamm.* **2020**, *17*, 320. [CrossRef]
77. Weissman, I.L. Translating stem and progenitor cell biology to the clinic: Barriers and opportunities. *Science* **2000**, *287*, 1442–1446. [CrossRef]
78. Kersin, S.G.; Ozek, E. Breast milk stem cells: Are they magic bullets in neonatology? *Turk. Arch. Pediatr.* **2021**, *56*, 187–191. [CrossRef]
79. Briere, C.E.; McGrath, J.M.; Jensen, T.; Matson, A.; Finck, C. Breast Milk Stem Cells: Current Science and Implications for Preterm Infants. *Adv. Neonatal. Care* **2016**, *16*, 410–419. [CrossRef]
80. Cregan, M.D.; Fan, Y.; Appelbee, A.; Brown, M.L.; Klopcic, B.; Koppen, J.; Mitoulas, L.R.; Piper, K.M.E.; Choolani, M.A.; Chong, Y.-S.; et al. Identification of nestin-positive putative mammary stem cells in human breastmilk. *Cell Tissue Res.* **2007**, *329*, 129–136. [CrossRef]
81. Briere, C.E.; Jensen, T.; McGrath, J.M.; Young, E.E.; Finck, C. Stem-Like Cell Characteristics from Breast Milk of Mothers with Preterm Infants as Compared to Mothers with Term Infants. *Breastfeed. Med.* **2017**, *12*, 174–179. [CrossRef] [PubMed]
82. Aydın, M.Ş.; Yiğit, E.N.; Vatandaşlar, E.; Erdoğan, E.; Öztürk, G. Transfer and Integration of Breast Milk Stem Cells to the Brain of Suckling Pups. *Sci. Rep.* **2018**, *8*, 14289. [CrossRef]
83. Belkozhayev, A.M.; Al-Yozbaki, M.; George, A.; Ye Niyazova, R.; Sharipov, K.O.; Byrne, L.J.; Wilson, C.M. Extracellular Vesicles, Stem Cells and the Role of miRNAs in Neurodegeneration. *Curr. Neuropharmacol.* **2022**, *20*, 1450–1478. [CrossRef]
84. Davis, C.; Savitz, S.I.; Satani, N. Mesenchymal Stem Cell Derived Extracellular Vesicles for Repairing the Neurovascular Unit after Ischemic Stroke. *Cells* **2021**, *10*, 767. [CrossRef] [PubMed]
85. Chang, Y.-H.; Wu, K.-C.; Harn, H.-J.; Lin, S.-Z.; Ding, D.-C. Exosomes and Stem Cells in Degenerative Disease Diagnosis and Therapy. *Cell Transplant.* **2018**, *27*, 349–363. [CrossRef] [PubMed]
86. Lendahl, U.; Zimmerman, L.B.; McKay, R.D.G. CNS stem cells express a new class of intermediate filament protein. *Cell* **1990**, *60*, 585–595. [CrossRef] [PubMed]
87. Hosseini, S.M.; Talaei-Khozani, T.; Sani, M.; Owrangi, B. Differentiation of human breast-milk stem cells to neural stem cells and neurons. *Neurol. Res. Int.* **2014**, *2014*, 807896. [CrossRef]
88. Turnbaugh, P.J.; Ley, R.E.; Hamady, M.; Fraser-Liggett, C.M.; Knight, R.; Gordon, J.I. The human microbiome project. *Nature* **2007**, *449*, 804–810. [CrossRef]
89. Berg, G.; Rybakova, D.; Fischer, D.; Cernava, T.; Vergès, M.-C.C.; Charles, T.; Chen, X.; Cocolin, L.; Eversole, K.; Corral, G.H.; et al. Microbiome definition re-visited: Old concepts and new challenges. *Microbiome* **2020**, *8*, 103. [CrossRef]
90. Gavin, A.; Ostovar, K.; Gavin, A.; Ostovar, K. Microbiological Characterization of Human Milk (1). *J. Food Prot.* **1977**, *40*, 614–616. [CrossRef]
91. Jones, C.A. Maternal transmission of infectious pathogens in breast milk. *J. Paediatr. Child Health* **2001**, *37*, 576–582. [CrossRef] [PubMed]

92. Martín, R.; Langa, S.; Reviriego, C.; Jimínez, E.; Marín, M.L.; Xaus, J.; Fernández, L.; Rodríguez, J.M. Human milk is a source of lactic acid bacteria for the infant gut. *J. Pediatr.* **2003**, *143*, 754–758. [CrossRef] [PubMed]
93. Collado, M.; Delgado, S.; Maldonado, A.; Rodríguez, J. Assessment of the bacterial diversity of breast milk of healthy women by quantitative real-time PCR. *Lett. Appl. Microbiol.* **2009**, *48*, 523–528. [CrossRef] [PubMed]
94. Hunt, K.M.; Foster, J.A.; Forney, L.J.; Schütte, U.M.E.; Beck, D.L.; Abdo, Z.; Fox, L.K.; Williams, J.E.; McGuire, M.K.; McGuire, M.A. Characterization of the diversity and temporal stability of bacterial communities in human milk. *PLoS ONE* **2011**, *6*, e21313. [CrossRef] [PubMed]
95. Yi, D.Y.; Kim, S.Y. Human Breast Milk Composition and Function in Human Health: From Nutritional Components to Microbiome and MicroRNAs. *Nutrients* **2021**, *13*, 3094. [CrossRef]
96. Moossavi, S.; Sepehri, S.; Robertson, B.; Bode, L.; Goruk, S.; Field, C.J.; Lix, L.M.; de Souza, R.J.; Becker, A.B.; Mandhane, P.J.; et al. Composition and Variation of the Human Milk Microbiota Are Influenced by Maternal and Early-Life Factors. *Cell Host Microbe* **2019**, *25*, 324–335.e4. [CrossRef]
97. Zimmermann, P.; Curtis, N. Breast milk microbiota: A review of the factors that influence composition. *J. Infect.* **2020**, *81*, 17–47. [CrossRef]
98. Damaceno, Q.S.; Souza, J.P.; Nicoli, J.R.; Paula, R.L.; Assis, G.B.; Figueiredo, H.C.; Azevedo, V.; Martins, F.S. Evaluation of Potential Probiotics Isolated from Human Milk and Colostrum. *Probiotics Antimicrob. Proteins* **2017**, *9*, 371–379. [CrossRef]
99. Solís, G.; de los Reyes-Gavilan, C.G.; Fernández, N.; Margolles, A.; Gueimonde, M. Establishment and development of lactic acid bacteria and bifidobacteria microbiota in breast-milk and the infant gut. *Anaerobe* **2010**, *16*, 307–310. [CrossRef]
100. Khodayar-Pardo, P.; Mira-Pascual, L.; Collado, M.C.; Martínez-Costa, C. Impact of lactation stage, gestational age and mode of delivery on breast milk microbiota. *J. Perinatol.* **2014**, *34*, 599–605. [CrossRef]
101. Dahaban, N.M.; Romli, M.F.; Roslan, N.R.; Kong, S.S.-S.; Cheah, F.-C. Bacteria in expressed breastmilk from mothers of premature infants and maternal hygienic status. *Breastfeed. Med.* **2013**, *8*, 422–423. [CrossRef] [PubMed]
102. Boix-Amorós, A.; Collado, M.C.; Mira, A. Relationship between Milk Microbiota, Bacterial Load, Macronutrients, and Human Cells during Lactation. *Front. Microbiol.* **2016**, *7*, 492. [CrossRef] [PubMed]
103. Hermansson, H.; Kumar, H.; Collado, M.C.; Salminen, S.; Isolauri, E.; Rautava, S. Breast Milk Microbiota Is Shaped by Mode of Delivery and Intrapartum Antibiotic Exposure. *Front. Nutr.* **2019**, *6*, 4. [CrossRef] [PubMed]
104. Simpson, M.R.; Avershina, E.; Storrø, O.; Johnsen, R.; Rudi, K.; Øien, T. Breastfeeding-associated microbiota in human milk following supplementation with Lactobacillus rhamnosus GG, Lactobacillus acidophilus La-5, and Bifidobacterium animalis ssp. lactis Bb-12. *J. Dairy Sci.* **2018**, *101*, 889–899. [CrossRef]
105. Gueimonde, M.; Laitinen, K.; Salminen, S.; Isolauri, E. Breast milk: A source of bifidobacteria for infant gut development and maturation? *Neonatology* **2007**, *92*, 64–66. [CrossRef]
106. Cabrera-Rubio, R.; Collado, M.C.; Laitinen, K.; Salminen, S.; Isolauri, E.; Mira, A. The human milk microbiome changes over lactation and is shaped by maternal weight and mode of delivery. *Am. J. Clin. Nutr.* **2012**, *96*, 544–551. [CrossRef]
107. Li, S.-W.; Watanabe, K.; Hsu, C.-C.; Chao, S.-H.; Yang, Z.-H.; Lin, Y.-J.; Chen, C.-C.; Cao, Y.-M.; Huang, H.-C.; Chang, C.-H.; et al. Bacterial Composition and Diversity in Breast Milk Samples from Mothers Living in Taiwan and Mainland China. *Front. Microbiol.* **2017**, *8*, 965. [CrossRef]
108. Grönlund, M.-M.; Gueimonde, M.; Laitinen, K.; Kociubinski, G.; Grönroos, T.; Salminen, S.; Isolauri, E. Maternal breast-milk and intestinal bifidobacteria guide the compositional development of the Bifidobacterium microbiota in infants at risk of allergic disease. *Clin. Exp. Allergy* **2007**, *37*, 1764–1772. [CrossRef]
109. Olivares, M.; Albrecht, S.; De Palma, G.; Ferrer, M.D.; Castillejo, G.; Schols, H.A.; Sanz, Y. Human milk composition differs in healthy mothers and mothers with celiac disease. *Eur. J. Nutr.* **2015**, *54*, 119–128. [CrossRef]
110. Ajeeb, T.T.; Gonzalez, E.; Solomons, N.W.; Koski, K.G. Human milk microbial species are associated with infant head-circumference during early and late lactation in Guatemalan mother-infant dyads. *Front. Microbiol.* **2022**, *13*, 908845. [CrossRef]
111. Rutayisire, E.; Huang, K.; Liu, Y.; Tao, F. The mode of delivery affects the diversity and colonization pattern of the gut microbiota during the first year of infants' life: A systematic review. *BMC Gastroenterol.* **2016**, *16*, 86. [CrossRef] [PubMed]
112. Pannaraj, P.S.; Li, F.; Cerini, C.; Bender, J.M.; Yang, S.; Rollie, A.; Adisetiyo, H.; Zabih, S.; Lincez, P.J.; Bittinger, K.; et al. Association Between Breast Milk Bacterial Communities and Establishment and Development of the Infant Gut Microbiome. *JAMA Pediatr.* **2017**, *171*, 647–654. [CrossRef]
113. Vuong, H.E. Intersections of the microbiome and early neurodevelopment. *Int. Rev. Neurobiol.* **2022**, *167*, 1–23. [CrossRef] [PubMed]
114. Lu, J.; Drobyshevsky, A.; Lu, L.; Yu, Y.; Caplan, M.S.; Claud, E.C. Microbiota from Preterm Infants Who Develop Necrotizing Enterocolitis Drives the Neurodevelopment Impairment in a Humanized Mouse Model. *Microorganisms* **2023**, *11*, 1131. [CrossRef]
115. Xia, J.; Claud, E.C. Gut Microbiome-Brain Axis as an Explanation for the Risk of Poor Neurodevelopment Out-come in Preterm Infants with Necrotizing Enterocolitis. *Microorganisms* **2023**, *11*, 1035. [CrossRef]
116. Indrio, F.; Martini, S.; Francavilla, R.; Corvaglia, L.; Cristofori, F.; Mastrolia, S.A.; Neu, J.; Rautava, S.; Spena, G.R.; Raimondi, F.; et al. Epigenetic Matters: The Link between Early Nutrition, Microbiome, and Long-term Health Development. *Front. Pediatr.* **2017**, *5*, 178. [CrossRef]
117. Tognini, P. Gut Microbiota: A Potential Regulator of Neurodevelopment. *Front. Cell. Neurosci.* **2017**, *11*, 25. [CrossRef] [PubMed]

118. Laue, H.E.; Coker, M.O.; Madan, J.C. The Developing Microbiome from Birth to 3 Years: The Gut-Brain Axis and Neurodevelopmental Outcomes. *Front. Pediatr.* **2022**, *10*, 815885. [CrossRef]
119. Ihekweazu, F.D.; Versalovic, J. Development of the Pediatric Gut Microbiome: Impact on Health and Disease. *Am. J. Med Sci.* **2018**, *356*, 413–423. [CrossRef]
120. Valicenti-McDermott, M.; McVicar, K.; Rapin, I.; Wershil, B.K.; Cohen, H.; Shinnar, S. Frequency of gastrointestinal symptoms in children with autistic spectrum disorders and association with family history of autoimmune disease. *J. Dev. Behav. Pediatr.* **2006**, *27*, S128–S136. [CrossRef]
121. Hsiao, E.Y.; McBride, S.W.; Hsien, S.; Sharon, G.; Hyde, E.R.; McCue, T.; Codelli, J.A.; Chow, J.; Reisman, S.E.; Petrosino, J.F.; et al. Microbiota modulate behavioral and physiological abnormalities associated with neurodevelopmental disorders. *Cell* **2013**, *155*, 1451–1463. [CrossRef] [PubMed]
122. Lu, J.; Claud, E.C. Connection between gut microbiome and brain development in preterm infants. *Dev. Psychobiol.* **2019**, *61*, 739–751. [CrossRef] [PubMed]

nutrients

Systematic Review

Association of Breastfeeding and Early Childhood Caries: A Systematic Review and Meta-Analysis

Sheetal Kiran Shrestha [1,2,*], Amit Arora [1,2,3,4,5], Narendar Manohar [2,6], Kanchana Ekanayake [7] and Jann Foster [8,9,10,*]

1 School of Health Sciences, Western Sydney University, Locked Bag 1797, Penrith, NSW 2751, Australia
2 Health Equity Laboratory, Campbelltown, NSW 2560, Australia
3 Discipline of Child and Adolescent Health, The Children's Hospital at Westmead Clinical School, Faculty of Medicine and Health, The University of Sydney, Westmead, NSW 2145, Australia
4 Translational Health Research Institute, Western Sydney University, Campbelltown, NSW 2560, Australia
5 Oral Health Services, Sydney Local Health District and Sydney Dental Hospital, NSW Health, Surry Hills, NSW 2010, Australia
6 Blackdog Institute, Hospital Road, Randwick, NSW 2031, Australia
7 University of Sydney Library, The University of Sydney, Camperdown, NSW 2006, Australia
8 School of Nursing and Midwifery, Western Sydney University, Locked Bag 1797, Penrith, NSW 2751, Australia
9 School of Nursing and Midwifery, University of Canberra, Bruce, ACT 2617, Australia
10 Ingham Research Institute, Liverpool, NSW 2170, Australia
* Correspondence: 20499440@student.westernsydney.edu.au (S.K.S.); j.foster@westernsydney.edu.au (J.F.)

Abstract: Early childhood caries (ECC) is a growing public health concern worldwide. Although numerous systematic reviews have been published regarding the association between breastfeeding and early childhood caries (ECC), the results remain inconclusive and equivocal. This systematic review synthesises the evidence on the association between breastfeeding and ECC. Five electronic databases and backward citation chasing were performed from inception until May 2023. A total of 31 studies (22 cohort studies and 9 case-control studies) were included in this review. The meta-analysis of the case-control studies showed statistically significant fewer dental caries in children who were breastfed for < 6 months compared to those who were breastfed for ≥6 months (OR = 0.53, 95% CI 0.41–0.67, $p < 0.001$). There was a statistically significant difference in dental caries between children who were breastfed for <12 months and those who were breastfed for ≥12 months (RR = 0.65, 95% CI 0.50–0.86, $p < 0.002$). Similarly, there was a statistically significant difference in dental caries in children who were breastfed for <18 months compared to those who were breastfed for ≥18 months (RR = 0.41, 95% CI 0.18–0.92, $p = 0.030$). Nocturnal breastfeeding increases the risk of ECC compared with no nocturnal breastfeeding (RR = 2.35, 95% CI 1.42–3.89, $p < 0.001$). The findings suggest breastfeeding for more than 12 months and nocturnal breastfeeding increase the risk of ECC.

Keywords: breastfeeding; early childhood caries; preschool children; oral health; dental caries

1. Introduction

Oral health is the state of well-being of the mouth and its associated structures that enable individuals to perform their essential functions without any pain or discomfort, as well as maintain their psychosocial health [1]. About 3.5 billion people in the world suffer from oral diseases, including dental caries [1]. Early childhood caries (ECC) is the most common oral disease among children [2]. The American Academy of Paediatric Dentistry (AAPD) defines ECC "as the presence of one or more decayed (non-cavitated or cavitated lesions), missing (due to caries), or filled tooth surfaces in any primary tooth in a child 71 months of age or younger" [3]. Globally, 514 million children, constituting 43% of the paediatric population, suffer from dental caries in their primary teeth [1]. Dental caries among young children is a widespread issue, with 21% of American children aged two to five years experiencing dental caries [4]. Similarly, a quarter of English children exhibit dental caries before starting school [5]. Likewise, the Australian National Child Oral Health

Study reported that 34.3% of children between the ages of five and six experience dental caries in their primary teeth, with 26.1% of those cases left untreated [6]. The plight of ECC in the developing world is worse. For example, in India, approximately one in two children suffers from ECC [7].

Early childhood caries develops along the gingival (gum) margin as a white spot lesion [8] and may progress quickly, resulting in health adversities such as toothache and infection [5]. Furthermore, in severe cases of ECC, surgery and/or hospital admission may be required for treatment, thus affecting not only the child but also the family [9].

ECC has a multifactorial aetiology [10]. ECC is strongly influenced by socioeconomic status (SES) and is more prevalent in children from families with low SES and in developing countries [7]. Other factors, such as a mother's education, attitude towards oral health, the presence of enamel defects, high levels of mutans streptococci, and feeding habits, increase the risk of ECC [11]. Feeding habits such as breastfeeding [12] and the age at which free sugars, including those naturally occurring in fruit juices or honey, are introduced, as well as the frequency of their consumption, play a crucial role in the development of ECC [13].

The association between breastfeeding and ECC is one of the most debated risk factors for ECC. Several studies have indicated that prolonged and exclusive breastfeeding does not contribute to the development of ECC in preschool children [14–17]. However, several other studies have reported that breastfeeding beyond 12 months and nocturnal breastfeeding increase the risk of ECC. This conundrum has kept the association between breastfeeding and oral health debatable and inconclusive. As a result, medical and dental organisations provide different recommendations, as outlined below. The World Health Organisation (WHO) recommends that all infants be exclusively breastfed for 6 months and complementary breastfeeding continue for 2 years or more [18]. In Australia, the National Health and Medical Research Council (NHMRC) recommends exclusive breastfeeding until around 6 months of age and continuing complementary breastfeeding until 12 months of age and beyond, provided that both the mother and child wish to do so [19]. The American Association of Paediatric Dentistry (AAPD) advocates breastfeeding for a duration of 12 months to promote optimum health and developmental outcomes for the infant and establish psychosocial wellbeing in infants [20]. However, the AAPD cautions against unrestricted nocturnal breastfeeding following the eruption of the first primary tooth, arguing that nocturnal feeding can increase the risk of ECC. Likewise, some studies suggest that children who are breastfed may exhibit a higher likelihood of developing dental caries than children who do not breastfeed [12,21].

Several systematic reviews [22–29] have explored the association of breastfeeding and ECC (Table S1). However, the evidence was assessed to be inconclusive and equivocal. Moreover, most of the above reviews were deemed to be of low quality, except for one [26], which was of moderate quality (Table S1). Moynihan et al. (2019) [26] did not conduct any meta-analysis, nor was it solely focused on breastfeeding and ECC. Most of the reviews included observational studies, including cross-sectional studies, which do not establish any causal evidence [22–26,28,29]. This systematic review emphasises scientific rigour by incorporating only longitudinal observational studies, specifically cohort and case-control studies, which are considered to possess a higher level of evidence among the observational studies [30]. Therefore, this review is designed to assess and consolidate the available evidence from cohort and case-control studies to provide a high-quality, comprehensive synthesis on the effect of breastfeeding on ECC among preschool children. Additionally, this review aims to investigate the prevalence of dental caries (ECC) in preschool children who were breastfed for different durations ($<$4 months, $<$6 months, $<$12 months, $<$18 months, $<$24 months, $\geq$24 months) and those who received nocturnal breastfeeding.

Hence, this review and meta-analyses address the following research questions:

1. Is there any association between breastfeeding and ECC?
2. Is the prevalence of ECC different among children breastfed for different durations?
3. Does nocturnal breastfeeding increase the risk of ECC?

2. Methods

This systematic review followed the JBI methodology for systematic reviews of aetiology and risk [31], and the results were presented as per the PRISMA 2020 guidelines [32]. The protocol of this systematic review has been registered in the PROSPERO International Prospective Register of Systematic Reviews (CRD42023442205).

2.1. Eligibility Criteria

The studies included in the review were of cohort (prospective and retrospective) and case-control design. Randomised controlled trials (RCTs), quasi-experimental studies, cross-sectional studies, and single case reports were excluded. Furthermore, grey literature, systematic reviews, literature reviews, umbrella reviews, and scoping reviews were also excluded from this review. The eligibility criteria are outlined in detail in Table 1.

Table 1. List of inclusion and exclusion criteria according to P(I/E)CO criteria.

	Inclusion Criteria	Exclusion Criteria
Population	• Children under 6 years of age (preschool children) • Any gender, race, geographical location, or socioeconomic status • Without any systemic disease or disability	• Children who are 6 years or older • Children with any systemic disease or disability
Exposure	• Preschool children (<6 years old) who are breastfed (exclusive or partial)	
Comparator	• Preschool children (<6 years old) who are not breastfed	
Outcome	• Studies reporting the prevalence of dental caries (as reported by a qualified dental practitioner or trained and calibrated non-dental personnel) • Studies reporting dental caries only on primary teeth in preschool children • First dental examination before the age of six	• Studies not reporting dental caries • Self-reported or unvalidated dental caries measures • Studies reporting dental caries in permanent teeth • First dental examination at 6 years or older
Study design	• Cohort studies • Case-control studies • Cohort and case-control studies nested in other study designs	• Randomised controlled trials (RCTs) • Quasi-experimental studies • Cross-sectional studies • Single case reports • Grey literature • Systematic reviews, literature reviews, umbrella reviews, and scoping reviews

2.2. Information Sources

The search was conducted in five databases without any date restrictions: MEDLINE (Ovid), Scopus, Web of Science (ISI), Embase (Ovid), and CINAHL (EBSCO). The search was conducted until 13 May 2023. The reference lists of the included studies and relevant past published systematic reviews were searched manually to ensure the inclusion of all relevant studies.

2.3. Search Strategy

The reviewers (SS, JF, and AA) devised the research question and search terms based on the P(I/E)CO (Population Intervention/Exposure Comparator Outcome) criteria. A logic grid was drafted using medical subject headings (MeSH) terms and keywords in collaboration with a health sciences librarian (KE). A preliminary search was conducted on MEDLINE (Ovid). The search strategy was adapted and modified for the remaining databases (Supplementary Materials S2).

2.4. Study Selection

Studies were identified through searching the five databases and were imported into Covidence. Two reviewers (SS and JF) independently screened the titles and abstracts of the imported articles against the inclusion criteria. Additional information from study authors was sought for studies with uncertain eligibility. In cases where there were no responses from the study authors after three attempts, the study was screened based on the available information. Any article with ambiguous eligibility was discussed between the two reviewers to reach a conclusion. In any instance where the two reviewers could not come to an agreement, a third reviewer (AA) was involved to seek a resolution. Duplicates identified in Covidence were removed. The reference lists of studies included in the full-text review were also screened for additional studies. A list of the excluded studies with reasons for their exclusion is provided in Supplementary Materials S6. The study selection process followed the PRISMA checklist, and the flow diagram is presented as Figure 1.

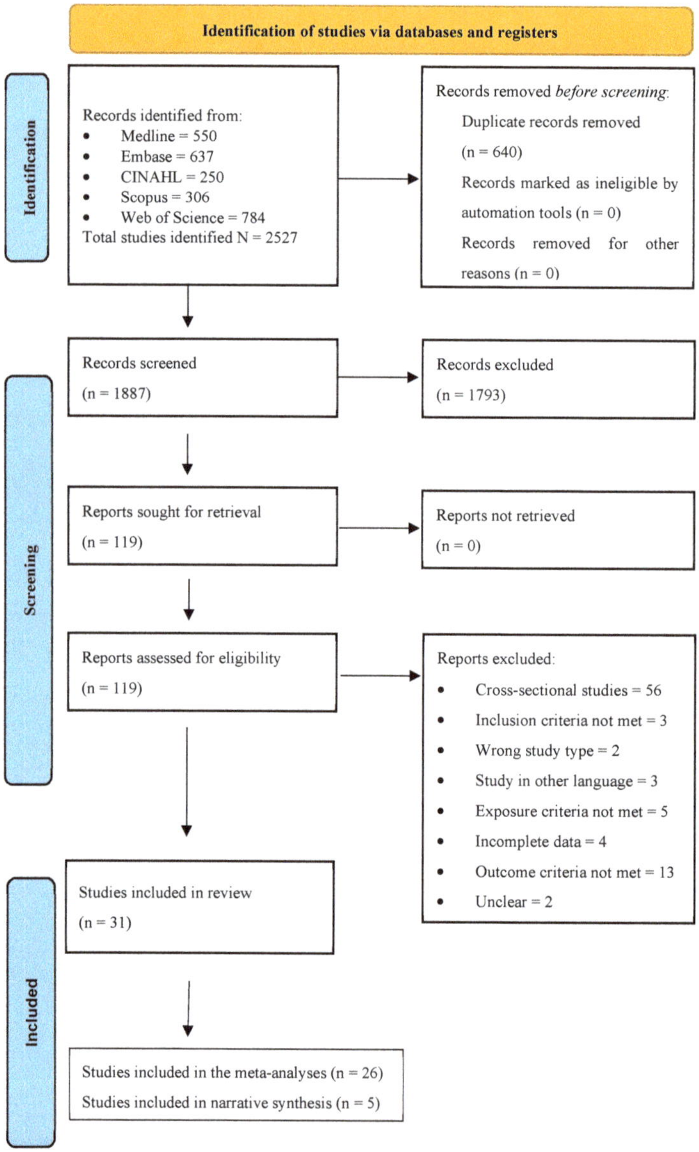

Figure 1. PRISMA flow diagram exhibiting steps in the selection process.

2.5. Data Collection Process and Data Items

The data were extracted using JBI SUMARI data extraction tools. Two reviewers (SS and JF) calibrated the information collected from two studies to ensure consistency in data extraction. The same two reviewers then extracted the data independently from the selected studies (Table S4). The information extracted from the included studies was the name of the authors and publication year, study design, setting and sample size, country, demography of the participants, breastfeeding data (method, duration, and timing), follow-up time, dental caries measures (dmft index, dmfs, index, dfs, ICDAS), study results, funding, and conclusion. A maximum of 3 attempts were made to contact the authors of potentially eligible studies for any unclear or missing information.

2.6. Data Synthesis

Cohort studies and case-control studies were included in this review. Effect sizes were expressed as risk ratios, odds ratios, or prevalence ratios for dichotomous data, and their 95% confidence intervals (CI) were calculated for analysis. Cohort estimates were presented as risk ratios with a 95% CI, and case-control estimates were presented as odds ratios with a 95% CI. Meta-analyses were conducted comparing children who were breastfed and those who were not; children breastfed for different durations (<4 months vs. ≥4 months; <6 months vs. ≥6 months; <12 months vs. ≥12 months; <18 months vs. ≥18 months; <24 months vs. ≥24 months); and those who received nocturnal breastfeeding vs. those who did not.

The meta-analyses were conducted using the statistical software "Review Manager" (RevMan Web Version 7.9.0). A fixed-effect model for meta-analysis was used in the first instance to combine the data where possible. When the heterogeneity was substantial, a random effects model was used. Heterogeneity was evaluated using the Chi^2 test and I^2 analysis. For the Chi^2 test, a p value of less than 0.10 was considered for heterogeneity. The I^2 value was considered according to the *Cochrane Handbook for Systematic Reviews of Interventions* [33] and the *JBI Manual for Evidence Synthesis* [34], where 0% to 40% was considered not important, 30% to 60% represented moderate heterogeneity, 50% to 90% represented substantial heterogeneity, and 75% to 100% represented considerable heterogeneity [33]. Studies that were inappropriate to be included in the meta-analysis due to their study design or reporting of the outcome measures were analysed, interpreted individually, and reported narratively.

2.7. Quality Assessment and Risk of Bias

Each study included in this review was independently assessed for their methodological quality by two reviewers (SS and JF) utilising the Joanna Briggs Institute critical appraisal tool for cohort studies (retrospective and prospective) and case-control studies [31]. The results of the JBI quality assessments are reported in Tables S2 and S3. All the studies were included in the review, regardless of their methodological quality. The third reviewer (AA) was consulted to seek a resolution in case of any disagreements.

3. Results

A total of 2527 studies were identified from the initial search. After 640 duplicates were removed, 1887 studies were screened. After removing 1793 records post title and abstract screening, a total of 118 studies were screened for full-text eligibility. After the exclusion of 88 studies (Supplementary Materials S6), 31 studies matching the inclusion criteria were included in this review. A total of 26 studies were included in the meta-analysis, and five were reported narratively (Figure 1). All the studies were in English and were published between 1994 and 2023. A total of 15,236 pre-school children were analysed.

3.1. Study Characteristics

Out of the 31 studies, 22 were cohort studies [35–56], and 9 were case-control studies [57–65]. Among the cohort studies, six were nested studies, one was nested within a cross-sectional study [36], and the remaining five were nested in randomised controlled trials [38,40–42,51]. Four of the cohort studies were retrospective in design [43,45,49,53]. Due to the high heterogeneity among the studies, most of the results were presented using random effects.

Eleven studies carried out dental examinations in clinical settings of dental clinics, hospitals, or universities [35,36,43–47,53,57,60,62]. Fourteen studies carried out dental examinations in field settings [37,38,40,42,48–51,54,55,58,59,61,64]. Four studies were unclear about their setting for dental examinations [39,56,63,65].

3.2. *Study Settings*

Seventeen studies [35,36,38,40,41,43,48–51,54,58–63] were conducted in middle-income countries [66] whereas fourteen [37,39,42,44–47,52,53,55–57,64,65] were carried out in high-income countries.

Most of the studies were conducted in Brazil [35,36,38,40,41,43,49,51]. Five studies were conducted in Japan [47,52,53,55,56]. Four studies were conducted in Australia [39,42,46,64]. Two studies were conducted in India [58,59], and two were conducted in Thailand [48,50]). Among the high-income countries, one study was conducted in the USA [44], one was conducted in Canada [65], one was undertaken in Italy [45], one in Scotland [37], and one in the Czech Republic [57]. Refs. [61,63] were undertaken in Tanzania and South Africa, respectively, while [54,62] were conducted in China and Myanmar, respectively.

3.3. *Early Childhood Caries*

The main outcome, ECC, was reported and classified differently amongst the studies. The outcomes for ECC were reported as dmfs (decayed, missing, and filled surfaces), dmft (decayed, missing, and filled teeth), dft (decayed, filled teeth), and dfs (decayed, filled surface). S-ECC (severe early childhood caries) was also reported and refers to one or more decayed, missing (due to caries), or filled tooth surfaces in the primary (baby) maxillary (upper) and anterior (front) teeth.

Eight studies [37,39,43,48,58,60,61,65] reported dental caries as dmfs ECC. Five studies [38,46,50,51,63] reported dental caries as dmfs S-ECC. Seven studies [35,42,47,49,52,55,64] reported dmft ECC. Two studies [53,56] reported ECC as the presence or absence of dental caries (cavitated and non-cavitated lesions). Two studies [40,41] reported ECC and S-ECC as modified dmft and dmfs. One study [44] reported dfs ECC. One study [54] only reported ECC as a frank cavitation. Barosso et al. (2021), Ganesh et al. (2022), and Majorana et al. (2014) [36,45,59] were the only three studies reporting ECC based on the International Caries Detection Assessment System (ICDAS) criteria.

3.4. *Methodological Quality and Risk of Bias Assessment*

The quality assessments of the 21 cohort studies and 9 case-control studies were conducted using appropriate JBI tools for cohort studies and case-control studies, respectively [31]. The critical appraisals for the studies are presented in Tables S2 and S3. The critical appraisal was conducted by two reviewers separately (SS and JF). Any differences were resolved through discussion until agreement was reached.

3.5. *Cohort Studies*

Chaffee et al. (2014), Devenish et al. (2020), Manohar et al. (2021), Nirunsittirat et al. (2016), Peltzer et al. (2015), and Yokoi et al. (2020) [38,39,46,48,50,55] were the only studies that fulfilled all the criteria among the cohort studies (Table S2). The similarity between the two groups (Q1), the similarity (Q2), and the validity (Q3) of the exposure were addressed by all the studies except Yonezu et al. (2006) [56], which was unclear for Q1 and Q3.

Confounding factors (Q4) were addressed by all the studies except Majorana et al. (2014), where it was unclear, and Yonezu et al. (2006) did not address the criteria. All studies mentioned the strategies to address confounders (Q5) except for Abanto et al. (2023), Feldens et al. (2010), and Majorana et al. (2014) [35,40,45], which were unclear, and Yonezu et al. (2006) [56] did not address the criteria. A third of the cohort studies [36,37,47,49,53,54,56] were either unclear or failed to mention if the participants were free of the outcome at the start of the study (Q6); the participants in the remaining two-thirds of the studies were free of the outcome at the start of the study.

Except for Yonezu et al. (2006) [56], the outcomes in all the studies were measured in a valid way (Q7). The follow-up time was adequate in all the studies (Q8). All but five studies [36,37,44,50,56] completed follow-up or addressed the loss of follow-up (Q9). All studies except Bernabé et al. (2017), Hong et al. (2014), and Peres et al. (2017) [37,44,51] addressed Q10 (strategies to deal with loss to follow up), while Majorana et al. (2014), Tanaka et al. (2013), and Yonezu et al. (2006) [45,52,56] were rated unclear. All the studies utilised appropriate statistical analysis (Q11). Overall, the studies were of moderate to high quality (Table S2).

3.6. *Case-Control Studies*

For the case-control studies, Ganesh et al. (2022) [59] and Lima et al. (2016) [60] were the only studies to fulfil all the criteria. All studies except Matee et al. (1994) [61] and Seow et al. (2009) [64] fulfilled Q1 (participants were comparable other than the presence of disease). The cases and controls were appropriately matched (Q2) in all the studies except in Matee et al. (1994) [61], whereby it was unclear. All the studies [58–65] addressed Q3, except for Cvanova et al. (2022) [57], and all the studies [57,59–61,64,65], except Dabawala et al. (2017) [58], Qin et al. (2008) [62], and Roberts et al., (1994) [63], addressed Q4.

All the studies addressed Q5–Q10, except Matee et al. (1994) [61]. It did not mention any strategies to deal with confounders (Q7). Overall, the majority of the studies were of moderate to high quality (Table S3).

3.7. *Effects of Breastfeeding on Early Childhood Caries*

3.7.1. Children Who Were Breastfed versus Children Who Were Not Breastfed

Fifteen studies [37,39,41,42,45,46,49,50,53,56,58,62–65] compared dental caries in children who were breastfed and children who were not breastfed and were included in the meta-analysis. Two separate analyses were conducted based on the study design. Of these fifteen studies, ten were of cohort design [37,39,41,42,45,46,49,50,53,56], and five were case-control studies [58,62–65].

In terms of cohort studies, the pooled estimates (Figure 2) show no statistically significant difference for dental caries between breastfed and non-breastfed children (RR 0.98, 95% CI 0.77 to 1.26; participants = 8506; studies = 10; I^2 = 91%, p = 0.89). To investigate the sensitivity, five studies [37,41,45,53,56] were removed. The heterogeneity was reduced to 0% (p = 0.048), and the pooled estimate suggested breastfeeding may be protective against ECC compared to no breastfeeding (RR = 0.82, 95% CI 0.71 to 0.95) (not shown in the figure). However, the result should be interpreted with caution due to the high heterogeneity among the studies.

In terms of case-control studies, the pooled estimates (Figure 3) show no significant difference in the dental caries experience between breastfed and non-breastfed children (OR 1.04, 95% CI 0.78 to 1.38; participants = 1022; studies = 5; I^2 = 14%, p = 0.81).

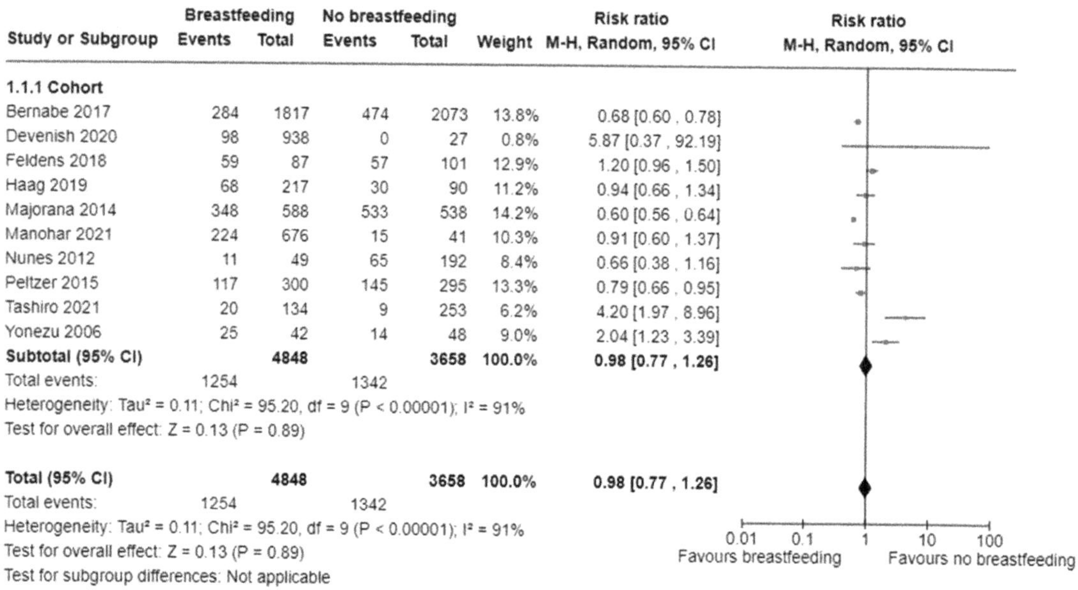

Figure 2. Breastfeeding versus no breastfeeding and the risk of dental caries: cohort studies [37,39,41, 42,45,46,49,50,53,56].

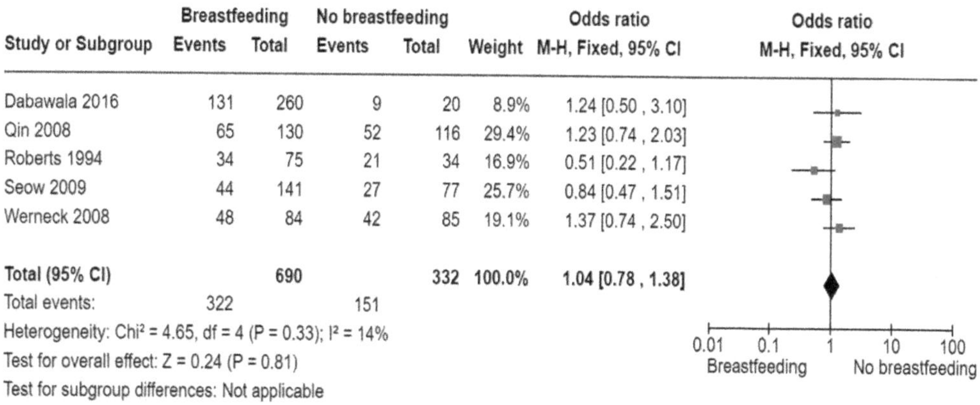

Figure 3. Breastfeeding versus no breastfeeding and the risk of dental caries: case-control studies [58,62,64,65].

3.7.2. Children Who Were Breastfed at Night versus Children Who Were Not

Seven studies reported nocturnal breastfeeding [39,47,50,54,59–61], and only three cohort studies [39,47,54] were able to be included in the meta-analysis. The pooled estimate for these cohort studies showed nocturnal breastfeeding could increase the risk of ECC compared with no nocturnal breastfeeding (RR 2.35, 95% CI 1.42 to 3.89; participants = 1590; studies = 3; $I^2 = 86\%$, $p = 0.0008$). After excluding the study with the possible risk of bias [39], the heterogeneity was found to be not important ($I^2 = 33\%$, $p= 0.22$) and the pooled estimate showed higher risk for the nocturnal breastfeeding group (RR = 3.05, 95% CI 2.40 to 3.87, $p < 0.0001$) The I^2 indicates substantial heterogeneity and therefore the result should be interpreted with caution. See Figure 4.

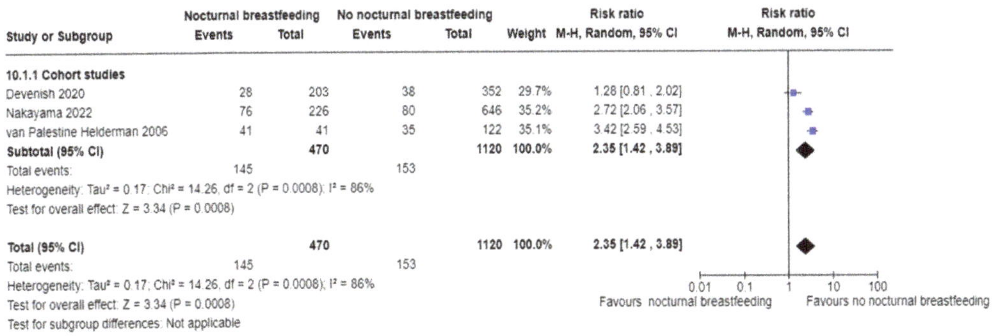

Figure 4. Nocturnal breastfeeding versus no nocturnal breastfeeding and the risk of dental caries [39,47,54].

The following four studies were not able to be included in the meta-analysis due to the study design or method of reporting the outcome, and their results were provided narratively. Ganesh et al. (2022) [59] was the only study dedicated to sleep-time feeding (both nighttime and daytime) practices. The study reported on ECC in children with various modes of feeding (breast, bottle, or other) during the beginning of sleep, early morning hours of sleep, and course of sleep. The aOR for breastfeeding at the beginning of sleep, during sleep, and in the early morning hours of sleep were found to be 6.7, 6.5, and 3.7, respectively (p = 0.001). The study found a strong association between sleep-time feeding and ECC. Lima et al. (2016) [60] found that children who were no longer breastfeeding during the night at 16 months were less likely to be diagnosed with ECC compared to children who engaged in nocturnal breastfeeding at 16 months (OR 0.51 (CI = 0.39–0.65), $p < 0.001$). Similarly, Matee et al. (1994) [61] found a strong association between ECC and night feeding habits with the breast nipple in the mouth of the sleeping infant (0 versus 5, OR = 17.8 (6.3–50.3), p = 0.0001). Peltzer and Mongkolchati (2015) [50] found nocturnal breastfeeding at 12 months (suckle to sleep when going to bed) to be associated with S-ECC (251/563 children). No other data were provided.

3.8. Association between Dental Caries and Breastfeeding Duration

3.8.1. Duration of Breastfeeding: <4 Months and ≥4 Months

Two studies [46,50] compared dental caries in children who were breastfed < 4 months and ≥4 months (Figure 5). No significant difference was found in the analysis (RR 0.95, 95% CI 0.80 to 1.13; participants = 1017; studies = 2; I^2 = 26%, p = 0.58).

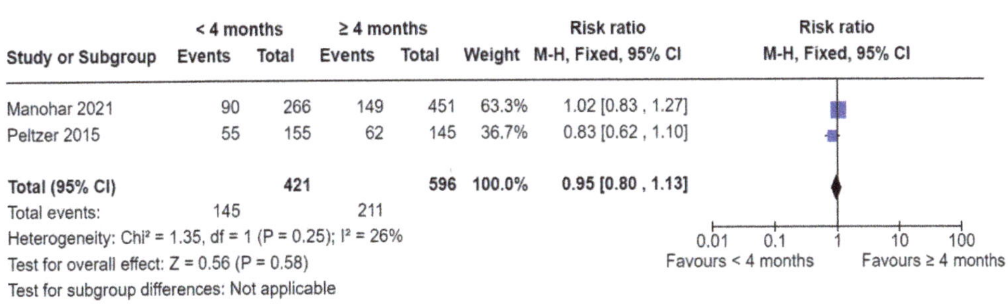

Figure 5. Breastfeeding < 4 months vs. breastfeeding ≥ 4 months and the risk of dental caries: cohort studies [46,50].

3.8.2. Duration of Breastfeeding: <6 Months and ≥6 Months

Nine studies [37,39,44,46,48,52,57,60,62] compared dental caries in children who were breastfed < 6 months and ≥ 6 months (Figures 6 and 7). Of these, six studies were of cohort design [37,39,44,46,48,52] and were included in the meta-analysis. No significant difference was found in the analysis (RR 0.97, 95% CI 0.88 to 1.06; participants = 4850; studies = 6; $I^2 = 0\%$, $p = 0.48$).

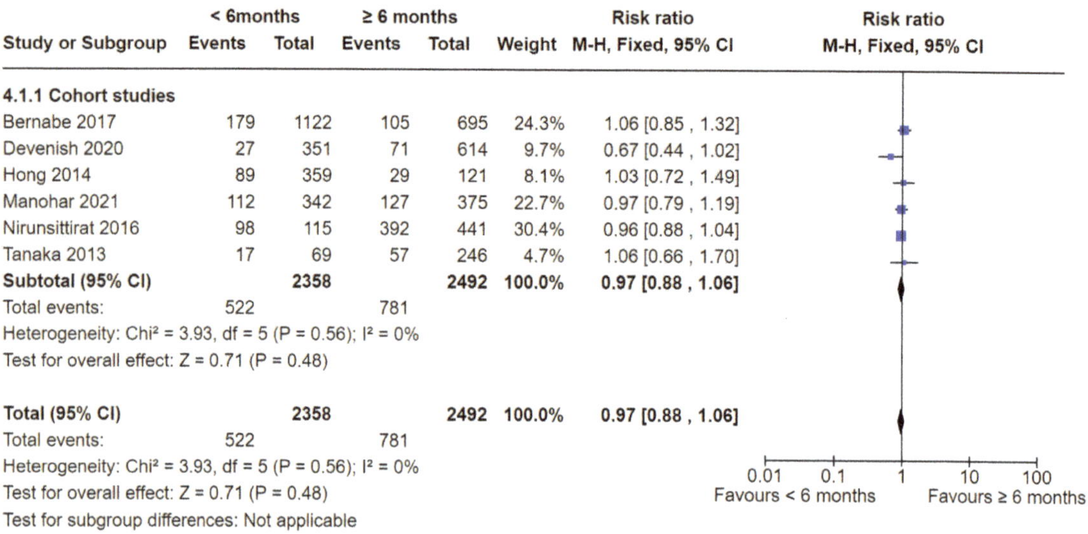

Figure 6. Breastfeeding < 6 months vs. breastfeeding ≥ 6 months and the risk of dental caries: cohort studies [37,39,44,46,48,52].

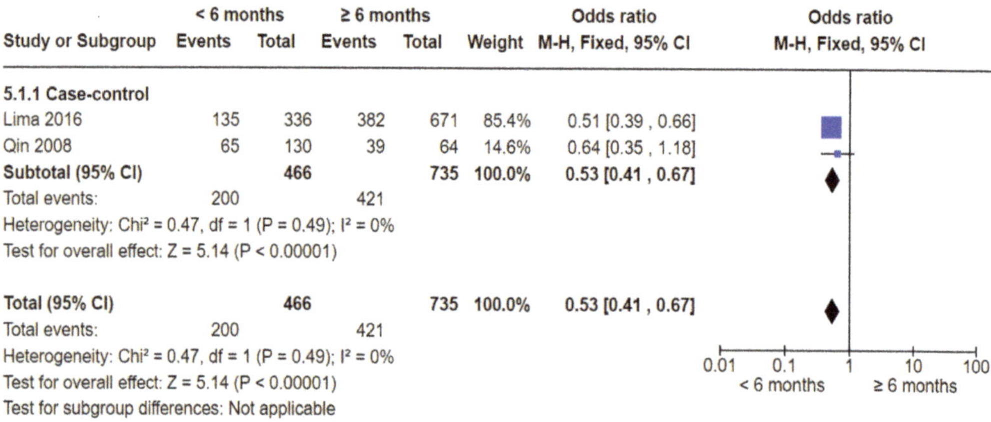

Figure 7. Breastfeeding < 6 months vs. breastfeeding ≥ 6 months and the risk of dental caries: case-control studies [60,62].

However, meta-analysis of two case-control studies [60,62] showed statistically significant fewer dental caries in the <6 months group compared to the ≥6 months group (OR 0.53, 95% CI 0.41 to 0.67; participants = 1201; studies = 2; $I^2 = 0\%$, $p < 0.00001$).

The results of the Cvanova et al. (2022) [57] study are presented narratively due to the method of reporting the outcome. The authors found statistically significant more cases of dental caries in children breastfed for ≤6 months compared to children breastfed > 6 months [OR (multivariate) = 2.71; 95% CI 1.45 to 5.07].

3.8.3. Duration of Breastfeeding: <12 Months and ≥12 Months

Eight studies comparing the duration of breastfeeding for <12 months and ≥12 months were able to be included in the meta-analysis [35,38–40,42,46,48,52]. All the studies were of cohort design and showed a statistically significant difference in dental caries between the <12 months group and the ≥12 months group (RR 0.65, 95% CI 0.50 to 0.86; participants = 4365; studies = 8; $I^2 = 90\%$, $p < 0.002$). The I^2 indicates substantial heterogeneity, and therefore the result should be interpreted with caution. See Figure 8. Three studies [35,42,48] were removed during sensitivity analysis, where the heterogeneity dropped to 0% ($p = 0.61$). The result was still statistically significant (RR = 0.70, 95% CI 0.62 to 0.80, $p < 0.0001$).

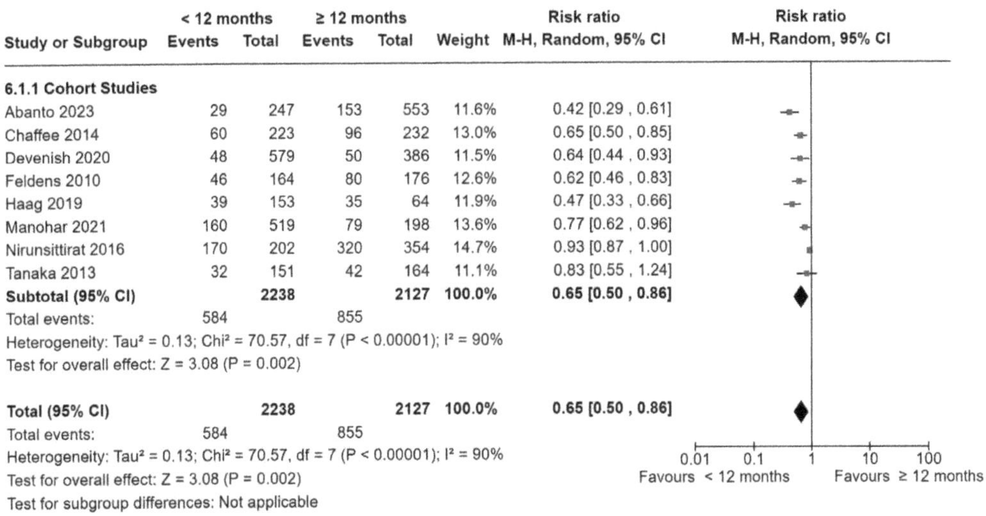

Figure 8. Breastfeeding < 12 months vs. breastfeeding ≥ 12 months and the risk of dental caries: cohort studies [35,38–40,42,46,48,52].

3.8.4. Duration of Breastfeeding: <18 Months and ≥18 Months

Six cohort studies [47,48,52,53,55,56] reported breastfeeding for <18 months and breastfeeding ≥ 18 months. Five cohort studies comparing the duration of breastfeeding for <18 months and ≥18 months were able to be included in the meta-analysis [47,48,52,53,56]. There were statistically significant fewer dental caries in the <18 months group compared to the ≥ 18 months group (RR 0.41, 95% CI 0.18 to 0.92; participants = 2332; studies = 5; $I^2 = 93\%$, $p = 0.03$) (Figure 9). After removing two studies [48,52] during sensitivity analysis, there was no heterogeneity among the studies ($I^2 = 0\%$, $p = 0.45$) and the pooled estimate remained statistically significant, favouring breastfeeding for <18 months (RR = 0.26, 95% CI 0.16 to 0.42).

Due to the method of reporting of the outcomes, the result of Yokoi et al. (2020) [55] is reported narratively. They observed prolonged breastfeeding significantly increases risk of ECC [OR = 1.71; 95% CI (1.15–2.55), $p < 0.001$].

Study or Subgroup	<18 months Events	<18 months Total	≥ 18 months Events	≥ 18 months Total	Weight	Risk ratio M-H, Random, 95% CI
7.1.1 Cohort Studies						
Nakayama 2022	14	608	16	248	20.0%	0.36 [0.18 , 0.72]
Nirunsittirat 2016	318	368	172	188	23.4%	0.94 [0.89 , 1.00]
Tanaka 2013	51	246	23	69	22.1%	0.62 [0.41 , 0.94]
Tashiro 2021	9	244	20	114	19.5%	0.21 [0.10 , 0.45]
Yonezu 2006	4	205	5	42	14.9%	0.16 [0.05 , 0.58]
Subtotal (95% CI)		**1671**		**661**	**100.0%**	**0.41 [0.18 , 0.92]**
Total events:	396		236			
Heterogeneity: Tau² = 0.74; Chi² = 60.84, df = 4 (P < 0.00001); I² = 93%						
Test for overall effect: Z = 2.16 (P = 0.03)						
Total (95% CI)		**1671**		**661**	**100.0%**	**0.41 [0.18 , 0.92]**
Total events:	396		236			
Heterogeneity: Tau² = 0.74; Chi² = 60.84, df = 4 (P < 0.00001); I² = 93%						
Test for overall effect: Z = 2.16 (P = 0.03)						
Test for subgroup differences: Not applicable						

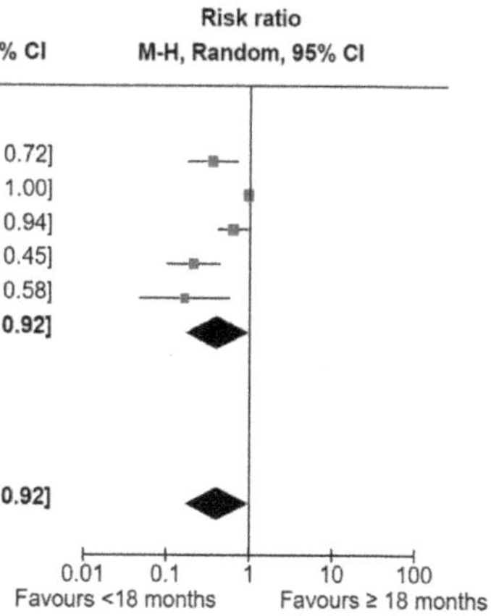

Figure 9. Breastfeeding < 18 months vs. breastfeeding ≥ 18 months and the risk of dental caries: cohort studies [47,48,52,53,56].

3.8.5. Duration of Breastfeeding: <24 Months and ≥24 Months

Four studies comparing the duration of breastfeeding (<24 months and ≥24 months) were able to be included in the meta-analysis [35,36,42,51]. There was no statistically significant difference in dental caries in the <24 months group compared to the ≥24 months group (RR 0.59, 95% CI 0.33 to 1.05; participants = 2271; studies = 4; I^2 = 92%, p = 0.07) (Figure 10). However, after removing Peres et al. (2017) during sensitivity analysis, the heterogeneity reduced significantly (I^2 = 6%, p = 0.34). The pooled estimates showed that children breastfed for <24 months had significantly fewer caries compared with children who were breastfed for ≥24 months (RR = 0.49, 95% CI 0.39 to 0.62).

The results of the Hartwig et al. (2019) [43] study are presented narratively due to the method of reporting the outcome. The authors found a statistically significant increase in dental caries in children breastfed for ≥24 months compared to those who were breastfed for less than 6 months or not breastfed (aRR = 8.29; 95% CI 1.82–37.72).

Study or Subgroup	<24 months Events	<24 months Total	≥ 24months Events	≥ 24months Total	Weight	Risk ratio M-H, Random, 95% CI
8.1.1 Cohort studies						
Abanto 2023	139	686	43	114	26.3%	0.54 [0.41 , 0.71]
Barroso 2021	11	66	33	66	21.7%	0.33 [0.18 , 0.60]
Haag 2019	52	188	16	29	24.7%	0.50 [0.34 , 0.75]
Peres 2017	382	866	96	256	27.3%	1.18 [0.99 , 1.40]
Subtotal (95% CI)		**1806**		**465**	**100.0%**	**0.59 [0.33 , 1.05]**
Total events:	584		188			
Heterogeneity: Tau² = 0.31; Chi² = 39.89, df = 3 (P < 0.00001); I² = 92%						
Test for overall effect: Z = 1.79 (P = 0.07)						
Total (95% CI)		**1806**		**465**	**100.0%**	**0.59 [0.33 , 1.05]**
Total events:	584		188			
Heterogeneity: Tau² = 0.31; Chi² = 39.89, df = 3 (P < 0.00001); I² = 92%						
Test for overall effect: Z = 1.79 (P = 0.07)						
Test for subgroup differences: Not applicable						

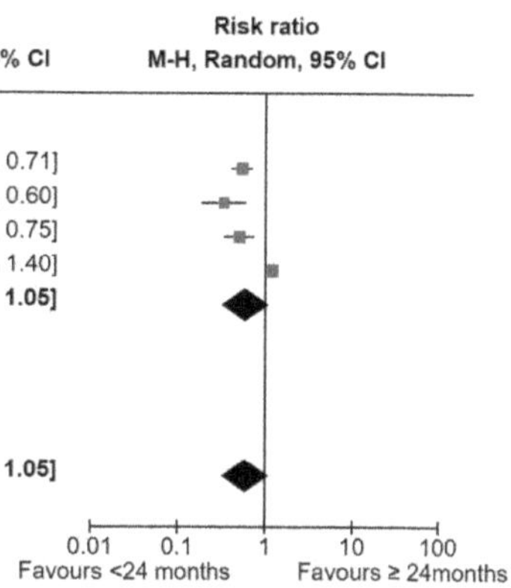

Figure 10. Breastfeeding < 24 months vs. breastfeeding ≥ 24 months and the risk of dental caries: cohort studies [35,36,42,51].

4. Discussion

The meta-analyses of the cohort and case-control studies failed to demonstrate a statistically significant difference in dental caries rates between breastfed and non-breastfed groups. However, the systematic review by Cui et al. (2017) [24] found breastfed children had a decreased risk of ECC compared with the children who were never breastfed. Similarly, the systematic review by Avila et al. (2015) [22] found breastfeeding was more protective against ECC than bottle feeding. Similarly, Klaiban et al. (2021) [25] concluded breastfeeding to be protective against ECC in a sufficiently breastfed group compared to a less sufficiently breastfed group. The systematic review by Tham et al. (2015) [28] was inconclusive about whether breastfeeding was associated with ECC. Bagher et al. (2013) [23] indicated exclusive breastfeeding is not associated with caries; however, they postulated that there was a possible protective effect of breastfeeding against ECC. The exclusion of studies with critical bias in the present review reduced heterogeneity, with the sensitivity analysis indicating potential protective effects of breastfeeding against ECC.

Despite breastfeeding being a personal choice, it is profoundly influenced by culture and society [67,68]. Mothers in low-income countries [68] tend to follow the WHO guidelines for breastfeeding, which are exclusive breastfeeding for 6 months and continuing breastfeeding for 2 years or more [18]. Likewise, in countries like Brazil, breastfeeding is culturally expected from mothers, whereas in developed countries like France, it is considered a personal choice. The potential inverse association between breastfeeding and ECC contributes to the broader health benefits of breastfeeding, potentially encouraging increased breastfeeding rates, especially in developed nations where rates are declining [68].

The frequency and duration of breastfeeding may also be influenced by the geographical location of birth, as indicated by studies by Odeniyi et al. (2020) [69] and Pastorelli et al. (2019) [67]. In many countries, the practice of on-demand or frequent breastfeeding [70,71] is prevalent, yet there is often insufficient emphasis on oral hygiene. The frequent exposure to fermentable carbohydrates, such as breast milk, and a lack of effective methods to remove the exposure from the oral cavity are the perfect amalgamation for the development of dental caries. This especially holds true for nocturnal breastfeeding, where there is pooling of breast milk inside the infant's mouth [27] and decreased salivary flow to wash out the substrate (milk). Thus, exposing the teeth for a prolonged duration to the acid produced by the cariogenic bacteria of the oral cavity results in dental caries. Nocturnal breastfeeding, identified as a risk factor for ECC in this review, has been consistently associated with increased caries risk in preschool children in various studies [50,57,60,61,72] and reviews [28,73].

A study conducted in Cambodia reported that most mothers believed that sucking at night helped children sleep, and more than half of the children who engaged in nocturnal suckling experienced ECC [74]. Similarly, van Palenstein Helderman et al. (2006) [54] observed that all the children who went to sleep with the breast nipple in their mouth experienced ECC. This highlights the need for increased awareness and education regarding the importance of oral hygiene practices, especially in the context of breastfeeding practices, to mitigate the risk of dental caries in preschool children.

Oral hygiene practices should ideally commence from birth, involving the cleaning of gums after each feeding [75]. Special attention to oral hygiene becomes crucial as primary teeth erupt (around 6 months) [76] or when infants start consuming solid food (around 6 months of age). Although cohort studies in this review did not show significant differences in the prevalence of ECC among children in the 4-month or 6-month groups, the meta-analysis of the two case-control studies [60,62] indicated that breastfeeding for less than 6 months is protective against caries. Notably, none of the identified systematic reviews have reported on the association between ECC and breastfeeding for less than or $\geq$6 months. Nonetheless, Branger et al. (2019) [77], Tham et al. (2015) [28], and Cui et al. (2017) [24] have indicated in their reviews that breastfeeding for < 12 months has a possible protective effect against dental caries. However, the protective association appears to diminish when breastfeeding extends beyond 12 months, and the current review aligns with these findings. Similar results were noticed in this review as well. Similarly, breastfeeding for less than 12 or 18 months may incur a protective effect against ECC, although this association seems to dissipate when the breastfeeding duration reaches 24 months. This outcome concurs with another systematic review [26] reporting that breastfeeding up to 24 months is not associated with a higher risk of ECC. Breast milk is known to inhibit the attachment of some bacteria, such as *Streptococcus mutans* and *Candida albicans* [78], which are known to cause dental caries [79]. However, it promotes the growth of other caries-causing *Streptococcus and Actinomyces* species [78]. Prolonged breastfeeding, therefore, could introduce bacteria that can cause ECC to the sensitive oral microbiome of the infant. There is also a possibility of vertical transmission of the oral pathogens from a mother with an active carious lesion.

Dental caries is a multifactorial disease influenced by host factors, oral bacteria, exposure time, and dietary habits. The escalating prevalence of ECC with age may be attributed to an increase in the number of teeth in the oral cavity [80] and the transition from an exclusive milk diet to a mixed diet incorporating solid foods [81]. Manohar et al. (2021) [82] noted that, beyond the age of two, as children gain autonomy, they tend to opt for unhealthy foods rich in saturated fat and free sugars, contributing to the development of ECC. This underscores the complex interplay of several factors in the aetiology of dental caries in early childhood. Nevertheless, the interpretation of the results of this review warrants caution due to the high heterogeneity observed among the included studies. The heterogeneity was expected due to the lack of homogeneity in the definition of both the exposure and outcome, as mentioned in several systematic reviews [22,23,27–29] as well as in some literature reviews [70,77].

5. Strengths and Limitations

The strengths of this review are a comprehensive search of five databases without any date or language restrictions and the inclusion of only the cohort and case-control studies, which are considered high-quality studies after experimental studies. Due to the nature of the study, it was determined a priori that RCTs would not be included as breastfeeding should not be randomised as it was deemed unethical by the authors. The critical appraisal was conducted by two reviewers using JBI SUMARI. This review provides evidence from ten meta-analyses showing the association between breastfeeding and ECC.

There were a few limitations while conducting this systematic review. Even though the search was conducted without any language restrictions, due to the limited resources, only the studies in English were included. Due to the exclusion of grey literature and studies in other languages, selection bias cannot be denied. Furthermore, the studies included in this review were mostly conducted in high- or middle-income countries. The search did not identify any studies included in low-income countries, which could result in publication bias. Another possible limitation is the utilisation of unadjusted data in instances where adjusted data were unavailable, which could impact the robustness of the findings. However, the inclusion of adjusted and unadjusted data in the meta-analysis could, in effect, introduce another source of bias.

One of the challenges while conducting this review was the lack of homogeneity of the included studies. Studies used different methods to measure exposure (breastfeeding) and outcomes (dental caries). Valaitis et al. (2000) [29], Peres et al. (2018) [70], and Branger et al. (2019) [77] voiced similar challenges in their reviews. The heterogeneity in the designs of the studies and methods for reporting the outcome measures presumably contributed to the high heterogeneity in several of the meta-analyses. For example, some limitations in the included studies may affect the outcome of the studies and hence influence their interpretation. Most of the challenges were centred upon the definition of the exposures—breastfeeding frequency, duration, and time—and outcomes (dental caries (ECC or S-ECC)). Additionally, the included studies were not clear about exclusive breastfeeding and predominant breastfeeding. Even though most of the studies used WHO criteria to define dental caries, some modifications were also noted. Some did not consider the initial white lesion as caries; some did not consider missing teeth (due to caries); and some only considered frank cavitation. There were inconsistencies regarding how the dental examinations were conducted as well. Some of the studies dried the tooth before examination (showing initial white lesions), while some utilised a visual aid (mouth mirror) only to detect caries (cannot differentiate between stains and caries or caries covered in plaque or food might not be visible), and there were others that used dental probes as well. Some of the dental examinations were conducted in clinical settings, and some were conducted in field settings. All these factors result in an underestimation or overestimation of the findings. Therefore, the results of this review should be interpreted with caution. It was also noted that some of the studies did not differentiate between the genders of the participants. While this lack of information did not affect the result of this review, it could be a possible limitation for anyone who would want to compare the prevalence of ECC between the sexes.

6. Recommendations for Future Policy, Practice, and Research

Based on the findings of this systematic review, it is recommended to use standardised definitions regarding duration, frequency, and type of breastfeeding, as well as standardised measurements (without variations) for dental caries assessment, including trained and calibrated dental professionals. Furthermore, clearly defining the minimum intra- and inter-examiner Cohen's kappa coefficient would help improve the quality of the data collected. A universal and standard method for dental examinations that can be applied in high-income as well as low-income settings would help in maintaining the quality of the studies in different settings.

During this review, it was noted that there was a lack of standard methods for measuring breastfeeding (duration, frequency, and type) in the included studies. Hence, the authors believe following one standard method (without any variations) to diagnose dental caries in future studies would provide a more comprehensive result regarding breastfeeding and ECC. It is also recommended that all the confounders related to breastfeeding and ECC be identified and adjusted to present more valid and reliable results. There is also a need for prospective birth cohort studies in low-income countries to fill the missing gap in the relationship between breastfeeding and ECC.

The findings of this review recommend that policy makers develop a comprehensive oral health promotion programme that includes behavioural modification (like wiping the gums after feeding or offering water after feeding to rinse out milk) to ensure optimum oral health outcomes for preschool children without compromising the nutritional and developmental benefits of breastfeeding. Health professionals such as general practitioners, midwives, and community health nurses should be trained to educate parents on proper oral hygiene from infancy. Since these health professionals take care of the mother and the baby during the antenatal and postnatal stages, oral health awareness can be effectively disseminated among families, particularly the mothers. Dental caries depends on exposure time. Hence, it is recommended to follow good oral hygiene practices as well as behaviour modifications such as minimising on-demand nocturnal feeding and sleeping with a breast nipple in the mouth. Cleaning the teeth with a wet cloth or offering water (to infants > 6 months old) after each feed could also minimise the exposure time. Visiting a dental professional after the child's first birthday could enhance the parents' oral health knowledge.

7. Conclusions

Even though the meta-analyses failed to demonstrate any statistically significant difference in the risk of ECC between the breastfed and non-breastfed children, they exhibited that breastfeeding for less than 24 months does not appear to increase the risk of ECC; in fact, it may exert a protective effect against ECC. However, it is crucial to note that breastfeeding nocturnally elevates the risk of dental caries in preschool children. Nonetheless, caution needs to be exercised while interpreting the results of this review due to the high heterogeneity. To establish a more comprehensive understanding of the relationship between breastfeeding and ECC, further research is required, employing consistent methods and addressing all the confounders. Until the results of such studies are published, which can provide a more assertive answer regarding the relationship between breastfeeding and ECC, health professionals should follow the recommended guidelines of the WHO and the guidelines of their local health ministry. They should encourage mothers to continue to breastfeed as long as they desire to provide the infants with the benefits of breastmilk, as well as provide oral health education to the mothers that focuses on good oral hygiene practices for the baby and healthy food practices to decrease the risk of ECC.

Supplementary Materials: The following supporting information can be downloaded at: https://www.mdpi.com/article/10.3390/nu16091355/s1, Table S1. Summarised assessment table of previous systematic reviews; Table S2. Critical appraisal of cohort studies; Table S3. Critical appraisal of case-control studies; Table S4. Description of cohort and case-control studies.

Author Contributions: Conceptualisation, S.K.S., J.F. and A.A.; methodology, S.K.S., J.F. and A.A.; software, S.K.S.; validation, S.K.S. and N.M.; formal analysis, S.K.S.; investigation, S.K.S., J.F., N.M. and A.A.; resources, J.F. and A.A.; data curation, S.K.S., J.F., K.E., N.M. and A.A.; writing—original draft preparation, S.K.S. and N.M.; writing—review and editing, S.K.S., J.F. and A.A.; visualisation, S.K.S.; supervision, J.F. and A.A.; project administration, A.A.; funding acquisition, none. All authors have read and agreed to the published version of the manuscript.

Funding: This research received no external funding.

Acknowledgments: The authors thank Lily Collison, School of Science and Health Librarian at Western Sydney University, for her ongoing support in the development of the search strategy.

Conflicts of Interest: The authors declare no conflicts of interest.

References

1. World Health Organization. *Oral Health*; World Health Organization: Geneva, Switzerland, 2023. Available online: https://www.who.int/news-room/fact-sheets/detail/oral-health#:~:text=Globally,%20an%20estimated%202%20billion, from%20caries%20of%20primary%20teeth (accessed on 11 November 2023).
2. Chen, K.J.; Gao, S.S.; Duangthip, D.; Lo, E.C.M.; Chu, C.H. Prevalence of early childhood caries among 5-year-old children: A systematic review. *J. Investig. Clin. Dent.* **2019**, *10*, e12376. [CrossRef]
3. Sharifi, M.; Pourseyedi, A.; Nejad, J.H.; Aftabi, R.; Hatami, N.; Poureslami, H. The Relationship between Weaning Method and its Time and Severe Early Childhood Caries. *Prev. Care Nurs. Midwifery J.* **2021**, *11*, 40–45. [CrossRef]
4. Fleming, E.; Afful, J. *Prevalence of Total and Untreated Dental Caries among Youth: United States, 2015–2016*; NCHS Data Brief, no 307; National Center for Health Statistics: Hyattsville, MD, USA, 2018; pp. 1–8.
5. Kotha, S.B. Lift the lip: A screening guide among the dental professionals. *Front. Oral Health* **2023**, *4*, 1177251. [CrossRef]
6. Ha, D.H.; Roberts-Thomson, K.F.; Arrow, P.; Peres, K.G.; Do, L.G. *Oral Health of Australian Children: The National Child Oral Health Study 2012–2014*; Do, L.G., Spencer, A.J., Eds.; University of Adelaide Press: Adelaide, Australia, 2016.
7. Devan, I.; Ramanarayanan, V.; Janakiram, C. Prevalence of early childhood caries in India: A systematic review and meta-analysis. *Indian J. Public Health* **2022**, *66*, S3–S11. [CrossRef] [PubMed]
8. Radha, S.; Kayalvizhi, G.; Prathima, G.S.; Ezhumalai, G.; Radha, S.; Adimoulame, S.; Muthusamy, K.; Jagadesaan, N. Comparative Evaluation of the Remineralizing Efficacy of Fluoride Varnish and its Combination Varnishes on White Spot Lesions in Children with ECC: A Randomized Clinical Trial. *Int. J. Clin. Pediatr. Dent.* **2020**, *13*, 311–317. [CrossRef]
9. Bencze, Z.; Mahrouseh, N.; Andrade, C.A.S.; Kovács, N.; Varga, O. The Burden of Early Childhood Caries in Children under 5 Years Old in the European Union and Associated Risk Factors: An Ecological Study. *Nutrients* **2021**, *13*, 455. [CrossRef] [PubMed]
10. Arora, A.; Schwarz, E.; Blinkhorn, A.S. Risk factors for early childhood caries in disadvantaged populations. *J. Investig. Clin. Dent.* **2011**, *2*, 223–228. [CrossRef]
11. Kirthiga, M.; Murugan, M.; Saikia, A.; Kirubakaran, R. Risk Factors for Early Childhood Caries: A Systematic Review and Meta-Analysis of Case Control and Cohort Studies. *Pediatr. Dent.* **2019**, *41*, 95–112.
12. Kato, T.; Yorifuji, T.; Yamakawa, M.; Inoue, S.; Saito, K.; Doi, H.; Kawachi, I. Association of breast feeding with early childhood dental caries: Japanese population-based study. *BMJ Open* **2015**, *5*, e006982. [CrossRef] [PubMed]
13. Tinanoff, N.; Baez, R.J.; Diaz Guillory, C.; Donly, K.J.; Feldens, C.A.; McGrath, C.; Phantumvanit, P.; Pitts, N.B.; Seow, W.K.; Sharkov, N. Early childhood caries epidemiology, aetiology, risk assessment, societal burden, management, education, and policy: Global perspective. *Int. J. Paediatr. Dent.* **2019**, *29*, 238–248. [CrossRef] [PubMed]
14. Beckett, D.; Wheeler, B.; Loch, C.; Mahoney, E.; Drummond, B.; Broadbent, J. Dental health in a cohort of six-year-old New Zealand children who were breastfed as infants–a comprehensive descriptive study. *NZ Dent. J.* **2022**, *118*, 5–13.

15. Kramer, M.; Vanilovich, I.; Matush, L.; Bogdanovich, N.; Zhang, X.; Shishko, G.; Muller-Bolla, M.; Platt, R. The Effect of Prolonged and Exclusive Breast-Feeding on Dental Caries in Early School-Age Children: New Evidence from a Large Randomized Trial. *Caries Res.* **2007**, *41*, 484–488. [CrossRef]
16. Park, Y.H.; Choi, Y.Y. Feeding Practices and Early Childhood Caries in Korean Preschool Children. *Int. Dent. J.* **2022**, *72*, 392–398. [CrossRef] [PubMed]
17. Setiawati, F.; Amalliah, I.; Ramadhani, A.; Maharani, D.A. Associated Factors of Early Childhood Caries (ECC) Among 24–42-Month-Old-Children in Jakarta: A Cross-Sectional Study. *J. Int. Dent. Med. Res.* **2021**, *14*, 1573–1579.
18. World Health Organization. *Breastfeeding*; World Health Organization: Geneva, Switzerland, 2023. Available online: https://www.who.int/health-topics/breastfeeding#tab=tab_1 (accessed on 11 November 2023).
19. National Health and Medical Research Council. *Infant Feeding Guidelines: Summary*; National Health and Medical Research Council: Canberra, Australia, 2013. Available online: https://www.eatforhealth.gov.au/sites/default/files/files/the_guidelines/n56_infant_feeding_guidelines_summary_150916.pdf (accessed on 11 November 2023).
20. American Academy of Pediatric Dentistry. *The Reference Manual of Pediatric Dentistry*; American Academy of Pediatric Dentistry: Chicago, IL, USA, 2023.
21. van Meijeren-van Lunteren, A.W.; Voortman, T.; Elfrink, M.E.; Wolvius, E.B.; Kragt, L. Breastfeeding and Childhood Dental Caries: Results from a Socially Diverse Birth Cohort Study. *Caries Res.* **2021**, *55*, 153–161. [CrossRef]
22. Avila, W.M.; Pordeus, I.A.; Paiva, S.M.; Martins, C.C. Breast and Bottle Feeding as Risk Factors for Dental Caries: A Systematic Review and Meta-Analysis. *PLoS ONE* **2015**, *10*, e0142922. [CrossRef]
23. Bagher, S.M.; Sabagh, H.J.; Mohammed, A.A.; Baghlaf, K.K. The Relationship between Breastfeeding and Dental Caries in Preschool Children in Saudi Arabia: A Systematic Review. *J. King Abdulaziz Univ.-Med. Sci.* **2013**, *20*, 53–66. [CrossRef]
24. Cui, L.; Li, X.; Tian, Y.; Bao, J.; Wang, L.; Xu, D.; Zhao, B.; Li, W. Breastfeeding and early childhood caries: A meta-analysis of observational studies. *Asia Pac. J. Clin. Nutr.* **2017**, *26*, 867–880.
25. Klaiban, M.; Asrar, M.; Bakhashwain, D.; Alsubaie, A.; Alghamdi, F.; Asrar, N.; Alzuhairi, W. Risk of Dental Caries and Breastfeeding: Systematic Review and Meta-analysis. *Ann. Med. Health Sci. Res.* **2021**, *11*, 1173–1177.
26. Moynihan, P.; Tanner, L.; Holmes, R.; Hillier-Brown, F.; Mashayekhi, A.; Kelly, S.; Craig, D. Systematic Review of Evidence Pertaining to Factors That Modify Risk of Early Childhood Caries. *JDR Clin. Transl. Res.* **2019**, *4*, 202–216. [CrossRef]
27. Sukmana, B.I.; Huldani Achmad, H.; Hidayah, N.; Putra, A.P.; Ramadhany, S.; Gadisha, S.B. A Review of Breastfeeding in Infants: Relation to the Occurrence of Early Childhood Caries (ECC). *Syst. Rev. Pharm.* **2020**, *11*. [CrossRef]
28. Tham, R.; Bowatte, G.; Dharmage, S.; Tan, D.; Lau, M.; Dai, X.; Allen, K.; Lodge, C. Breastfeeding and the risk of dental caries: A systematic review and meta-analysis. *Acta Paediatr.* **2015**, *104*, 62–84. [CrossRef]
29. Valaitis, R.; Hesch, R.; Passarelli, C.; Sheehan, D.; Sinton, J. A Systematic Review of the Relationship Between Breastfeeding and Early Childhood Caries. *Can. J. Public Health* **2000**, *91*, 411–417. [CrossRef] [PubMed]
30. Joanna Briggs Institute. *JBI Levels of Evidence*; The Joanna Briggs Institute: Adelaide, Australia, 2013.
31. Moola, S.; Munn, Z.; Tufanaru, C.; Aromataris, E.; Sears, K.; Sfetcu, R.; Currie, M.; Lisy, K.; Qureshi, R.; Mattis, P.; et al. Chapter 7: Systematic reviews of etiology and risk. In *JBI Manual for Evidence Synthesis*; Aromataris, E., Munn, Z., Eds.; JBI: Sydney, Australia, 2020. [CrossRef]
32. Page, M.J.; Moher, D.; Bossuyt, P.M.; Boutron, I.; Hoffmann, T.C.; Mulrow, C.D.; Shamseer, L.; Tetzlaff, J.M.; Akl, E.A.; Brennan, S.E.; et al. PRISMA 2020 explanation and elaboration: Updated guidance and exemplars for reporting systematic reviews. *BMJ* **2021**, *372*, n160. [CrossRef] [PubMed]
33. Higgins JP, T.; Thomas, J.; Chandler, J.; Cumpston, M.; Li, T.; Page, M.J.; Welch, V.A. *Cochrane Handbook for Systematic Reviews of Interventions*, 2nd ed.; John Wiley & Sons, Incorporated: Hoboken, NJ, USA, 2019. [CrossRef]
34. Aromataris, E.; Munn, Z. (Eds.) *JBI Manual for Evidence Synthesis*; Joanna Briggs Institute: Adelaide, Australia, 2020. Available online: https://synthesismanual.jbi.global (accessed on 8 November 2023).
35. Abanto, J.; Maruyama, J.M.; Pinheiro, E.; Matijasevich, A.; Antunes, J.L.F.; Bönecker, M.; Cardoso, M.A.; The MINA-Brazil Study Group. Prolonged breastfeeding, sugar consumption and dental caries at 2 years of age: A birth cohort study. *Community Dent. Oral Epidemiol.* **2023**, *51*, 575–582. [CrossRef]
36. Barroso, H.H.; Mourão, P.S.; Gomes, R.L.; de Almeida, M.T.P.; Silva, T.S.; Ramos-Jorge, J.; Ramos-Jorge, M.L.; Fernandes, I.B. Influence of breastfeeding duration on the incidence of dental caries in preschoolers: A cohort study. *Rev. Bras. Saúde Matern. Infant.* **2021**, *21*, 227–238. [CrossRef]
37. Bernabé, E.; MacRitchie, H.; Longbottom, C.; Pitts, N.; Sabbah, W. Birth weight, breastfeeding, maternal smoking and caries trajectories. *J. Dent. Res.* **2017**, *96*, 171–178. [CrossRef] [PubMed]
38. Chaffee, B.W.; Feldens, C.A.; Vítolo, M.R. Association of long-duration breastfeeding and dental caries estimated with marginal structural models. *Ann. Epidemiol.* **2014**, *24*, 448–454. [CrossRef] [PubMed]
39. Devenish, G.; Mukhtar, A.; Begley, A.; Spencer, A.J.; Thomson, W.M.; Ha, D.; Do, L.; A Scott, J. Early childhood feeding practices and dental caries among Australian preschoolers. *Am. J. Clin. Nutr.* **2020**, *111*, 821–828. [CrossRef]
40. Feldens, C.; Giugliani, E.; Vigo, Á.; Vítolo, M. Early feeding practices and severe early childhood caries in four-year-old children from southern Brazil: A birth cohort study. *Caries Res.* **2010**, *44*, 445–452. [CrossRef]
41. Feldens, C.A.; Rodrigues, P.H.; de Anastácio, G.; Vítolo, M.R.; Chaffee, B.W. Feeding frequency in infancy and dental caries in childhood: A prospective cohort study. *Int. Dent. J.* **2018**, *68*, 113–121. [CrossRef] [PubMed]

42. Haag, D.G.; Jamieson, L.M.; Hedges, J.; Smithers, L.G. Is there an association between breastfeeding and dental caries among three-year-old Australian Aboriginal children? *Nutrients* **2019**, *11*, 2811. [CrossRef] [PubMed]
43. Hartwig, F.P.; Loret de Mola, C.; Davies, N.M.; Victora, C.G.; Relton, C.L. Breastfeeding effects on DNA methylation in the offspring: A systematic literature review. *PLoS ONE* **2017**, *12*, e0173070.
44. Hong, L.; Levy, S.M.; Warren, J.J.; Broffitt, B. Infant breast-feeding and childhood caries: A nine-year study. *Pediatr. Dent.* **2014**, *36*, 342–347.
45. Majorana, A.; Cagetti, M.G.; Bardellini, E.; Amadori, F.; Conti, G.; Strohmenger, L. Guglielmo Campus Feeding and smoking habits as cumulative risk factors for early childhood caries in toddlers, after adjustment for several behavioral determinants: A retrospective study. *BMC Pediatr.* **2014**, *14*, 45. [CrossRef] [PubMed]
46. Manohar, N.; Hayen, A.; Scott, J.A.; Do, L.G.; Bhole, S.; Arora, A. Impact of Dietary Trajectories on Obesity and Dental Caries in Preschool Children: Findings from the Healthy Smiles Healthy Kids Study. *Nutrients* **2021**, *13*, 2240. [CrossRef] [PubMed]
47. Nakayama, Y.; Ohnishi, H. Risk Factors for Early Childhood Caries in Three-Year-Old Japanese Children: A Prospective Cohort Study. *Pediatr. Dent.* **2022**, *44*, 346–354. [PubMed]
48. Nirunsittirat, A.; Pitiphat, W.; McKinney, C.M.; DeRouen, T.A.; Chansamak, N.; Angwaravong, O.; Patcharanuchat, P.; Pimpak, T. Adverse birth outcomes and childhood caries: A cohort study. *Community Dent. Oral Epidemiol.* **2016**, *44*, 239–247. [CrossRef]
49. Nunes, A.M.M.; Alves, C.M.C.; de Araújo, F.B.; Ortiz, T.M.L.; Ribeiro, M.R.C.; da Silva, A.A.M.; Ribeiro, C.C.C. Association between prolonged breast-feeding and early childhood caries: A hierarchical approach. *Community Dent. Oral Epidemiol.* **2012**, *40*, 542–549. [CrossRef]
50. Peltzer, K.; Mongkolchati, A. Severe early childhood caries and social determinants in three-year-old children from Northern Thailand: A birth cohort study. *BMC Oral Health* **2015**, *15*, 108. [CrossRef]
51. Peres, K.G.; Nascimento, G.G.; Peres, M.A.; Mittinty, M.N.; Demarco, F.F.; Santos, I.S.; Matijasevich, A.; Barros, A.J.D. Impact of prolonged breastfeeding on dental caries: A population-based birth cohort study. *Pediatrics* **2017**, *140*, e20162943. [CrossRef] [PubMed]
52. Tanaka, K.; Miyake, Y.; Sasaki, S.; Hirota, Y. Infant feeding practices and risk of dental caries in Japan: The osaka maternal and child health study. *Pediatr. Dent.* **2013**, *35*, 267–271. [PubMed]
53. Tashiro, A.; Yonezu, T.; Kumazawa, K.; Sakurai, A.; Shintani, S. Caries and its association with infant feeding and oral health-related behavior in 18-month and 3-year-old Japanese children. *Bull. Tokyo Dent. Coll.* **2021**, *62*, 71–87. [CrossRef] [PubMed]
54. Palenstein Helderman, W.H.; Soe, W.; van't Hof, M.A. Risk factors of early childhood caries in a southeast asian population. *J. Dent. Res.* **2006**, *85*, 85–88. [CrossRef] [PubMed]
55. Yokoi, A.; Takeuchi, N.; Ekuni, D.; Morita, M. Association between the incidence of early childhood caries and attending childcare among toddlers in a rural area of Japan: A prospective cohort study. *Acta Odontol. Scand.* **2021**, *79*, 118–123. [CrossRef] [PubMed]
56. Yonezu, T.; Ushida, N.; Yakushiji, M. Longitudinal study of prolonged breast- or bottle-feeding on dental caries in Japanese children. *Bull. Tokyo Dent. Coll.* **2006**, *47*, 157–160. [CrossRef] [PubMed]
57. Cvanova, M.; Ruzicka, F.; Kukletova, M.; Lipovy, B.; Gachova, D.; Holla, L.I.; Danek, Z.; Hola, V.; Bartosova, M.; Jarkovsky, J.; et al. Candida species and selected behavioral factors co-associated with severe early childhood caries: Case-control study. *Front. Cell. Infect. Microbiol.* **2022**, *12*, 943480. [CrossRef] [PubMed]
58. Dabawala, S.; Suprabha, B.S.; Shenoy, R.; Rao, A.; Shah, N. Parenting style and oral health practices in early childhood caries: A case–control study. *Int. J. Paediatr. Dent.* **2017**, *27*, 135–144. [CrossRef] [PubMed]
59. Ganesh, A.; Muthu, M.; Padmanabhan, R.; Nuvvula, S. Association of Sleep-Time Feeding Practices with Early Childhood Caries: A Case-Control Study. *Caries Res.* **2022**, *56*, 399–406. [CrossRef]
60. Lima, M.D.D.M.; Brito-Neto, Z.S.; Amaral, H.O.; Lima, C.C.B.; de Moura, M.S.; Moura, L.D.F.A.d.D. Risk factors associated with early childhood caries—A case control study. *Rev. Odonto Ciência* **2016**, *31*, 83–88. [CrossRef]
61. Matee, M.; Hof, M.V.; Maselle, S.; Mikx, F.; Helderman, W.v.P. Nursing caries, linear hypoplasia, and nursing and weaning habits in Tanzanian infants. *Community Dent. Oral Epidemiol.* **1994**, *22*, 289–293. [CrossRef]
62. Qin, M.; Li, J.; Zhang, S.; Ma, W. Risk factors for severe early childhood caries in children younger than 4 years old in Beijing, China. *Pediatr. Dent.* **2008**, *30*, 122–128.
63. Roberts, G.J.; Cleaton-Jones, P.E.; Fatti, L.P.; Richardson, B.D.; Sinwel, R.E.; Hargreaves, J.A.; Williams, S.; Lucas, V.S. Patterns of breast and bottle feeding and their association with dental caries in 1-to 4-year-old South African children. 2. A case control study of children with nursing caries. *Community Dent. Health* **1994**, *11*, 38–41.
64. Seow, W.K.; Clifford, H.; Battistutta, D.; Morawska, A.; Holcombe, T. Case-control study of early childhood caries in Australia. *Caries Res.* **2009**, *43*, 25–35. [CrossRef]
65. Werneck, R.; Lawrence, H.P.; Kulkarni, G.V.; Locker, D. Early childhood caries and access to dental care among children of Portuguese-speaking immigrants in the city of Toronto. *J. Can. Dent. Assoc.* **2008**, *74*, 805.
66. Hamadeh, N.; van Rompaey, C.; Metreau, E. World Bank Group Country Classifications by Income Level for FY24 (July 1, 2023–June 30, 2024). 2023. Available online: https://blogs.worldbank.org/opendata/new-world-bank-group-country-classifications-income-level-fy24 (accessed on 31 October 2023).
67. Pastorelli, P.; Oliveira, E.; Silva, L.; Silva, L.; Silva, M. Meaning and cultural experiences of breastfeeding among women from two countries. *Rev. Enferm. UERJ* **2019**, *27*, 1–7.
68. Prentice, A.M. Breastfeeding in the modern world. *Ann. Nutr. Metab.* **2022**, *78* (Suppl. S2), 29–38. [CrossRef]

69. Odeniyi, A.O.; Embleton, N.; Ngongalah, L.; Akor, W.; Rankin, J. Breastfeeding beliefs and experiences of African immigrant mothers in high-income countries: A systematic review. *Matern. Child Nutr.* **2020**, *16*, e12970. [CrossRef] [PubMed]
70. Peres, K.; Chaffee, B.; Feldens, C.; Flores-Mir, C.; Moynihan, P.; Rugg-Gunn, A. Breastfeeding and Oral Health: Evidence and Methodological Challenges. *J. Dent. Res.* **2018**, *97*, 251–258. [CrossRef]
71. Wassuna, D.; Opinya, G. Infant Feeding, Weaning Practices and Oral Hygiene Status of 3–5-Year-Old Children with Severe Early Childhood Caries and Children without Caries in Kisumu, Kenya. *Control. Trial Mod. App. Dent. Oral Health* **2018**, *2*, 128. [CrossRef]
72. Carrillo-Díaz, M.; Ortega-Martínez, A.R.; Ruiz-Guillén, A.; Romero-Maroto, M.; González-Olmo, M.J. Impact of breastfeeding and cosleeping on early childhood caries: A Cross-Sectional Study. *J. Clin. Med.* **2021**, *10*, 1561. [CrossRef] [PubMed]
73. Panchanadikar, N.T.; S, A.; Muthu, M.S.; H, S.; Jayakumar, P.; Agarwal, A. Breastfeeding and its Association with Early Childhood Caries—An Umbrella Review. *J. Clin. Pediatr. Dent.* **2022**, *46*, 75–85. [CrossRef] [PubMed]
74. Kubota, Y.; Pech, N.S.; Durward, C.; Ogawa, H. Early childhood caries status and its associated factors among young children in a rural area of Cambodia. *Pediatr. Dent. J.* **2020**, *30*, 17–23. [CrossRef]
75. Butera, A.; Maiorani, C.; Morandini, A.; Simonini, M.; Morittu, S.; Trombini, J.; Scribante, A. Evaluation of children caries risk factors: A narrative review of nutritional aspects, oral hygiene habits, and bacterial alterations. *Children* **2022**, *9*, 262. [CrossRef] [PubMed]
76. Xu, H.; Tian, B.; Shi, W.; Tian, J.; Wang, W.; Qin, M. Maturation of the oral microbiota during primary teeth eruption: A longitudinal, preliminary study. *J. Oral Microbiol.* **2022**, *14*, 2051352. [CrossRef] [PubMed]
77. Branger, B.; Camelot, F.; Droz, D.; Houbiers, B.; Marchalot, A.; Bruel, H.; Laczny, E.; Clement, C. Breastfeeding and early childhood caries. Review of the literature, recommendations, and prevention. *Arch. Pédiatrie* **2019**, *26*, 497–503. [CrossRef] [PubMed]
78. Nardi, G.M.; Grassi, R.; Ndokaj, A.; Antonioni, M.; Jedlinski, M.; Rumi, G.; Grocholewicz, K.; Dus-Ilnicka, I.; Grassi, F.R.; Ottolenghi, L.; et al. Maternal and Neonatal Oral Microbiome Developmental Patterns and Correlated Factors: A Systematic Review—Does the Apple Fall Close to the Tree? *Int. J. Environ. Res. Public Health* **2021**, *18*, 5569. [CrossRef] [PubMed]
79. Li, Y.; Huang, S.; Du, J.; Wu, M.; Huang, X. Current and prospective therapeutic strategies: Tackling Candida albicans and Streptococcus mutans cross-kingdom biofilm. *Front. Cell. Infect. Microbiol.* **2023**, *13*, 1106231. [CrossRef]
80. Olatosi, O.; Inem, V.; Sofola, O.; Prakash, P.; Sote, E. The prevalence of early childhood caries and its associated risk factors among preschool children referred to a tertiary care institution. *Niger. J. Clin. Pract.* **2015**, *18*, 493–501. [CrossRef]
81. Amezdroz, E.; Carpenter, L.; O'Callaghan, E.; Johnson, S.; Waters, E. Transition from milks to the introduction of solid foods across the first 2 years of life: Findings from an Australian birth cohort study. *J. Hum. Nutr. Diet.* **2015**, *28*, 375–383. [CrossRef]
82. Manohar, N.; Hayen, A.; Do, L.; Scott, J.; Bhole, S.; Arora, A. Early life and socio-economic determinants of dietary trajectories in infancy and early childhood—Results from the HSHK birth cohort study. *Nutr. J.* **2021**, *20*, 76. [CrossRef] [PubMed]

MDPI AG
Grosspeteranlage 5
4052 Basel
Switzerland
Tel.: +41 61 683 77 34

Nutrients Editorial Office
E-mail: nutrients@mdpi.com
www.mdpi.com/journal/nutrients

www.ingramcontent.com/pod-product-compliance
Lightning Source LLC
Chambersburg PA
CBHW061843210926
51850CB00006B/958
* 9 7 8 3 7 2 5 8 5 0 8 9 1 *